Prevention Across the Lifespan: A Review of Evidence-Based Interventions for Common Oral Conditions

Ann Eshenaur Spolarich, RDH, PhD, FSCDH
Professor and Director of Research
Arizona School of Dentistry and Oral Health
A.T. Still University
Mesa, AZ, USA

Fotinos S. Panagakos, DMD, PhD
Global Director, Scientific Affairs
Colgate-Palmolive Company
Piscataway, NJ, USA

Prevention Across the Lifespan: A Review of Evidence-Based Interventions for Common Oral Conditions

Copyright © 2017 by the Colgate-Palmolive Company. All rights reserved.

No part of this publication may be used or reproduced in any form or by any means, or stored in a database or retrieval system, without prior written permission of the Colgate-Palmolive Company. Making copies of any part of this book for any purpose other than your own personal use is a violation of United States copyright laws.

ISBN-10: 0966284917
ISBN-13: 978-0-9662849-1-1

Published by ...

Professional Audience Communications, Inc.
PO Box 39486
Charlotte, North Carolina 28278 USA

Editorial Quality Control/Proofreading: Teri S. Siegel
Copyediting: Donna Frassetto
Layout and Design: Horizons Advertising & Graphic Design
Cover Design: Horizons Advertising & Graphic Design
Indexing: Allegheny Writing & Publishing Services, LLC
Publisher: Stephen M. Siegel

Printed in the United States of America

Last digit is the print number: 6 5 4 3 2 1

CONTRIBUTORS

P. Mark Bartold, BDS, BScDent(Hons) PhD, DDSc, FRACDS(Perio)
Professor of Periodontology, Director,
Colgate Australian Clinical Dental Research Centre
University of Adelaide Department of Dentistry
Adelaide, South Australia

Sharon M. Compton, DipDH, BSc, MA (Ed), PhD
Professor and Director
Dental Hygiene Undergraduate and Graduate Programs
School of Dentistry, Faculty of Medicine and Dentistry
University of Alberta
Alberta, Canada

Louis G. DePaola, DDS, MS
Assistant Dean of Clinical Affairs
Professor, Department of Oncology and Diagnostic Sciences
University of Maryland School of Dentistry
Baltimore, Maryland, USA

Zameera Fida, DMD
Department of Dentistry, Boston Children's Hospital
Director of Predoctoral Pediatric Dentistry
Instructor, Developmental Biology
Harvard School of Dental Medicine
Boston, Massachusetts, USA

Jacquelyn L. Fried, RDH, BA, MS
Associate Professor and Director of Interprofessional Initiatives
Associate Faculty, Schools of Nursing and Pharmacy
Department of Periodontics, Division of Dental Hygiene
University of Maryland School of Dentistry
Baltimore, Maryland, USA

JoAnn R. Gurenlian, RDH, MS, PhD
Professor and Graduate Program Director
Department of Dental Hygiene
Division of Health Sciences
Idaho State University
Pocatello, Idaho, USA

Phuu P. Han, DDS, PhD
Diplomate of the American Board of Orofacial Pain
Assistant Professor of Clinical Dentistry
Division of Dental Public Health and Pediatric Dentistry
Herman Ostrow School of Dentistry of USC
Los Angeles, California, USA

Yiming Li, DDS, MSD, PhD
Associate Dean for Research
Professor and Director, Center for Dental Research
Loma Linda University School of Dentistry
Loma Linda, California, USA

Mark S. Montana, DDS
Certificate in Prosthodontics
Private practice, Tempe, Arizona, USA

Antonio J. Moretti, DDS, MS
Associate Professor and Graduate Program Director
Department of Periodontology
University of North Carolina School of Dentistry
Chapel Hill, North Carolina, USA

Roseann Mulligan, DDS, MS
Fellow of the Gerontological Society of America
Director of the Online Programs in Geriatric Dentistry
Charles M. Goldstein Professor of Community Dentistry
Associate Dean, Community Health Programs and Hospital Affairs
Chair of the Division of Dental Public Health and Pediatric Dentistry
Herman Ostrow School of Dentistry of USC
Professor, USC Davis School of Gerontology
Los Angeles, California, USA

CONTRIBUTORS

Fotinos S. Panagakos, DMD, PhD
Global Director, Scientific Affairs
Colgate-Palmolive Company
Piscataway, New Jersey, USA

Philip M. Preshaw, BDS, FDS RCSEd, PhD
Professor of Periodontology
School of Dental Sciences and Institute
of Cellular Medicine
Newcastle University
Newcastle upon Tyne, United Kingdom

Professor Iain A. Pretty
Dental Health Unit, University
of Manchester
Manchester, England

Michael P. Rethman, DDS, MS
Associate Professor (adjunct), Baltimore
College of Dental Surgery,
University of Maryland
Assistant Professor (adjunct), College of
Dentistry, The Ohio State University
Prescott, Arizona, USA

Erik R. Roskam, DDS
Tandartsenpraktijk Santpoort Noord
The Netherlands

S.D. Shanti, DDS, MPH, PhD, CPH
Associate Professor of Public Health
Arizona School of Dentistry and Oral Health
College of Graduate Health Studies
A.T. Still University of Health Sciences
Mesa, Arizona, USA

Harlan Shiau, DDS, DMedSc
Diplomate, American Board of
Periodontology
Clinical Associate Professor, Department
of Periodontology
University of Maryland School of Dentistry
Baltimore, Maryland, USA

Marc Shlossman, DDS, MS
Assistant Professor and Interim Director,
Periodontics
Director, Clinical Research
Arizona School of Dentistry and Oral Health
A.T. Still University
Mesa, Arizona, USA

Ann Eshenaur Spolarich, RDH, PhD, FSCDH
Professor and Director of Research
Arizona School of Dentistry and
Oral Health
A.T. Still University
Mesa, Arizona, USA

Piedad Suarez-Durall, DDS
Section Chair, Geriatric and Special
Patients Clinic
Co-director of the Special Patients Clinic
Associate Professor of Clinical Dentistry
Division of Dental Public Health and
Pediatric Dentistry
Herman Ostrow School of Dentistry
of USC
Los Angeles, California, USA

J.M. ('Bob') ten Cate, PhD, Drhc
Emeritus Professor of Preventive
Dentistry
Academic Center for Dentistry Amsterdam
(ACTA)
The Netherlands

Rebecca S. Wilder, BSDH, MS
Professor and Director of Faculty
Development
Office of Academic Affairs
Director, Graduate Dental Hygiene
Education
University of North Carolina-Chapel Hill
Chapel Hill, North Carolina, USA

Mark S. Wolff, DDS, PhD
Associate Dean for Predoctoral
Clinical Education
Associate Dean for Development
Professor and Chair, Cariology and
Comprehensive Care
New York University College of Dentistry
New York, New York, USA

Minn N. Yoon, PhD
Assistant Professor, School of Dentistry
Faculty of Medicine and Dentistry
University of Alberta
Edmonton, Alberta, Canada

From the Editors

Dear Reader:

We are delighted to present the textbook *Prevention Across the Lifespan: A Review of Evidence-Based Interventions for Common Oral Conditions*. It is very appropriate that this book is being published at a time when prevention is front and center within oral healthcare, both in education and professional practice.

In this textbook, we have structured the material so that it can be used by those early in their educational journey as well as seasoned practitioners. It will provide the reader with practical information regarding the prevention of the most common oral health indications, with a special emphasis on age-related considerations. This text focuses on the current best evidence available to support decision making for recommended preventive interventions. This book is not intended to be a comprehensive review of the science around diagnosis and treatment for each of these indications – there are numerous resources available from experts in the field if one is interested in diving deeper in areas such as caries, periodontal disease, or dry mouth. Rather, it is our intention to emphasize how practitioners can help patients prevent disease from occurring, recurring, or progressing.

This book is the result of a 12-month process based on the most contemporary thinking behind what the literature suggests regarding prevention of oral disease. A unique feature in many of the chapters is the addition of case reviews that bring to life the content in the chapter. The reader will be able to use these cases to reinforce what they just read. Students will find these cases useful in incorporating the content into the broader learning process in which they are engaged. Finally, dental faculty will find these cases useful in their respective courses.

We would like to express our deep appreciation to the chapter authors. It was through their knowledge of these vitally important subjects, their professional relationships with the two of us, and their backgrounds as highly regarded researchers and educators in dentistry, that we are able to bring you this significant work.

Since the launch of its first toothpaste in 1873, the Colgate-Palmolive Company has been a world leader in oral care, both through cutting-edge therapeutics, as well as important educational services to the dental professions. This book, *Prevention Across the Lifespan: A Review of Evidence-Based Interventions for Common Oral Conditions*, which has been produced and distributed through an educational grant from the company (by which the company provided funding to the publisher), is a prime example of Colgate's continuing commitment to ensuring education for dental professionals.

Ann E. Spolarich

Fotinos A. Panagakos

CONTENTS

CHAPTER 1
Adopting an Evidence-Based Philosophy of Practice
Ann Eshenaur Spolarich and Fotinos Panagakos 1

CHAPTER 2
Behavioral Science
S.D. Shanti 23

CHAPTER 3
Risk Assessment
JoAnn R. Gurenlian 37

CHAPTER 4
Dental Caries
J.M. ("Bob") ten Cate and Erik R. Roskam 57

CHAPTER 5
Gingival Diseases
Rebecca Wilder and Antonio Moretti 71

CHAPTER 6
Preventing Damage to Oral Hard and Soft Tissues
Marc Shlossman and Mark Montana .... .97

CHAPTER 7
Head and Neck Cancers
Jacquelyn Fried 121

CHAPTER 8
Oral Malodor
P. Mark Bartold 146

CONTENTS

CHAPTER 9
Dentin Hypersensitivity
Yiming Li 160

CHAPTER 10
Dry Mouth
Sharon Compton and Minn Yoon 175

CHAPTER 11
Orofacial Injuries
Zameera Fida 192

CHAPTER 12
Prevention in the Context of Oral–Systemic Health
Philip M. Preshaw 207

CHAPTER 13
Preventive Considerations in Special Care Dentistry
Roseann Mulligan, Phuu Pwint Han, and Piedad Suarez-Durall 221

CHAPTER 14
Fluorides
I. A. Pretty 235

CHAPTER 15
Non-Fluoride Remineralization Therapies
Mark S. Wolff and Michael P. Rethman 246

CHAPTER 16
Chemotherapeutic Agents
Harlan J. Shiau and Louis G. DePaola 257

INDEX 272

Chapter 1
Adopting an Evidence-Based Philosophy of Practice

Ann Eshenaur Spolarich and Fotinos Panagakos

Evidence-based dentistry (EBD) is a philosophical approach to practice that facilitates the clinician's decision making about patient care. Decisions should be patient centered, tailoring care to each individual's treatment needs, while taking into consideration the clinician's expertise and experiences, as well as the patient's needs, preferences, and desires. Clinical decisions are based on knowledge of current best evidence obtained by accessing and critically appraising published studies in the scientific literature. The clinician must carefully weigh the patient's general and oral healthcare needs and determine how the evidence may be applied to address those needs. Clinicians must also help patients make treatment decisions utilizing this knowledge when considering options for care, while taking into account the patient's values, expectations, and unique clinical circumstances. Social, cultural, and behavioral factors may influence the patient's willingness to accept the proposed plan of treatment as well as compliance with professional recommendations. Practicing with this type of philosophy is not easy and demands certain skills and due diligence to be successful. Ultimately, the goal is to improve the consistency and quality of care delivered while improving patient outcomes[1-3] (see Figure 1).

Since the evidence-based decision-making (EBDM) discussion began, there has been a stronger emphasis on the strength of the science than on the clinician and on the patient. There is a mystical view that evidence is "all knowing" and that the evidence alone is the most critical factor that drives decision making. However, the objective of EBDM is to improve the probability of making the "best" decision. In a true evidence-based model of care, the clinician's judgment should be regarded as being at least as, if not more, important as the science. Clinicians are the end-users of this information and must be able to interpret and apply that knowledge to the best of their abilities with the best of intentions for a successful outcome. In this chapter, we explore the challenges encountered when trying to incorporate this model of care into daily practice.

Figure 1. Evidence-Based Practice Model

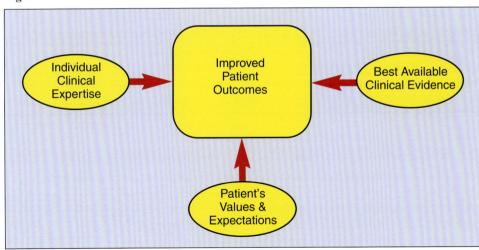

Source: Adapted from http://www.lonestar.edu/departments/libraries/kingwood-library/ebp_illus.jpg.

CHALLENGES IN ADOPTING AN EVIDENCE-BASED PHILOSOPHY OF PRACTICE

Keeping Up with the Literature

Clinicians may face many challenges when choosing to adopt an evidence-based philosophy of practice. It can be overwhelming to learn how to navigate the sheer volume of information that is available to clinicians in the scientific literature. More than two million articles are published annually, including over 500 clinical trials published across 50 journals representing all the dental specialties.[4,5] The challenge of finding time to read only those papers that are most relevant to the clinician's area of expertise is daunting. Most clinicians find it difficult to keep up with the latest findings from research because of the lack of time needed to read. Thus, clinicians may be tempted to read only those publications to which they subscribe, and then may briefly peruse the article or simply read the abstract and conclusions of the paper. Readers should know that abstracts do not always accurately portray the content of the paper, leading them to miss important nuances about the study design or additional results that may influence how the study outcomes may be interpreted. Conclusions stated in the abstract are often too limited to reflect all that has been learned from reported results.

Accessing Information

Difficulty in gaining access to information is also a common frustration. The lack of access to full text articles discourages clinicians' attempts to locate best evidence. Some publishers offer access to full text articles for a fee, which is collected for downloading individual papers online or for electronic access to all journals within the publisher's library with payment of an annual subscription fee. Professional organizations offer access to articles published in their respective journals—print or electronic format, or both—as a benefit of membership. Studies that are publicly funded through the National Institutes of

Table 1. Locating Best Evidence

Database	Web Address
The Cochrane Library	http://www.cochranelibrary.com
Database of Abstracts of Reviews of Effects (DARE); University of York Centre for Reviews and Dissemination	http://www.york.ac.uk/crd
Turning Research Into Practice (TRIP) Database	http://www.tripdatabase.com
PubMed (National Library of Medicine)	https://www.ncbi.nlm.nih.gov/pubmed
PubMed Health (National Library of Medicine)	https://www.ncbi.nlm.nih.gov/pubmedhealth
PubMed Clinical Queries	https://www.ncbi.nlm.nih.gov/pubmed/clinical
Google Scholar	https://scholar.google.com
National Information Center on Health Services Research and Health Care Technology (NICHSR)	https://www.nlm.nih.gov/nichsr
Health Technology Assessment Database	http://www.dimdi.de/static/en/db/dbinfo/inahta.htm
Embase	https://www.elsevier.com/solutions/embase-biomedical-research
PscyINFO (American Psychological Association)	http://www.apa.org/pubs/databases/psycinfo/index.aspx
CINAHL (Cumulative Index of Nursing and Allied Health Literature)	https://health.ebsco.com/products/the-cinahl-database/allied-health-nursing
LILACS (Literature from Latin America and the Caribbean)	http://lilacs.bvsalud.org/en
SciELO (Scientific Electronic Library Online, in Spanish)	http://www.scielo.org/php/index.php

Health (NIH) are available through an open-access mechanism after 1 year. There are an increasing number of open-access journals, but as with all journals, the reader must be able to critically evaluate the studies that appear in these publications.

Locating Best Evidence
Clinicians must learn how to locate the information that is needed to guide their decision making. Skills necessary for navigating electronic databases to locate best evidence can be developed through practice or may be obtained through participation in a training program. Numerous databases are available to clinicians to assist with information retrieval (see Table 1). While developing good database searching skills may help improve the clinician's confidence in locating information, possessing these skills alone is not enough to answer the many questions that arise in daily practice. Clinicians must also possess the necessary skills to critically appraise the literature, which requires an understanding of research methodology and criteria used to determine the quality of the evidence.

Understanding Research Methodology
To practice with an evidence-based philosophy, clinicians must possess at least some basic knowledge about research design. Lack of training in research methods while in school significantly challenges many clinicians when reading and interpreting a published study. The following section is intended to introduce the reader to some basic elements for consideration of various study designs. This section is not intended to be a comprehensive review; the reader is referred elsewhere for more detailed information about specific study designs. There is a hierarchy of research designs reflecting the levels of evidence (see Figure 2).

INTRODUCTION TO STUDY DESIGNS
Self-Reported Data: Surveys and Interviews
Surveys are used to collect self-reported data from individual participants using questionnaires or an interview. Surveys provide an easy, cost-effective, and time-efficient way to gather information, especially when information is needed from a large number of

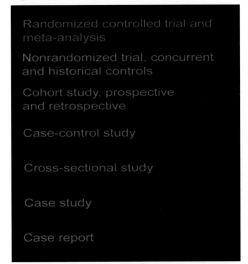

Figure 2. Hierarchy of Research Designs

Source: http://valueanalysismag.com/wp-content/uploads/2013/04/use-this-one-now.jpg with permission.

people. Interviews allow for gathering more detailed information, which can later be verified by patient records, including laboratory tests. An important limitation is that self-reported data are subject to recall bias, meaning that participants may not always accurately report their answers. An advantage of conducting interviews is that trained interviewers record participants' responses, which helps ensure that answers are accurate and complete. Surveys can also be used to gather sensitive information that otherwise might not be disclosed, especially when participant identity can remain anonymous.

Self-reported data may be supplemented with anthropometric measures, such as height, weight, waist/hip circumference, mid-/upper arm circumference, or body fat percentage. Physiological measures may include vital signs or tests of biological specimens, such as urinalysis, blood tests, salivary tests, or tests of physical fitness. Other measures may be obtained from a clinical examination or diagnostic imaging.[6]

For example, individuals may be asked to complete a survey about their perceptions about their own oral health status and oral hygiene habits. These responses could then be supplemented with findings from dental and radiographic examinations. A response to a question about whether the person believes that he or she has periodontal disease could be verified using pocket depths and clinical attachment loss measures, as well as radiographic evidence of bone loss. The additional measures give greater insight about the self-reported information on the survey.

Case Series

Case series studies are observational studies, the goal of which is to gather a collection of reports to describe the treatment of a group of individuals with the same clinical condition[6] (see Figure 3). Similarly, a *case report* is used to document a single individual. Case series designs can be used to capture information about a given aspect of a condition, an approach to treatment, or adverse events associated with treatment. Case reports and case series are easy to understand and are often very useful sources of information for busy clinicians when they encounter a patient who has a clinical condition with which they are unfamiliar. The limitation of this type of design is that there is no control group, so it is not possible to compare this information against another set of treated or untreated individuals.

Cross-Sectional Survey

The goal of a cross-sectional survey is to determine exposure or disease status in a population. These surveys are commonly used in epidemiological research. The investigator assesses what proportion of the population has had exposure to or has a given disease.[6-8] These studies are also known as *prevalence* studies. Cross-sectional studies collect a "snapshot" of information, meaning that all data are collected at one time-point (see Figure 4). The purpose of conducting this type of study is to identify correlations, or relationships, between risk factors and diseases. It is important to remember that a correlation is not the same as cause and effect.[8] These studies are relatively easy to conduct, but are limited in usefulness.

For example, an investigator decides to study work-related musculoskeletal disorders (WRMD) among 1,500 practicing dental hygienists. In the study sample, 1,450 of the participants are female. All participants complete a questionnaire to assess the number of areas on the body where the individual self-reports chronic pain. Other variables assessed include self-reported age, sex, race, height, and weight. Among the study results are strong correlations between age and sex with the number of areas that are reported to be painful. Study results must be interpreted with caution, as risk for painful musculoskeletal disorders, such as arthritis and tendonitis, tends to increase with age in the general population. The study does not account for other possible causes for musculoskeletal pain, such as sports injuries or history of motor vehicle accidents, so it is difficult to determine whether clinical findings are solely related to WRMD. It would be incorrect to conclude that female dental

Figure 3. Case Report/Case Series Design

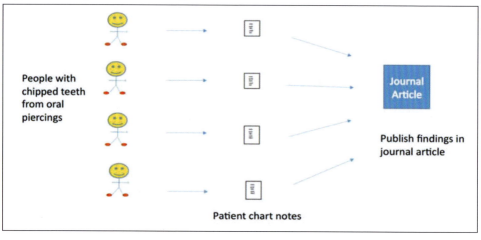

Figure 4. Cross-Sectional Design

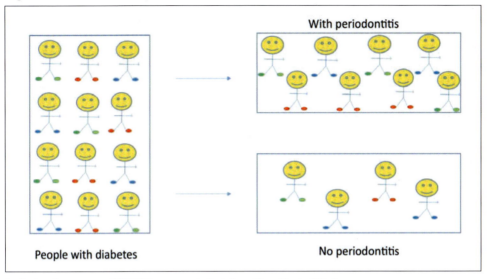

hygienists have more WRMD, as most dental hygienists are disproportionately female, both in this study sample and in the general population of dental hygienists. To assess the relationship between sex and WRMD, there should be an equal number of male dental hygienists as participants in the study.

In another example, an epidemiological study reports that among 600 people examined in a small rural community, triclosan metabolites were reported to be present in urine samples collected from 95% of subjects. The investigators conclude that the community is being exposed to triclosan; however, the source, dose, and frequency of use cannot be determined. Lack of understanding about the limitations of this type of study design and misinformation create a perceived risk for a harmful health outcome based solely on the presence of a metabolite, although no adverse health effects are documented. The study results do not address the possibility that metabolites in the urine may actually indicate that any triclosan that was ingested has been adequately metabolized by the liver and removed from the body by the kidneys. Normal triclosan exposure is topical, not systemic. Behaviors related to triclosan use change because of a perceived negative association and incomplete information.

Case-Control Study
Case-control studies are also observational studies, the goal of which is to compare exposure histories in people with disease (cases) to people without disease (controls).[7,9] People are selected to be in the study based upon their diagnosis. This design is used to identify likely risk factors for a disease, especially for uncommon conditions that are only present in a select number of individuals in the general population. The investigator asks, "Do cases and controls have different exposure histories?"[6] Typically, this design is *retrospective*. People with the disease and a control group of people without the disease are selected, and then the investigator determines the proportion of cases who were exposed to risk factors in the past and compares that to the proportion of people exposed in the control group. For example, this design may be used to determine whether exposure to radiation is a risk factor for thyroid cancer (see Figure 5). The investigator would compare the radiation exposure history of people with thyroid cancer (cases) with the radiation exposure history of those without thyroid cancer (controls). The hypothesis may be that patients with thyroid cancer have greater odds of frequent or large dosages of radiation exposure than those without thyroid cancer.

Figure 5. Case-Control Study Design

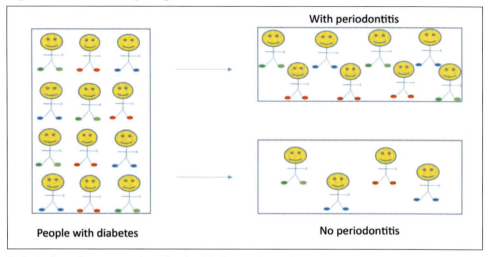

A limitation of case-control studies is risk for *recall bias*. Subjects are often asked to recall events that occurred a long time ago or the sequence of events as they occurred. Also, this type of study cannot be used to determine absolute risk for a negative outcome from exposure, as the study population is usually not representative of the general population as a whole.[7] Although the prevalence of the disease in the exposed population in the study may be high, the prevalence in the general population from which the cases were recruited may be relatively rare. Thus, these studies cannot be used to calculate rates of disease among the exposed and not exposed. Rather, they are used to determine the *odds* of exposure among the diseased and not diseased.[7] A measure of association, known as an odds ratio (OR), is used to report the results. An OR reflects the odds of exposure in cases to the odds of exposure in controls. Investigators must provide a clear case definition to identify the appropriate subjects for the study population, have a source of cases to study, and determine whether it will be useful to "match" the cases and controls. Matching as many similar characteristics as possible between cases and controls results in populations that have similar distributions for age, sex, socioeconomic status, and so on, allowing for greater confidence in study findings.

Cohort Study

The goal of a cohort study is to compare rates of new disease in a group of similar people with different exposure histories or to follow a population prospectively across time to look for new disease.[6,7,9] As the goal is to look for new disease, none of the participants can have the disease in question at the start of the study. Participants must be similar in their characteristics except for their exposure histories. Cohort studies often require patients to be followed for months or years and require large numbers of subjects. This design is not a good choice for determining rare outcomes. Results of cohort studies are reported using a measure of association known as the *rate ratio* (RR), which is also known as the *relative rate*, *risk ratio*, or *relative risk*. The RR compares the incidence rate among the exposed to the incidence rate in the unexposed.[6,7]

A *prospective* design allows an investigator to assess the baseline exposure and disease status of all participants and then conduct follow-up assessments to determine how many people develop the new disease after the initial examination.[6] In Figure 6, the investigator examines subjects who all have prosthetic joints, who are free of joint infection, and are patients of record in the same large community health center. The study will be used to determine whether use of antibiotics prior to invasive medical and dental procedures influences the development of prosthetic joint infection. For this study, patients are not randomly assigned to receive prophylactic antibiotics or not; the investigator does not control the exposure history (antibiotic use). Patients report whether they take prophylactic antibiotics when the investigator tracks the patients every 6 months as they undergo a variety of invasive procedures over 3 years. At the end of the study period, the investigator can sort the patients who develop prosthetic joint infection by reported prophylactic antibiotic use or not, as well as identify when an infection occurred during the study period, and type of invasive procedures performed prior to the onset of the infection. In this illustrated example, the outcome of prosthetic joint infection did not differ among participants, regardless of antibiotic use. The incidence rate was the same in the exposed and unexposed; this means that the exposure was not associated with the disease (RR = 1). Limitations of this design include risk for dropouts or information bias (e.g., examining patients who did not take prophylactic antibiotics more vigorously to check for signs of infection). To reduce risk for information bias, subjects should undergo the same examination procedures at baseline and at all follow-up appointments.

A cohort study may also be *retrospective*, when a source of individuals with the disease is already available and the investigator is trying to learn about the events (risks) that may have contributed to development of the disease.[6,7,10] Retrospective studies use documented information to establish baseline status and track members of the cohort to a point in the past or to the present. A critical consideration is that the outcome of interest is not present at baseline in any members of the cohort.[10] In Figure 7, the investigator already has access to a group of subjects with prosthetic joint infection. The investigator conducts a chart review to identify risk factors that may have contributed to the development of prosthetic joint infection going back to the time of prosthetic placement. Limitations of this design include missing data from incomplete documentation and missing records. In this illustrated example, the investigator sorts the cases, identifying those who took prophylactic antibiotics prior to invasive procedures from those who did not.[11,12]

Longitudinal cohort studies also follow a group of people across time. However, members of the cohort are recruited because they belong to a well-defined population pool, which differs from a prospective study, where recruitment is based on participant exposure status. At baseline, participants are assessed for many exposures and diseases and are tracked across time to determine the incidence rate for new disease(s).[11,12] There are several variations in design themes for longitudinal studies using different measurement schemes at different time-points.[7,10]

Figure 6. Cohort Study: Prospective Design

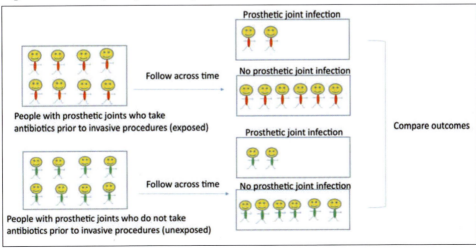

Nonexperimental Intervention Study

The nonexperimental intervention study is also known as a pretest/posttest design. This type of design is most often used to assess the impact of an educational intervention on knowledge, attitudes, and beliefs of study participants. All participants undergo the same study procedures. Figure 8 depicts a study in which the investigator wants to assess the knowledge of schoolchildren about caries risk related to dietary choices, with the goal of helping the children make better food choices to improve their dental health. The investigator designs a simple pretest using supplied response questions that are appropriate to the age and literacy level of the children. After the pretest has been administered and collected, the children attend an educational training program about cariogenic foods and strategies to improve their behaviors related to food choices and risk reduction following consumption of cariogenic foods. After the training program, the children complete the posttest, which contains the same items as the pretest. Scores on the pretest are compared with those from the posttest. Test scores can be compared for each individual child or as a group. Results may be influenced by many factors, including differences in learning styles, susceptibility to distraction during the training or testing process, attitudes towards the trainer, willingness to participate, or cognitive ability.

Experimental Study

The goal of an experimental study is to compare outcomes in people who have been assigned to

Figure 7. Cohort Study: Retrospective Chart Review

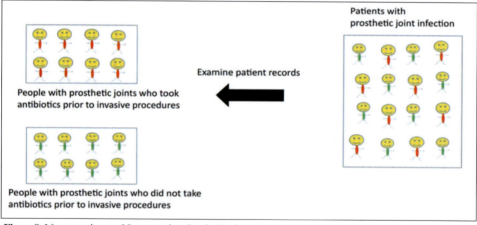

Figure 8. Nonexperimental Intervention Study Design

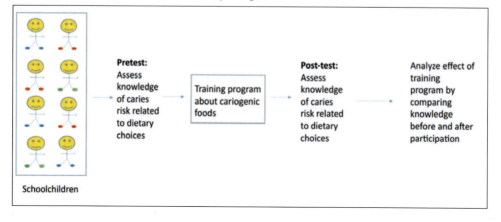

receive an intervention (experimental group) compared to people who have not received the intervention (controls). This design is used to establish a cause-and-effect relationship. The investigator examines whether exposed people are more likely than unexposed people to have a prespecified outcome.[6] These studies are known as randomized controlled trials (RCTs). Members of the experimental group may also be referred to as the treatment group, who receive the intervention under investigation. Members of the control group receive either standard treatment or no treatment (placebo). Patients are randomly assigned to either group to reduce bias and to help increase the probability that differences in the study outcome between the groups can be attributed to the intervention under study.

RCTs are considered the gold standard for clinical research and are primarily used to evaluate treatment effectiveness. Figure 9 depicts an RCT using a placebo. In this study, patients with self-reported dental anxiety are randomly assigned to receive either a benzodiazepine prior to dental treatment or a placebo. The placebo tablet is the same color, shape, and size as the benzodiazepine so that neither the investigator nor the subject knows which drug is being taken. This is known as a *double-blind design*, which is the most rigorous of all research designs. It reduces risk of bias and any potential placebo effect, and increases confidence that the treatment is, in fact, responsible for the outcome. The subjects are asked to rate their level of dental anxiety before and after taking their assigned drug. The hypothesis for this study is that pretreatment benzodiazepine use will reduce the level of self-reported dental anxiety. Differences in self-reported dental anxiety should be greater in the benzodiazepine (experimental) group.

Single-blind design may be used when it is not possible for the subject to be unaware of the type of intervention being used, but the investigator can remain blinded. For example, an investigator wants to assess differences in efficacy of supragingival plaque removal by comparing use of a power toothbrush with a manual toothbrush. Subjects could still be randomly assigned to a toothbrush group, but would be trained in brushing technique by another member of the research team. Then the investigator would only interact with the subject during the clinical examination to record plaque scores, while remaining unaware of the type of toothbrush being used.

Sometimes, RCTs compare two or more interventions, all of which produce effects; this approach is also known as head-to-head comparison studies. In this case, the alternate interventions are known as active controls. This type of design is frequently used in dental studies to evaluate differences in product effectiveness, such as mouthwash studies in which each mouthwash contains a different active ingredient that has demonstrated efficacy for supragingival plaque and gingivitis reduction. The purpose of this type of study would be to determine which mouthwash performs "best" by comparing scores on standardized plaque and gingival indices.

Figure 9. Randomized Controlled Trial: Placebo Control Design

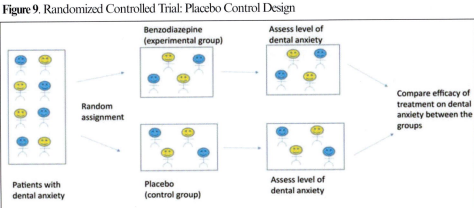

Alternately, an RCT may use an active control when it is not ethical to withhold an intervention that is deemed necessary for the health of the individual. Human subject review boards do not approve studies when the risk for compromising health status in participants is too great. Figure 10 depicts an RCT in patients who are about to begin radiation therapy for a newly diagnosed head and neck cancer. Because caries risk is well-documented to be very high for this population, it would not be ethical to withhold fluoride therapy for any participants in this group. The investigator in this study wants to determine if the method of fluoride application influences the formation of new caries in this at-risk population. The standard of care for fluoride application in this population is with use of custom trays, which becomes the intervention that subjects who are randomly assigned to the control group will receive. Thus, controls will not be at increased risk as nothing is being taken away or withheld from them. Participants who are randomly assigned to the experimental group will apply fluoride using a toothbrush. Both groups are receiving fluoride and their rates of new caries formation will be assessed at regular intervals across the study period.

Qualitative Study
The goal of a qualitative study is to understand how individuals, communities, and populations perceive, interpret, and make sense of phenomena and their experiences.[6,13] Qualitative methods are used to study human behavior, communication, and emotions in the context of cultural, societal, and environmental situations. Qualitative studies often use many different types of methods to gather information, including observation and interviews, using *purposeful* sampling, selecting individuals who are representative of the group or topic under investigation. Among the most common methods used to collect data are interviews and focus groups.[13,14] During in-depth or semi-structured interviews, the investigator poses open-ended questions to participants and is allowed to ask more in-depth questions to gain a better understanding of subjects' perspectives.[6,13] Focus groups are comprised of small numbers of participants led by a facilitator who is often a member of the research team.[14] The purpose of the focus group is to study how members interact with one another and to identify shared viewpoints and controversies. The lead investigator will observe the focus group, often out of view, or via a videotaped or audiotaped recording of the session. Session transcripts from interviews and focus groups are studied to capture both verbal and nonverbal communications, which are coded and scored for interpretation.[6,15] Qualitative research may be used along with quantitative research.

Systematic Review
A systematic review is conducted to synthesize existing knowledge to answer a very specific question.[16] The goal is to compare findings from previously published studies to draw a conclusion.[6] It is much more rigorous than a literature review. A systematic review is conducted according to a very detailed

Figure 10. Randomized Controlled Trial: Active Control Design

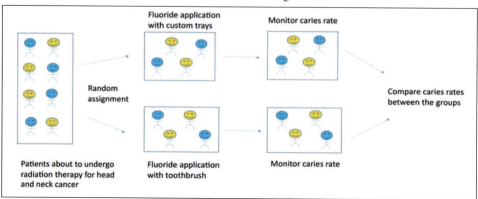

process, which the authors disclose in their published review. This disclosure helps the reader to understand which articles have been included in the review and why.

The first step in conducting a systematic review is to identify a very narrow and focused question. The investigators then define criteria as part of the strategy that is used to search the literature. This may include the use of specific search terms, time frames during which the papers were published, studies with specific types of research designs, and studies with a minimum number of subjects.[6] Studies that do not meet these criteria are automatically excluded. The investigators then *systematically* search multiple databases to locate possible studies for inclusion. Each article is read in its entirety to determine eligibility for inclusion. A systematic review is also unique in that investigators may also choose to include unpublished data if it meets the criteria and is relevant to the question. Afterward, the investigators identify a count of the final number of papers included for review.

The investigators then critically appraise each of the included articles, and results from the individual studies are combined for analysis. Studies that find no statistically significant findings are also included with those that do not. These results are also disclosed in the review. For example, the investigators may report that, "Of the 150 articles that were identified in the search, 30 studies met the criteria for inclusion. Of those 30 studies, 13 studies show that use of Drug A significantly reduced the level of postoperative dental pain while 17 studies found that there were no differences between using Drug A and placebo on degree of postoperative dental pain."

In the context of a systematic review, the *quality* of the included articles reflects the degree of confidence that the estimates of the treatment effect are correct. Systematic reviews are at risk for *publication bias*, meaning that articles that demonstrate statistically significant findings are more likely to be published than those that do not.[6,17,18] There is also a risk that a systematic review is based on only a small number of studies due to a limited number of available published papers on the topic. The reader must also be mindful of the time frame used for study inclusion. A systematic review may influence a reader to believe that an intervention is not appropriate for a given patient population, when in fact many other studies that support the intervention as a favorable choice have been published after the time frame for inclusion has ended. Clinicians should be aware that other publications, speakers, and marketing materials frequently cite findings from a systematic review long after the review has become outdated, especially if the review can be used to endorse a particular product. As with all studies, as new information becomes available, systematic reviews need to be continuously updated.[19]

Meta-Analysis

A meta-analysis is also conducted to synthesize existing knowledge, but with a different strategy from a systematic review.[6,20] A meta-analysis merges

Figure 11. Meta-Analysis

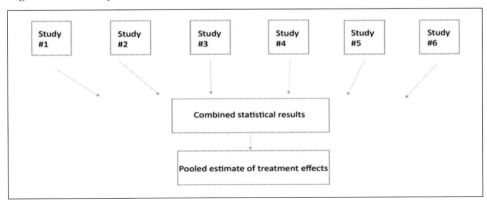

the results from previously published studies pooling the statistics to obtain an estimate of treatment effectiveness (see Figure 11). Data are typically from RCTs, although data can also be combined from case control and cohort studies.[20,21]

Only results from studies with the same research design, similar statistics used for analysis, and those using the same intervention, type of control, and study populations may be pooled. Similar studies are known as *homogeneous* studies. Studies that are too different (*heterogeneous*) are not appropriate for inclusion. The investigators are responsible for demonstrating that the results from studies are comparable and therefore appropriate for inclusion.

Meta-analyses answer questions not posed by individual studies. As with systematic reviews, there is also risk for publication bias with this type of study.[22,23] Quality of the findings of the meta-analysis is based on the quality of the design of the included studies. Meta-analyses should reflect the highest level of evidence available to support clinical decision making.

Registering Systematic Reviews and Meta-Analyses

There has been a widespread effort to encourage investigators to register their protocols for systematic reviews to promote collaboration and to avoid duplication of efforts by multiple research teams who are interested in answering the same question. These registries include the Campbell Collaboration, which produces systematic reviews of the effects of social interventions (https://www.campbellcollaboration.org);

Table 2. Resources to Assist with Critically Appraising the Literature

Resource	
Critical Appraisal Skills Programme (CASP)	http://www.casp-uk.net/checklists
Appraisal of Guidelines Research and Evaluation (AGREE)	http://www.agreetrust.org/wp-content/uploads/2013/12/AGREE-II-GRS-Instument.pdf
University of South Australia Critical Appraisal Tools	http://www.unisa.edu.au/Research/Sansom-Institute-for-Health-Research/Research/Allied-Health-Evidence/Resources/CAT
University of Oxford Critical Appraisal Tools	http://www.cebm.net/critical-appraisal
CONSORT	http://www.consort-statement.org
STARD	http://www.equator-network.org/reporting-guidelines/stard
STROBE	http://www.strobe-statement.org/index.php?id=strobe-home
MOOSE	https://www.editorialmanager.com/jognn/account/MOOSE.pdf
COREQ	http://cdn.elsevier.com/promis_misc/ISSM_COREQ_Checklist.pdf
RECORD	http://www.record-statement.org/
INSPIRE	http://inspiresim.com/simreporting
TREND	http://www.cdc.gov/trendstatement/Index.html
PRISMA	http://prisma-statement.org
Stichting Center for Evidence-Based Management (CEBMa)	https://www.cebma.org/resources-and-tools/what-is-critical-appraisal
Richards D, Clarkson J, Matthews D, Niederman R. *Evidence-based Dentistry: Managing Information for Better Practice.*	[Textbook] London, England: Quintessence Publishing Company; 2008. ISBN: 13:978-1-85097-126-9
Frantsve-Hawley J. *Evidence-Based Dentistry for the Dental Hygienist.*	[Textbook] Chicago, IL: Quintessence Publishing Company; 2014. ISBN: 978-0-86715-646-1

the Cochrane Collaboration, an international group that produces and disseminates systematic reviews of healthcare interventions (http://www.cochrane.org); and PROSPERO, an international prospective register of systematic reviews (http://www.crd.york.ac.uk/prospero).[24-26]

Guidelines for Reporting
Guidelines have been developed to improve the quality of reporting study methods and results in the literature. The purpose of these guidelines is to help the reader better understand how the studies were designed and conducted and to aid with interpretation of the results.[27] Use of these guidelines is helpful when clinicians critically appraise published papers to determine relevancy and usefulness to help answer clinical questions. There are guidelines to authors for reporting RCTs (CONSORT), diagnostic tests (STARD), observational studies (STROBE), meta-analyses of observational studies (MOOSE), qualitative studies (COREQ), observational routinely collected health data (RECORD), healthcare simulation research (INSPIRE), non-randomized designs (TREND), and systematic reviews and meta-analyses (PRISMA).[28-38] The International Committee of Medical Journal Editors (ICMJE) also has requirements for authors to follow when submitting papers for publication to biomedical journals.[39] Clinicians are encouraged to use available resources, found in Table 2, to assist with critically appraising a published paper.

STEPS OF EVIDENCE-BASED PRACTICE
Evidence-based practice involves these five steps:
1. Asking answerable questions (*Ask*)
2. Searching for best evidence (*Acquire*)
3. Critically appraising the evidence (*Appraise*)
4. Applying the evidence (*Apply*)
5. Evaluating the outcome (*Assess*)[40] (see Figure 12)

It is important to ask good questions that are searchable. To begin this process, clinicians should ask
- "What is the most important issue for this patient now?"
- "What issue should I address first?"
- "Which question, when answered, will help me most?"[41]

Questions should be framed following the PICO format:[41]
P = Patient or population or presenting symptom
I = Intervention or exposure
C = Control or comparison
O = Outcome

For example, "In adult smokers (**P**), does brushing with an antibacterial toothpaste (**I**) as compared to brushing with a whitening toothpaste (**C**) reduce more supragingival plaque (**O**)?"

LEVELS OF EVIDENCE
After the clinician forms the question to *Ask*, the next step is to *Acquire* the information needed to

Figure 12. The Five Steps of Evidence-Based Medicine

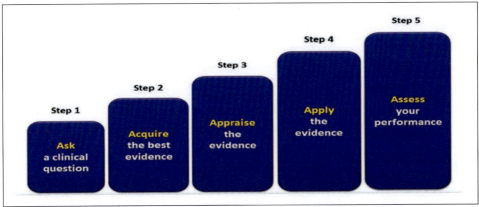

Source: https://www.healthcatalyst.com/wp-content/uploads/2015/09/five-steps-evidence-based-medicine.png with permission.

answer the question. With so many published papers to choose from, clinicians may struggle with deciding which type of information is most current and most useful. As previously discussed, the ability to both search and locate the information that is being sought are skills unto themselves that can directly impact which papers the clinician accesses to read. Further, a decision must be made about whether the information is truly useful, which largely depends on the methodology of the study. As can be seen from the preceding discussion, not all methodology is equally reliable. Today, it is rare for a clinician to seek sources from *primary research*, meaning the original, individual studies about a topic of interest. Many clinicians also depend upon expert opinion, which is considered the lowest level of evidence. Primary sources include the laboratory, observational, experimental, and qualitative studies that have been published, which are the important building blocks for what is known as *secondary, or preappraised, research*.

Preappraised evidence reflects information that has been critically appraised, or filtered, for quality. Preappraised sources consist of critically evaluated journal articles, systematic reviews, meta-analyses, synopses and critical summaries, and clinical practice guidelines, all of which are less time-consuming to read and contain key findings from the original sources. Critical summaries published in evidence-based abstraction journals can be very helpful resources for clinicians, as they provide 1- to 2-page summaries of studies and systematic reviews, allowing for quick access to useful information[42] (see Table 3). Using preappraised resources will increase the chances of efficiently finding high-quality, current evidence that is relevant to practice. The 6S pyramid reflects the hierarchy of preappraised evidence that appears in order of usefulness to busy clinicians[43] (see Figure 13).

Table 3. Helpful Resources that Support Clinical Decision Making

Resource	Web Address
Evidence-Based Dentistry (journal subscription)	http://www.nature.com/ebd/index.html
Evidence-Based Dentistry website	http://www.nature.com/ebd/site_features.html
Journal of Evidence-Based Dental Practice (subscription)	http://www.jebdp.com
International Journal of Evidence-Based Practice for the Dental Hygienist	http://www.quintpub.com/journals/ebh/about.php
DHNet (National Center for Dental Hygiene Research & Practice)	http://dent-web01.usc.edu/dhnet
Medscape	http://www.medscape.com
ACP Journal Club	http://acpjc.acponline.org

Figure 13. The 6S Hierarchy of Preappraised Evidence

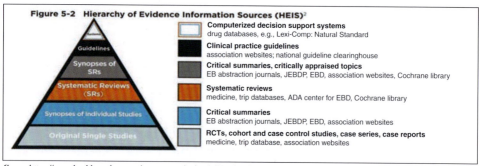

Source: https://www.healthcatalyst.com/wp-content/uploads/2015/09/five-steps-evidence-based-medicine.png.
© Forrest & Miller, EBDM in Action: Developing Competence in EB Practice

CLINICAL PRACTICE GUIDELINES

Clinical practice guidelines (CPGs) are among the easiest of resources for clinicians to locate and use to support their practice. Guidelines represent best available evidence, preferably obtained from systematic reviews and meta-analyses. Information contained within the guidelines has usually undergone the first three steps of the evidence-based process (*Ask, Acquire, Appraise*), and some guidelines include recommendations about when and how they should be applied and how the user should assess outcomes, reflecting the last two steps of the process (*Apply, Assess*).[40]

Use of CPGs promotes consistency of care and best practices. The recommendations included in CPGs are often broad enough to allow clinicians to deviate within an "acceptable framework of variation."[44] Variation occurs for a variety of reasons, encouraging clinicians to exercise their judgment, tailor interventions to a patient's individual needs, and weigh risks versus benefits. These actions reflect the underlying premise of practicing with an evidence-based philosophy: scientific evidence alone is not sufficient to support clinical decision making.[45,46] From this perspective, CPGs should not be viewed as a "one-size-fits-all" approach to care, but instead as a guide to promote the delivery of quality, patient-centered care. Patients, too, may access information about CPGs on the Internet, empowering them to engage in discussions with their care providers to participate in the planning and evaluation of their treatment and expected outcomes.[47] CPGs should not be misconstrued as rules or as legal documents, although if widely adopted and endorsed by key stakeholders in dentistry, they may reflect the current standard of care. Finally, CPGs help to identify additional needs for research using better methodologies to answer clinical questions.[44] Table 4 provides a list of resources for locating clinical practice guidelines.

GRADING SCIENTIFIC EVIDENCE
(*APPRAISE*)

One of the most challenging aspects of reviewing and interpreting the scientific evidence is assigning or ascribing some sort of value to the evidence. Putting aside personal bias, it is often challenging

Table 4. Locating Clinical Practice Guidelines

Organization	Web Address
National Guideline Clearinghouse (part of AHRQ)	http://www.guideline.gov
AHRQ Search for Research Summaries, Reviews, and Reports	http://www.effectivehealthcare.ahrq.gov/index.cfm/search-for-guides-reviews-and-reports/
American College of Physicians	https://www.acponline.org/clinical-information/guidelines
Canadian Medical Association Infobase: Clinical Practice Guidelines Database	https://www.cma.ca/En/Pages/clinical-practice-guidelines.aspx
American Dental Association Center for Evidence-Based Dentistry	http://ebd.ada.org
American Academy of Pediatric Dentistry	http://www.aapd.org/policies
Centers for Disease Control and Prevention: Oral Health Home	http://www.cdc.gov/oralhealth/guidelines.htm
U.S. Preventive Services Task Force	https://www.uspreventiveservicestaskforce.org/BrowseRec/Index/browse-recommendations
Scottish Intercollegiate Guidelines Network (SIGN)	http://www.sign.ac.uk/guidelines/published/index.html#Dentistry
Scottish Dental Clinical Effectiveness Programme (SDCEP)	http://www.sdcep.org.uk
National Institute for Health and Care Excellence (NICE)	https://www.nice.org.uk

for the clinician, who is not directly involved with reviewing the science, to determine the quality of the information contained in the article he or she just read. Fortunately, there are groups that focus on evaluating and grading the scientific literature. These groups are a superb resource when the clinician is searching for quality evidence regarding a clinical question. These groups are well established and respected, and the reviews they create are often used by policy makers and others in the provision of care. Understanding the grading systems used by these groups allows any clinician to apply one of these approaches to the scientific information under review and determine the strength of the evidence.

Centre for Evidence-Based Medicine
(http://www.cebm.net)
The Centre for Evidence-Based Medicine (CEBM) is located on the campus of the University of Oxford, UK. CEBM is a nonprofit organization that focuses on three important areas related to evidence-based medicine: research, teaching, and information dissemination. CEBM has a large staff, who work with a wide variety of individuals throughout the world, producing high-quality systematic reviews meant to improve clinical practice. The Centre also teaches courses in evidence-based medicine at all levels—from undergraduate students to seasoned clinicians—via workshops and courses. Finally, the Centre also publishes its findings in a publicly accessible database.

CEBM has created a set of very useful tables that allow a numerical grade to be given to a type of evidence. The Centre has prepared these tables based on the overall type of evidence that is being evaluated:

- Therapy, prevention, etiology, and harm (see Table 5)
- Diagnosis (see Table 6)

Table 5. CEBM Table for Therapy, Prevention, Etiology, Harm

1a	Systematic reviews (with homogeneity) of randomized controlled trials
1b	Individual randomized controlled trials (with narrow confidence interval)
1c	All or none randomized controlled trials
2a	Systematic reviews (with homogeneity) of cohort studies
2b	Individual cohort study or low-quality randomized controlled trials (e.g., < 80% follow-up)
2c	"Outcomes" research; ecological studies
3a	Systematic review (with homogeneity) of case-control studies
3b	Individual case-control study
4	Case series (and poor quality cohort and case-control studies)
5	Expert opinion without explicit critical appraisal, or based on physiology, bench research, or "first principles"

Table 6. CEBM Table for Diagnosis

1a	Systematic review (with homogeneity) of Level 1 diagnostic studies; or a clinical decision rule with 1b studies from different clinical centers
1b	Validating cohort study with good reference standards; or clinical decision rule tested within one clinical center
1c	Absolute SpPins And SnNouts*
2a	Systematic review (with homogeneity) of Level > 2 diagnostic studies
2b	Exploratory cohort study with good reference standards; clinical decision rule after derivation, or validated only on split-sample or databases
3a	Systematic review (with homogeneity) of 3b and better studies
3b	Nonconsecutive study; or without consistently applied reference standards
4	Case-control study, poor or nonindependent reference standard
5	Expert opinion without explicit critical appraisal, or based on physiology, bench research or "first principles"

*An Absolute SpPin is a diagnostic finding whose Specificity is so high that a Positive result rules in the diagnosis. An Absolute SnNout is a diagnostic finding whose Sensitivity is so high that a Negative result rules out the diagnosis.

• Prognosis (see Table 7)

How the evidence is graded is similar in each table, with subtle differences based on the type of evidence. These systems are often used by independent researchers conducting systematic reviews to evaluate and grade evidence that is included in the review.

GRADE (http://www.gradeworkinggroup.org)
Another group that has attempted to bring some order to the evaluation and assessment of evidence is the GRADE working group. Created in 2000, GRADE (Grading of Recommendations, Assessment, Development, and Evaluation) focuses on bringing together individuals with an interest in grading scientific evidence, who are also concerned with the deficiencies in some of the systems being used. The group has developed a simple and straightforward approach to assessing the scientific evidence (see Table 8). It is not as complex or detailed as the CEBM system, but the utility of the GRADE system lies in its simplicity. By extension, the GRADE working group has also provided tools by which evidence, once it is evaluated, can be converted into clinical guidelines. To facilitate its use, the GRADE working group offers training and development courses, and has provided an online resource, called GRADEPro (https://gradepro.org), which has software that allows the development of summary findings from a review, and the conversion into guidelines.

Agency for Healthcare Research and Quality
(http://www.ahrq.gov)
The Agency for Healthcare Research and Quality

Table 7. CEBM Table for Diagnosis

1a	Systematic review (with homogeneity) of inception cohort studies; or a clinical decision rule validated in different populations.
1b	Individual inception cohort study with > 80% follow-up; or a clinical decision rule validated on a single population
1c	All or none case series
2a	Systematic review (with homogeneity) of either retrospective cohort studies or untreated control groups in randomized controlled trials.
2b	Retrospective cohort study or follow-up of untreated control patients in a randomized controlled trial; or derivation of a clinical decision rule or validated on split-sample only
2c	"Outcomes" research
3	Individual Case Control Study
4	Case series (and poor-quality prognostic cohort studies)
5	Expert opinion without explicit critical appraisal, or based on physiology, bench research, or "first principles"

Table 8. Grading of Recommendations, Assessment, Development, and Evaluation (GRADE)

Code	Quality of Evidence	Definition
A	High	Further research is very unlikely to change our confidence in the estimate of effect. • Several high-quality studies with consistent results • In special cases: one large, high-quality multicenter trial
B	Moderate	Further research is likely to have an important impact on our confidence in the estimate of effect and may change the estimate. • One high-quality study • Several studies with some limitations
C	Low	Further research is very likely to have an important impact on our confidence in the estimate of effect and is likely to change the estimate. • One or more studies with severe limitations
D	Very Low	Any estimate of effect is very uncertain. • Expert opinion • No direct research evidence • One or more studies with very severe limitations

(AHRQ) is a United States federal organization, part of the United States Department of Health and Human Services, which conducts research about healthcare evidence, with the goal of making care safer and of better quality. A main focus of AHRQ is to evaluate, measure, and track the US healthcare system, providing data to health professionals and policy makers on the performance of the system. AHRQ also has an important mission of producing high-quality resources that can be used to educate health professionals to improve the quality of care for their patients. AHRQ has adapted evidence-based approaches into its system of evidence reviews and how recommendations should be graded (see Tables 9 and 10).

Cochrane Collaboration
(http://www.cochrane.org)
Finally, the entity that is likely most recognizable to the reader is the Cochrane Collaboration, which was established in 1993 by Sir Iain Chalmers, a British health services researcher. This independent, nonprofit, and nongovernmental organization evolved in response to Dr. Archibald (Archie) Cochrane's advocacy for using RCTs to enhance the effectiveness and efficiency of medicine. Cochrane's book, *Effectiveness and Efficiency: Random Reflections on Health Service*, remains a staple for those in the field of evidence-based medicine.[48]

The Cochrane Collaboration was formed to review and organize medical research information using a systematic approach so that health professionals, policy makers, and even patients, can make informed decisions regarding health treatments and interventions according to established principles of evidence-based medicine. The strength of the organization comes from the more than 37,000 volunteers in over 130 countries who form the core that conducts the systematic reviews for which the Collaboration is famous. The Cochrane Collaboration publishes the results from these reviews in the Cochrane Library. Details about the Collaboration, how it is organized, and access to reviews can be found at the organization's website, listed earlier. Table 11 provides a succinct summary of the organization's guiding principles.

Table 9. AHRQ Levels of Scientific Evidence

Level	Type of Scientific Evidence (SE)
Ia	SE obtained from meta-analyses of randomized clinical trials.
Ib	SE obtained from at least one randomized clinical trial
IIa	SE obtained from at least one well-designed, nonrandomized controlled prospective study
IIb	SE obtained from at least one well-designed, quasi-experimental study
III	SE obtained from well-designed observational studies, such as comparative studies, correlation study, or case-control studies
IV	SE obtained from documents or opinions of expert committees, or clinical experiences of renowned opinion leaders, or both

Table 10. AHRQ Grades of Recommendation

Grade	Recommendation
A (Levels of SE Ia, Ib)	It requires at least one randomized clinical trial as part of the scientific evidence, with overall good quality and consistency in terms of the specific recommendation.
B (Levels of SE IIa, IIb, III)	It requires methodologically correct clinical trials that are not randomized clinical trials on the topic of recommendation. It includes studies that do not meet Criteria A or C.
C (Level of SE IV)	It requires documents or opinions of expert committees or clinical experiences of renowned opinion leaders, or both. It indicates the absence of high-quality, directly applicable clinical studies.

SE, scientific evidence.

Reviews by the Cochrane Collaboration follow a very specific format:
1. The review question must be well defined.
2. Criteria to guide those conducting the review must be developed, so that the reviewers can determine if a study should be included or not.
3. The reviewers conduct a search for all relevant studies.
4. Studies are selected and data is collected.
5. Risk of bias in studies that have been included in the review must be determined (this step is additional to the process of grading evidence previously discussed).
6. The data are analyzed and the meta-analysis is conducted.
7. A report is generated using a set Cochrane Collaboration format.
8. Following review and acceptance, the report is published.

Reviews, once published, consist of two formats. The full report, which is available to those who subscribe to the Cochrane Collaboration journal, and a shorter executive summary, are open source and freely accessible.

APPLYING EVIDENCE TO PRACTICE (*APPLY*)

Having found and appraised the best available evidence, the next step is to decide how the results of the search apply to the clinical question. The clinician should ask the following questions to assess the clinical relevance of a study.[49]

Is this form of care or treatment feasible in my clinical setting?

It is important to remember that replicating the conditions of an RCT, including practice setting, is extremely difficult. Further investigation may be needed to determine if the proposed intervention will work in the clinician's setting. Different equipment may be necessary, training may be required, or the cost of the intervention may make implementation unrealistic.

Are the patients in my clinical setting very different from those in this study?

Subjects in research studies may have very different

Table 11. Cochrane Collaboration Key Principles

1.	Collaboration	By fostering global cooperation, teamwork, and open and transparent communication and decision making
2.	Building on the enthusiasm of individuals	By involving, supporting, and training people of different skills and backgrounds
3.	Avoiding duplication of effort	By good management, coordination, and effective internal communications to maximize economy of effort
4.	Minimizing bias	Through a variety of approaches such as scientific rigor, ensuring broad participation, and avoiding conflicts of interest
5.	Keeping up to date	By a commitment to ensure that Cochrane Systematic Reviews are maintained through identification and incorporation of new evidence
6.	Striving for relevance	By promoting the assessment of health questions using outcomes that matter to people making choices in health and health care
7.	Promoting access	By wide dissemination of our outputs, taking advantage of strategic alliances, and by promoting appropriate access models and delivery solutions to meet the needs of users worldwide
8.	Ensuring quality	By applying advances in methodology, developing systems for quality improvement, and being open and responsive to criticism
9.	Continuity	By ensuring that responsibility for reviews, editorial processes, and key functions is maintained and renewed
10.	Enabling wide participation	In our work by reducing barriers to contributing and by encouraging diversity

characteristics than the patients seen in the clinician's work setting. Compliance with the proposed intervention may have been easier for the subjects, especially if they were closely monitored or rewarded in some way for their participation. Compliance is a critical consideration when asking any individual to try something new or "different" from what is currently being used.

Will my patient benefit more or less than the people in the study?
Ultimately, the clinician must decide if his or her patients will benefit more or less than those who were studied. Clinicians must look carefully at what was actually being tested in the study. In the case of an oral care product, it is important to know whether the study evaluated the actual product formulation or just an ingredient found in this and many other products. Clinicians should beware of statements such as "45 studies support the efficacy of this product." Ask to see a reference list of these cited studies.

Other important questions to ask include
- What was the duration of the study? Twenty-four hours? One week? One month? Three months?
- How long is "long enough?"
- Is the strength, dose, or concentration of the product the same as the product I will use with my patients?
- How big was the study sample?
- Are these pilot data?

Is there evidence of harm?
A particular challenge is that it is not easy to find information about possible harmful effects associated with an intervention. As previously mentioned, publication bias has resulted in a preponderance of published studies with positive outcomes. Clinicians need to know whether something is contraindicated or not the best choice for certain individuals. Potential harm is also an important consideration in weighing risk versus benefit and identifying alternative options when obtaining informed consent for treatment. Doing nothing may also be an option should no good alternative exist.

Will the potential benefits outweigh the potential harms of this form of care (or treatment) for my patients?
Clinicians need to be informed of both risks and benefits in order to make good decisions. This information is also needed to inform patients about reasonable, anticipated outcomes and what potential risks are involved if the proposed treatment is accepted. Clinicians are cautioned not to become overly affected by marketing claims made by product competitors, who may exaggerate benefits or suggest risk if the clinician chooses a product other than theirs. Clinicians should always refer back to published data that support product claims.

CONCLUSIONS

Adopting an evidence-based philosophy of practice requires a commitment to skill development in accessing, critically appraising, and applying the best information to support clinical decision making, lifelong learning, and professional development. Using research in daily practice may be challenging for the clinician; however, many online tools and resources are available to help with implementation. Keeping current with new research findings is of major importance in the delivery of quality patient care. Clinicians should be aware of interventions that are beneficial, as well as harmful, to patients so they can assist their patients with making choices about treatment options. Further, knowledge about the ineffectiveness of interventions is also helpful, so that clinicians can seek better alternatives for their patients and themselves. Finally, if there is no evidence available to answer a clinical question, clinicians can rely on their experience and judgment to guide their decision making.

REFERENCES

1. Sackett DL, Straus SE, Richardson WS, et al. *Evidence-Based Medicine: How to Practice and Teach EBM*. 2nd ed. Edinburgh, Scotland: Churchill Livingstone; 2000.
2. Sackett DL, Rosenberg WM, Gray JA, Haynes RB, Richardson WS. Evidence based medicine: what it is and what it isn't. *BMJ*. 1996;312:71–72.
3. Haynes RB, Devereaux PJ, Guyatt GH. Clinical expertise in the era of evidence-based medicine and patient choice. *Evid Based Med*. 2002;7:36–38.

4. Haines A, Donald A. *Getting Research Findings into Practice*. London, England: BMJ Publishing Group; 1998.
5. Niederman R. Evidence-based dentistry finds a new forum: Exelauno. *J Am Dent Assoc*. 2009;140:272–274.
6. Jacobsen KJ. *Introduction to Health Research Methods. A Practical Guide*. Sudbury, MA: Jones & Bartlett Learning; 2012.
7. Mann CJ. Observational research methods. Research design II: cohort, cross sectional, and case-control studies. *Emerg Med J*. 2003;20:54–60.
8. Lucas RM, McMichael AJ. Association or causation: evaluating links between "environment and disease." *Bull World Health Org*. 2005;83:792–795.
9. Black N. Why we need observational studies to evaluate the effectiveness of health care. *BMJ*. 1996;312(7040):1215–1218.
10. Rochon PA, Gurwitz JH, Sykora K, et al. Reader's guide to critical appraisal of cohort studies: 1. Role and design. *BMJ*. 2005;330(7496):895–897.
11. Mamdani M, Sykora K, Li P, et al. Reader's guide to critical appraisal of cohort studies: 2. Assessing potential for confounding. *BMJ*. 2005;330(7497):960–962.
12. Normand SL, Sykora K, Li P, Mamdani M, Rochon PA, Anderson GM. Reader's guide to critical appraisal of cohort studies: 3. Analytical strategies to reduce confounding. *BMJ*. 2005;330(7498):1021–1023.
13. Sofaer S. Qualitative research methods. *Int J Qual Health Care*. 2002;14:329–336.
14. Krueger RA, Casey MA. *Focus Groups. A Practical Guide for Applied Research*. Thousand Oaks, CA: Sage Publications; 2000.
15. Dixon-Woods M, Shaw RL, Agarwal S, et al. The problem of appraising qualitative research. *Qual Saf Health Care*. 2004;13:223–225.
16. Agency for Healthcare Research and Quality. Training modules for the systematic reviews methods guide. Available at: https://www.effectivehealthcare.ahrq.gov/search-for-guides-reviews-and-reports/?pageaction=displayproduct&productID=2351. Accessed December 3, 2016.
17. Dwan K, Gamble C, Williamson PR, Kirkham JJ, Reporting Bias Group: Systematic review of the empirical evidence of study publication bias and outcome reporting bias—an updated review. *PLoS ONE* 2013;8(7):e66844.
18. Page MJ, McKenzie JE, Kirkham J, et al. Bias due to selective inclusion and reporting of outcomes and analyses in systematic reviews of randomised trials of healthcare interventions. *Cochrane Lib*. 2014;(10):Art No.:MR000035. doi: 10.1002/14651858.MR000035.pub2.
19. Moher D, Tsertsvadze A. Systematic reviews: when is an update an update? *Lancet*. 2006;367:881–883.
20. Sacks HS, Reitman D, Pagano D, Kupelnick B. Meta-analysis: an update. *Mt Sinai J Med*. 1996;63:216–224.
21. Stewart LA, Clarke MJ. Practical methodology of meta-analyses (overviews) using updated individual patient data. Cochrane Working Group. *Stat Med*. 1995;14:2057–2079.
22. Sutton AJ. Evidence concerning the consequences of publication and related biases. In: Rothstein HR, Sutton AJ, Borenstein M, eds. *Publication Bias in Meta-Analysis—Prevention, Assessment and Adjustments*. Chichester, England: John Wiley; 2005:175–192.
23. Dickersin K. Publication bias: recognizing the problem, understanding its origins and scope, and preventing harm. In: Rothstein HR, Sutton AJ, Borenstein M, eds. *Publication Bias in Meta-Analysis—Prevention, Assessment and Adjustments*. Chichester, England: John Wiley; 2005:11–33.
24. Straus S, Moher D. Registering systematic reviews. *CMAJ*. 2010,182:13–14. doi: 10.1503/cmaj.081849.
25. Booth A, Clarke M, Ghersi D, Moher D, Petticrew M, Stewart L. An international registry of systematic-review protocols. *Lancet*. 2011;377(9760):108–109.
26. Booth A, Clarke M, Dooley G, Ghersi D, Moher D, Petticrew M, Stewart L: The nuts and bolts of PROSPERO: an international prospective register of systematic reviews. *Syst Rev*. 2012;1:2.
27. Sarkis-Onofre R, Cenci MS, Demarco FF, et al. Use of guidelines to improve the quality and transparency of reporting oral health research. *J Dent*. 2015;43:397–404.
28. Moher D, Schultz KF, Altman D. The CONSORT statement: revised recommendations for improving the quality of reports of parallel-group randomized trials. *JAMA*. 2001;285:1987–1991.
29. Rennie D. Improving reports of studies of diagnostic tests: the STARD initiative. *JAMA*. 2003;289:89–90.
30. Bossuyt PM, Cohen JF, Gatsonis CA, Korevaar DA; STARD group. STARD 2015: updated reporting guidelines for all diagnostic accuracy studies. *Ann Transl Med*. 2016;4:85. doi: 10.3978/j.issn.2305–5839.2016.02.06.
31. Vandenbroucke JP, von Elm E, Altman DG, et al. STROBE Initiative. Strengthening the Reporting of Observational Studies in Epidemiology (STROBE): explanation and elaboration. *Ann Intern Med*. 2007;147(8):W163–194.
32. von Elm E, Altman DG, Egger M, et al. STROBE Initiative. Strengthening the Reporting of Observational Studies in Epidemiology (STROBE) Statement: guidelines for reporting observational studies. *Int J Surg*. 2014;12:1495–1499.
33. Stroup DF, Berlin JA, Morton SC, et al. Meta-analysis of observational studies in epidemiology: a proposal for reporting Meta-analysis of Observational Studies in Epidemiology (MOOSE) group. *JAMA*. 2000;283:2008–2012.
34. Nicholls SG, Quach P, von Elm E, et al. The Reporting of Studies Conducted Using Observational Routinely-Collected Health Data (RECORD) statement: methods for arriving at consensus and developing reporting guidelines. *PLoS One*. 2015;10:e0125620.
35. Cheng A, Kessler D, Mackinnon R, et al. International

Network for Simulation-based Pediatric Innovation, Research, and Education (INSPIRE) reporting guidelines investigators. Reporting guidelines for health care simulation research: extensions to the CONSORT and STROBE statements. *Simul Healthc*. 2016;11:238–248.
36. Des Jarlais DC, Lyles C, Crepaz N. TREND Group. Improving the reporting quality of nonrandomized evaluations of behavioral and public health interventions: the TREND statement. *Am J Public Health*. 2004;94:361–366.
37. Moher D, Liberati A, Tetzlaff J, Altman DG. PRISMA Group. Preferred reporting items for systematic reviews and meta-analyses: the PRISMA statement. *BMJ*. 2009;339:b2535.
38. Moher D, Shamseer L, Clarke M, et al. PRISMA-P Group. Preferred reporting items for systematic review and meta-analysis protocols (PRISMA-P) 2015 statement. *Syst Rev*. 2015;4:1.
39. International Committee of Medical Journal Editors. Recommendations for the conduct, reporting, editing, and publication of scholarly work in medical journals. Available at: http://www.icmje.org/recommendations. Accessed December 3, 2016.
40. Richards D, Clarkson J, Matthews D, Niederman R. Evidence-based guidelines. In: *Evidenced-Based Dentistry: Managing Information for Better Practice*. London, England: Quintessence Publishing Co. 2008.
41. Richardson WS, Wilson MC, Nishikawa J, Hayward RS. The well-built clinical question: a key to evidence-based decisions. *ACP J Club*. 1995;123(3):A12–A13.
42. Abt E, Bader JD, Bonetti D. A practitioner's guide to developing critical appraisal skills: translating research into clinical practice. *J Am Dent Assoc*. 2012;143:386–390.
43. DiCenso A, Bayley L, Haynes RB. ACP Journal Club. Editorial: Accessing preappraised evidence: fine-tuning the 5S model into a 6S model. *Ann Intern Med*. 2009;151(6):JC3-2, JC3-3.
44. Sutherland SE, Matthews DC, Fendrich P. Clinical practice guidelines in dentistry. Part I. Navigating new waters. *J Can Dent Assoc*. 2001;67:379–383.
45. Kay E, Nuttall N. Clinical decision making—an art or a science? Part III: To treat or not to treat? *Br Dent J*. 1995;178:153–155.
46. Kay E, Nuttall N. Clinical decision making—an art or a science? Part II: Making sense of treatment decisions. *Br Dent J*. 1995;178:113–116.
47. Sutherland SE. Evidence-based dentistry: Part III: Searching for answers to clinical questions. Finding evidence on the Internet. *J Can Dent Assoc*. 2001;67:320–323.
48. Cochrane AL. *Effectiveness and Efficiency: Random Reflections on Health Service*. London, England: Nuffield Provincial Hospitals Trust; 1972.
49. Clinical Information Access Portal. Module 4: Integrating evidence into practice. Available at: http://www.ciap.health.nsw.gov.au/education/learning module4/intro.html. Accessed December 3, 2016.

Chapter 2
Behavioral Science
S. D. Shanti

THE BIOPSYCHOSOCIAL APPROACH TO PATIENT CARE

Dentistry originated with a focus on biological aspects of illness and health. This "biomedical" model of disease offered a limited perspective for understanding patient health. To expand this perspective Engel proposed the "biopsychosocial" approach, which takes into consideration the psychological, behavioral, and social aspects along with the biological aspects of health.[1] This conceptualization offers clinicians a deeper understanding of their patients' orientation toward health and wellness and the numerous factors that influence their health behaviors. Thus, this model can help illuminate why a patient might choose an action that differs from what the clinician recommends. For instance, a dental professional might suggest that the patient have root canal therapy and a crown, but if the patient is accustomed to extractions and this is the norm in his or her environment, he or she may not wish to spend the money on retaining the tooth. Similarly, if it is common for most children in a community to have extensive caries in primary teeth, parents may come to see this oral disease condition as inevitable and not accept recommendations for caries prevention.

It is important to bear in mind that patient behavior is a major determinant of oral health. In terms of general health, it is estimated that 40% of premature deaths can be attributed to behavioral patterns, putting patient behavior ahead of other causes such as genetic vulnerability, social circumstances, and experiences within the healthcare system.[2] Although this statistic applies to general health, one can extrapolate the implications for oral health. All dental professionals have encountered situations in which behavioral issues such as lack of self-care, improper diet, and tobacco contributed to oral disease.

The behavioral sciences offer instruments to help patients achieve optimal oral health; these instruments are in the form of theories. Theories are intended to serve as a guide or means of explaining phenomena and offer two major benefits:[3]
- A way to understand patients and the context of their actions (or inaction)
- A means to effectively intervene, either to promote a healthy behavior or to stop an unhealthy one

Dental clinicians often share health information with patients in the hopes of persuading them to adopt recommended behaviors. However, information alone is not enough to make a person change his or her behavior. If it were so, then most smokers would stop smoking, as they already know that it is harmful to their health. Simply giving patients more information and telling them what to do is an authoritarian way of interacting with patients and is not likely to bring about lasting change. Rather, patients must be encouraged to take responsibility for their own self-care. By communicating well with their patients, clinicians can help to identify barriers to behavioral change, such as a low level of health literacy or inability or unwillingness to engage in a behavior. The goal is to promote self-efficacy so that patients do not place the burden of their well-being entirely upon their clinicians. Successful behavioral change through improved partnerships between clinicians and patients are crucial for long-term health.

Health behavior is complex and varies among individuals. Clinicians may feel overwhelmed and frustrated when patients do not adopt their recommendations, and may be tempted to stop trying to help their patients change their behaviors. This chapter offers a means to help clinicians better understand patient behavior and to support clinicians in their quest to have patients adopt healthy behaviors.

KEY CONSIDERATIONS
Social Determinants of Health
Social determinants of health are the variables outside the healthcare system that exert an influence

on a person's health and well-being.[4] Also termed "the cause of causes," social determinants include income, education, and the social and political conditions under which people live. Clinicians may offer well-intended advice about optimal oral health, but when doing so, it is important to consider the social context of the patient's life and its impact on his or her health behavior.

Socioeconomic Gradient and Poverty
Poverty and related financial pressures are ubiquitous. In wealthier countries, there are poor people; in poorer countries, there are relatively wealthy people. The distribution of wealth and differences between members of a society are referred to as the social gradient, and these inequalities are manifested in differences in health status.[5] The higher a person is on the gradient, the more likely it is that he or she will be healthy as compared to someone at the lower end of the gradient.

Poverty is the single most important social determinant of health, affecting over a billion people.[6] Poverty limits access to resources and restricts the range of options for interventions related to health. Poverty is stressful because limited resources, often linked with marginalization in society, present a multitude of challenges related to basic necessities such as food, water, shelter, and health care.[7] Disease prevention is relevant to everyone, but is especially poignant when people at greatest risk for experiencing disease have difficulty affording a simple product such as toothpaste with fluoride.[8]

Quality of Life
Disease prevention and timely treatment are self-evident goals in patient care. However, the individual's subjective experience of health (or illness) and ability to function influences quality of life (QOL). Within dentistry, oral health is also measured as the patient's perceived oral health-related quality of life (OHRQOL).[9,10] The concept of OHRQOL encompasses such things as the patient's ability to chew, speak, eat foods without restrictions, and be free from pain and infections. OHRQOL provides a means of understanding the patient's perspective on how he or she experiences oral health.

As OHRQOL is a subjective experience, patients present with a range of perceptions. Yet, what is evident from research across different countries is that people report poorer quality of life when their oral health is suffering.[11-13] Negative life events can have an adverse effect on a person's OHRQOL.[14] Lower levels of parental education are also associated with lower levels of OHRQOL among children.[15] Taking a proactive stance toward one's oral health, as characterized by engaging in positive health behaviors and seeking regular dental care, have been found to increase a person's OHRQOL.[16]

Health Literacy
Health literacy encompasses basic literacy (i.e., the ability to read and write simple text) and additionally the ability to understand, evaluate, and apply health information.[17] Levels of health literacy vary widely, depending on age, education, attitudes toward health issues, and life experiences. Health literacy should not be underestimated in light of data indicating that half the adults in the United States lack the skills to understand print materials for everyday tasks.[18] The European Health Literacy Survey also found that half the Europeans in the study had "inadequate or problematic health literacy."[19] Lower levels of health literacy increase the likelihood that patients may not follow instructions and may fail to understand the importance of disease preventive practices.

Common Risk Factor Approach
In recent years, there has been a call in the dental profession for taking a "common risk factor approach" to preventing oral diseases.[20,21] This approach focuses on three major pathogenic elements—poor diet, alcohol misuse, and tobacco use—and seeks to place oral health within the larger context of overall health. These three elements are associated not only with oral disease, but also with diabetes and cardiovascular disease—which are among the leading chronic diseases throughout

the world. Although this approach has its origins in public health, it is also relevant to patient care as it underscores the connection between oral health and systemic health. In public health, reducing risk factors common to many diseases can benefit people on a population level, and in clinical practice, doing so enables the practitioner to develop an individualized plan for promoting both the oral and the systemic health of the patient.

Understanding and Influencing Health Behavior
Behavioral science theories and models are applied in both public health and clinical settings. They have influenced the development of behavior-based interventions—to both prevent disease and manage it. The repertoire of behavioral theories is vast and can overwhelm even the most ardent researcher. It is helpful to evaluate theories in connection with research outcomes, and to focus on the practical application of theory within clinical settings. Social cognitive theory, stress and coping theory, and the trans-theoretical model, along with the psychotherapeutic method of motivational interviewing are among the most relevant theories and techniques for dental care, especially with respect to disease prevention.[22-25]

Social Cognitive Theory
Social cognitive theory (SCT) contends that people exist in a reciprocal relationship with three elements: what is inside of them (e.g., thoughts, feelings, and motivation level); what they do (e.g., acting with intention); and the world around them (e.g., their environment, which comprises people, structures, and social and political forces). Because of the interconnectedness of these elements, all three offer entry points for initiating change (see Figure 1).

Using this model, it is possible for a person to change how he or she thinks or feels about oral health and, as a result, change behavior (e.g., by brushing with a fluoride toothpaste twice daily). It is also possible for a person to engage in self-care behavior, even if he or she does not initially feel like doing so. Once the action is underway and the

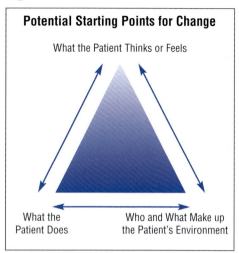

Figure 1.

individual is fully absorbed in the activity, ensuing changes in attitude or level of motivation can result. A person's environment can also have a major impact on oral health. For example, having candy easily accessible in the home or workplace serves as a cue to eat it. Modifying the environment—in this instance, removing the candy—will reduce the likelihood of a person eating it, as the cue for eating candy has been removed.

Self-efficacy is a major element within SCT; it refers to a person's confidence in his or her ability to achieve a goal and overcome impediments along the way. At first glance, the concept may seem simplistic, but the importance of self-efficacy has been borne out by a vast body of research that supports its validity across various domains, including dentistry.[26,27] Self-efficacy is malleable and can be increased in the following ways:
- Patients can look back at past challenges they have successfully dealt with and feel confident about future challenges.
- Patients can observe role models; that is, others who have successfully carried out the desired change.
- Patients can identify important people in their lives who can offer encouragement.

Lastly, it is important to remind patients not to judge their level of self-efficacy when they are tired, stressed, or feeling depleted, as these states hinder an accurate self-assessment of their capacity for change.

Goal setting, done in a collaborative manner, encompasses not only clear definitions of the goal, but also the necessary steps toward the goal (i.e., the subgoals). Often clinicians focus on the goal but do not address the subgoals. However, it is necessary to attend to subgoals, because what may seem like a simple request to the clinician can be experienced as something complex by the patient. Patients may be embarrassed or hesitant to admit that they cannot actually do what is asked of them because they lack the skills to do so. Taking time with patients to elaborate upon the subgoals helps them break down a complex task into small units that they can more readily take on.

Eating fewer sweets and flossing daily are common health recommendations made in dental settings. The likelihood of behavior change is increased by breaking each of these recommendations into small steps that are necessary for reaching the desired goal. Subgoals relevant to healthy eating include identifying healthy snacks to substitute for high sugar ones, writing a grocery list that includes healthy items and omits usual purchases of cookies or candy, structuring the patient's home and work environment to remove easily accessible sweets, and preparing a plan for refusing sweets when offered by others. Subgoals for flossing include discovering which kind of floss best suits the patient's situation; knowing how to floss correctly; making adaptations for physical limitations; identifying a time in the patient's day when the desired behavior can be implemented; linking the flossing to an existing habit such as toothbrushing, so the new habit can be tied to another behavior; and placing floss in a prominent area so it serves as a visual cue for the desired action.

Environments play an important role in influencing behaviors. While it is beyond the scope of the dental clinician to address major environmental factors, such as social and political processes that influence a patient's life, it is possible to address the patient's physical environment—in terms of the modifications that can be made in the home and workplace—in order to support the desired behavior. Previously described measures, such as omitting sweets in the home and placing floss where it is readily visible, are examples of how patients can modify their environment to support their behaviors. Other people in the patient's life are also a part of the environment that surrounds the individual and can influence his or her actions. For instance, a sleep-deprived parent who has to go to work early in the morning may insist that the other parent give a bottle at night to soothe a crying child. Friends who continue to smoke in the presence of the individual who is attempting to quit or friends who offer sweets to someone who is diabetic exemplify how behavior change efforts can be undermined by environmental factors, including other people.

Stress and Coping

Stress is something that every human being experiences, but when it is persistent or overwhelming, it has the potential to affect people's health in adverse ways.[28] Stress exerts direct physical effects on the body. People may also cope with stress in unhealthy ways—such as eating unhealthy foods, smoking, or drinking—and may forgo healthy habits during stressful times.

Stress is defined as a situation in which the demands placed on an individual exceed his or her resources. The process of evaluating the resources at hand and deciding how to respond to the stressors is referred to as appraisal, and it influences the coping process.[29] Events such as job loss and the death of a family member are categorized as major stressors. It is important not to underestimate what are called microstressors or daily hassles, as these are important in their own right and have been shown to have an impact on well-being. Microstressors include recurring events, such as problems with paying bills, difficulties with transportation, and neighborhood annoyances beyond one's control.[30]

Broadly speaking, there are two ways of coping with stress: emotion-focused coping and action-focused coping (also called problem-focused coping). Emotion-focused coping refers to the soothing of emotions associated with stress and encompasses such things as empathy and reassurance. Action-focused coping refers to active problem solving, and taking steps to deal with the stressor and ease the burden. These two forms of coping are not mutually exclusive, and the dental professional can draw upon both forms of coping to support patients. For instance, a father may have a job that prevents him from supervising his child's nightly toothbrushing. In such a situation, the clinician can be empathic toward the parent's dilemma and also brainstorm alternatives to direct supervision. Perhaps there are other adults who might be able to supervise brushing in such situations. Or, perhaps the parent can phone the child from work to check on the brushing behavior.

Other people in the patient's life can offer social support and, in doing so, help reduce the patient's stress. They can offer reassurance to soothe the individual or offer practical assistance with stressful tasks. Family members, friends, and other caring individuals can offer social support and can become involved in supporting the patient's healthy behaviors.

Transtheoretical Model

The transtheoretical model (TTM) arose out of Prochaska and DiClemente's examination of the process of change within the context of various psychological theories.[23] It offers a way of understanding patient behaviors—and underscores that people do not reach their desired goals in one step. Rather, before overt behavior change is visible, there are underlying steps that set the stage for carrying out the new behavior, or the ceasing of unwanted behaviors. Additionally, people do not simply move forward through stages of change in a linear manner, as they may also go back and forth among the stages.

The stages of change according to the TTM are
- **Precontemplation:** The person is neither aware of the need to change nor has plans to change, even if he or she knows that there is a need to change. Examples of this stage include a parent giving a child a bottle filled with milk at bedtime because he or she is unaware of the potential harm it can cause; or a smoker who is aware of the dangers of tobacco use but has no plans to quit.
- **Contemplation:** The person is thinking about changing his or her behavior but is weighing the cost versus the benefit of the new behavior. Using the earlier examples, this stage includes a parent who is thinking about stopping the child's bottle use at bedtime but doubts whether he or she can deal with the child crying when refused the bottle; or a smoker who is thinking about quitting reflects on the effort involved in cessation, and doubts whether he or she can be successful.
- **Preparation:** The person creates a plan of action to reach the desired goal. At this stage, individuals may acquire skills if needed to carry out the desired behavior. For example, the parent comes up with a list of responses to opposition from the child when not given the bottle; or the smoker identifies ways to modify his or her home environment so that cues for smoking are eliminated.
- **Action**: The person finally undertakes the desired behavior, and repetition of the behavior helps to strengthen the change. Examples include the parent not giving a milk-filled bottle to the child at bedtime; or the smoker refraining from smoking.
- **Termination (or Maintenance)**: This is the stage where action has taken hold and become a long-term habit. For example, the parent no longer feeds the child milk in a bottle at bedtime and has established a new routine, replacing the old one; or the smoker has stopped smoking, and furthermore has stopped craving cigarettes and no longer has the desire to smoke.

The TTM led to efforts to match interventions with the patient's stage in the change process. Although this approach appears logical, studies have shown that for patients enrolled in smoking cessation programs, the mere fact of being offered assistance with quitting was beneficial, even if the cessation intervention did not match the patient's particular stage of readiness.[31]

Motivational Interviewing
Motivational interviewing (MI) is a technique to help resolve ambivalence about the change process, and seeks to draw forth the patient's intrinsic motivation to help reach the goal. Key elements that contribute to its success include combining empathy with evoking the patient's own desire to change his or her behaviors. MI has emerged in the literature as a promising intervention in dental settings both for patients and for parents of pediatric patients.[32,33] This technique has also been found to be useful in addressing alcohol misuse and smoking cessation.[34,35] However, the originators of the method, Miller and Rollnick, caution against adopting a simplistic approach to MI.[36] Although free resources on the Internet offer training in MI, and various continuing education courses teach this technique, they advise that this technique be approached with caution. It is a sensitive intervention that needs to be carried out by people with proper training in the method. Without extensive training, it is difficult for dental professionals to replicate the precise methods used in research studies of MI; therefore, clinicians may not achieve the same results as reported in the scientific literature.

An important lesson from the body of work on MI is that it is natural for patients who are "stuck" to have ambivalence about the process of change. The best response in such situations is to reflect back to the patient with empathy while also striving to promote self-efficacy. For instance, if a patient says, "I'm not sure about quitting smoking; it's really difficult," the dental professional could respond by saying, "Tell me more about that. I'd like to understand what's going on." After the patient elaborates on the situation and feels understood, the clinician might reply, "I realize that it's not easy to quit, but it is possible. If you would like me to, I can share resources with you that you may find useful." Such a response from the clinician, couched in empathy and curiosity, invites dialogue and potential partnership. This is in contrast to an authoritarian response, such as, "You have to quit smoking, otherwise your gum disease will continue to progress and you also risk getting cancer." Often strong emotions, such as ambivalence, that surround a behavior change (e.g., quitting smoking) can override rational factors (e.g., that smoking is harmful to the patient's health). Therefore, it is necessary to address emotions in order to facilitate change.

APPLICATION TO CLINICAL PRACTICE
The Process of Disease Prevention
Despite advances in medical and dental research, it is not possible to entirely prevent disease. One may speak of disease prevention and predict the efficacy of a preventive measure on a population level. However, in clinical terms, it is impossible to predict with accuracy whether a person will develop a disease. As a result, while one can prevent disease on a population level, on a clinical level the dental professional can only reduce risk of disease occurrence for each individual.

Nevertheless, by adopting healthy behaviors and ending unhealthy ones, individuals can greatly increase their odds of being disease free. Sporadic behaviors have little to no impact in terms of improving a patient's health. In order to exert maximum benefits, healthy behaviors must be carried out on a regular basis. Making a behavior a habit and integrating the desired behavior into the patient's lifestyle are best. If the patient has unhealthy habits, such as tobacco use or improper diet, then these behaviors need to be eliminated from the patient's routines and replaced with healthy alternatives.

Disease Prevention Across the Lifespan
Children are dependent upon parents or other caregivers for their well-being. Thus, it is important to include both the child and the parent or caregiver when offering oral hygiene instructions. Many parents experience difficulty in motivating their children to brush their teeth regularly. The best way to encourage children to brush is to model the desired behavior.[37]

If parents or caregivers are stressed, they are less able to attend to the oral health needs of their child.[38] Depending on their social norms, parents may not view primary teeth as important, and thus may not be concerned about a healthy primary dentition. In such situations, the importance of primary teeth in the child's overall health and well-being should be explained to the parents, given that if left untreated, decayed primary teeth can lead to pain and potentially life-threatening infections.

Progression from childhood to adolescence is marked by the emergence of autonomy, which at times may lead patients to resist guidance about self-care. In such instances, the dental professional can attempt to establish rapport and take a collaborative approach with the patient. Additionally, it can be helpful to connect with the values and goals of the adolescent and his or her family. For instance, if the patient values looking good, one can link oral hygiene to appearances; or, if the patient values being a good son or daughter, then self-care can be linked to being virtuous. This is also a period when individuals begin experimenting with tobacco and alcohol use. Thus, it is necessary to inquire about substance use—and offer assistance in linking patients with resources to support responsible drinking and tobacco avoidance. Additional strategies for communicating with youth about alcohol and tobacco use include addressing ways to resist peer pressure to partake of these substances. It can be challenging to counsel an adolescent not to smoke, especially when his or her parents are smoking. In such instances, it is best to emphasize the health benefits of smoking cessation, and offer to help both the patient and his parents in stopping tobacco use.

Older adults may experience difficulty with oral hygiene because of physical limitations such as arthritis, neurodegenerative diseases or motor disorders, or mental challenges due to cognitive impairment. These situations impair the older adult's ability to effectively complete self-care, including oral care. Along with exploring how to adapt oral self-care behaviors according to the individual's ability, it is equally important to validate the person's expression of independence.

When caring for elderly patients who are not living independently, it becomes necessary to involve caregivers in oral hygiene instructions. In situations where patients present with complex medical conditions or cognitive impairment, it is necessary to use a collaborative, interdisciplinary approach to inform other healthcare providers and family members about the individual's oral healthcare needs.[39,40] Patients affected by dementia may engage fully in conversation, but may not recall health-related instructions later on. Visual cues and written instructions may provide prompts that allow the individual to participate in self-care, with assistance from others to ensure efficacy.

Common Risk Factors and Links to Systemic Health

The dental appointment presents an opportunity to link oral health with systemic health and to emphasize this connection to patients. It is a way of approaching oral health that underscores the fact that the mouth is situated within the body, and that what a patient does to his or her mouth (e.g., consumption of tobacco or sugar-sweetened beverages) has far-reaching effects beyond caries and aesthetics. These are sensitive issues for patients, and a nonjudgmental approach when inquiring about them is less likely to elicit a defensive response. If a patient indicates that he or she has a problem in one of these areas, it is beneficial to offer practical suggestions to stop the habit. If the patient expresses a desire to change but does not know how, he or she can be referred to online resources and in-person programs, for instance, for smoking cessation.

From Trying New Behaviors to Establishing Healthy Habits

For optimal health, it is necessary to regularly engage in health-promoting behavior. Introducing patients to new behavior is only the first step, and the greatest benefits are obtained when the behavior becomes a habit. A habit can be defined as something the patient does automatically in response to external cues.[41] For example, a red traffic light is an external cue to stop at an intersection, and likewise the process of getting dressed in the morning for school or work can become a cue for brushing one's teeth.

The following elements are helpful in turning a new or sporadic behavior into a lasting habit:
- Defining the desired behavior and goal clearly
- Stating an intention to carry out the behavior, or committing to the goal
- Bolstering the patient's self-efficacy
- Learning the desired behavior
- Repeating the desired behavior so it becomes automatic
- Integrating the behavior into existing routines so it becomes part of the patient's lifestyle
- Monitoring the repetition of the behavior by tracking the frequency with which the desired behavior is carried out
- Anticipating impediments in advance and planning ways to deal with them
- Rewarding efforts, especially through internal rewards such as feelings of accomplishment (versus external rewards such as gifts)
- Attending to the patient's environment to make modifications so that the environment is conducive to carrying out the new behavior
- Identifying people in the patient's life who can support and encourage the adoption of the new behavior. (It may also be necessary to identify people who might undermine the patient's efforts at behavior change, and develop a plan to address that challenge.)

These processes can be used not only to acquire a positive health behavior, but also to eliminate negative health habits. For example, a patient may state "not smoking cigarettes" as a goal.

Integrating Desired Behavior into Patient Lifestyles

Any change from a person's norms and routines has the potential to create discomfort. Patients may intellectually understand the benefits of disease-preventing behavior, such as eating less sugar and not smoking. However, asking them to change long-term habits can elicit stress and conflicting feelings, resulting in ambivalence. On the one hand, the patient may desire health, but on the other hand he or she may find it difficult to do what is required and thus dread the effort involved in behavior change. What may seem like an obvious choice of action for a dental professional can be experienced as a major stressor by the patient, or the parent of a child patient—for instance, when asking the parent not to feed the child with a bottle at bedtime. Patients may experience ambivalence and express doubts about their ability to adopt new behaviors or to let go of long-lasting ones.

Respectful inquiry can illuminate reasons for the patient's reluctance to adopt the recommended behavior. It is important to keep in mind that not all patients are ready to change behaviors immediately. Additionally, individuals who are experiencing stressful life situations, such as caring for a severely ill family member or dealing with unemployment, may hesitate to adopt a new behavior because they perceive it as yet another stressor, even if the benefits are apparent. In such instances, clinicians can let their patients know that they are available to help whenever they are ready to change, and offer to connect patients with supportive resources.

Interpersonal Communication

Interpersonal communication is a fundamental element of all dental appointments. It is the vehicle through which the psychological and social aspects of the appointment are manifested. It is important to maintain a caring and empathic tone when striving to build a partnership with patients, as they are sensitive to nuances of the clinician's voice.

A study of surgeons and their tone of voice found that it was possible to differentiate between those who had a history of malpractice and those who did not, solely on the basis of listening to 10-second snippets of conversations with their patients.[42] Surgeons who used a harsh tone of speech were more likely to have been sued for malpractice compared with those who used a warmer tone. Interpersonal communication also touches upon health literacy as it influences how one speaks and the words one uses.

Health Literacy in the Context of the Dental Appointment

In practical terms, attending to a patient's ability to comprehend and utilize medical information will yield better patient outcomes, and reduce frustration for both the patient and the clinician. Patients may not admit that they do not understand medical terms or instructions fully. They might be embarrassed to let the clinician know that they have not understood what they have been told. Even patients who hold advanced degrees may lack the capacity to understand medical and dental terminology, especially if their degrees are in another field.

Health literacy is closely linked with patient communication, and the following suggestions offer strategies to increase the likelihood that patients will more fully comprehend what is being said:

Respectful Patient Communication
- Do not "talk down" to the patient when he or she does not understand dental terminology, or has misconceptions.
- Be sensitive to the patient's gender, age, and culture.
- Engage in a dialogue and establish a partnership with the patient rather than speaking with an authoritarian tone.

Simplified Communication
- Use straightforward language to explain situations to patients.
- Avoid use of technical terms.
- Explain concepts using short sentences that allow the patient to closely follow what is being said.

Use the Teach-Back Method
- Ask the patient to repeat back in his or her words what the healthcare provider has said (e.g., details about a medication regimen).
- Ask the patient to demonstrate the self-care technique (e.g., flossing) to ensure that the patient has the necessary skills to carry out the behavior at home.

Common Psychological Conditions

Depression is one of the leading causes of disability around the world.[43] Although its manifestation can vary across cultures, the most common elements include feelings of hopelessness and diminished ability to engage in and enjoy life. It may also manifest as complaints of feeling unwell. One can think of depression as existing on a spectrum from mild to intense distress. From a practical point of view, it is important to consider whether the distress is interfering with the patient's functioning and whether a referral to a mental health professional might be indicated. Often depression is found as a comorbid condition among patients with chronic illnesses, such as heart disease and diabetes, and is associated with diminished self-care.[44]

In many cultures, there are negative attitudes toward depression and other psychological conditions. Unfortunately, these conditions are viewed as personal weaknesses rather than as an illness. It is important to be open-minded toward patients who may be depressed and make appropriate referrals for further care. Depression is associated with increased risk for suicide; thus, a timely mental health referral can benefit the patient greatly. In terms of preventing dental disease, it is important to explore ways of supporting the patient's self-care and draw upon individuals in the patient's life who might be able to help encourage compliance with recommended self-care regimens.

Anxiety is also a common psychological condition experienced around the world.[45] It can occur in a generalized form or as a specific phobia (e.g., dental phobia); it can also occur as post-traumatic stress disorder following a traumatic experience. Anxiety disorders vary in presentation and tend to be characterized by feelings of vulnerability, threat, or lack of a sense of safety. It is very important for care providers to reassure patients and not dismiss their concerns, or brand the patients as "excessive worriers." If the patient appears to be experiencing difficulty because of anxiety, referral to a mental health care professional may be beneficial. In situations where a mental health professional is not accessible, the dental professional might consider referring the patient to a primary care physician.

Supporting Patients in the Clinical Setting: A Chairside Checklist

The Chairside Checklist (Appendix 1) presented in this chapter draws upon theoretical constructs from the social and behavioral sciences, and aims to translate them into a practical instrument that dental professionals can use to enhance patient outcomes. It is hoped that this checklist will lessen dental professionals' frustration with patient challenges, and thereby enhance enjoyment of their work. The Chairside Checklist is intended to facilitate the application of the information presented in this chapter. It is a guide to help dental professionals support their patients in the adoption and maintenance of healthy behaviors. Additionally, it can also be applied to help patients stop unhealthy behaviors.

The checklist integrates practitioner and patient variables and can be used to enrich the patient appointment. Some items on the checklist may not be relevant to each patient or each appointment. The nature of the clinical encounter will dictate which items might be most applicable to a patient, and the clinician can choose those elements that are most relevant. Another value of the checklist is in understanding challenging patients, who might be variously referred to as "difficult," "uncooperative," "resistant," or "stubborn." In an ideal situation, the checklist can enhance the appointment. But in a difficult situation, the checklist can help to identify problems and identify potential solutions. Lastly, the checklist can be viewed as an instrument to help foster an atmosphere of patient-centered care.

SUMMARY

Good oral health is a component of overall well-being, and disease prevention is a goal shared by dental professionals around the world. What people eat and drink, and whether or not they use tobacco, will influence their oral health status. Convincing patients to develop health-promoting habits and eliminate harmful behavior is a challenge frequently encountered by dental professionals. Patients cannot be kept free of disease solely through biomedical agents, nor can health be guaranteed solely on the basis of procedures carried out in the clinical setting. Patients need to actively engage in self-care in an ongoing way. In many instances, clinicians give their patients health information with the expectation that patients will immediately adopt the recommended behavior. However, providing information is but one step within the larger process of eliciting and maintaining healthy behavior. Information alone is not enough to change behavior.

The behavioral sciences contain numerous theories that can explain patient behavior. Patient behavior must be understood in terms of internal influences (i.e., thoughts, feelings, motivations), as well as external influences (i.e., the environment, which comprises other people, physical structures, cultural norms, economics, and sociopolitical factors). Owing to practical considerations, it is not possible to explore all theories of potential relevance in this chapter. The theories and constructs discussed were selected because of the strong basis of support from research, and for their utility in the clinical setting and relevance to patients from varied cultures and socioeconomic levels.

The authoritarian approach to patient education is outmoded; it leads to frustration (for both the clinician and the patient) and hampers interpersonal communication. Dental professionals should not merely inform patients about strategies for disease prevention and hope that patients will automatically adopt their recommendations. The wealth of information from the behavioral sciences informs dental professionals about how to create an efficacious and meaningful partnership that facilitates the process of change. It *is* possible for patients to adopt new behavior leading to lasting habits; it is also possible to eliminate harmful behavior in the long term. The partnership between clinician and patient is the vehicle through which the process of change is facilitated, and the contents of this chapter, including the Chairside Checklist, are intended to guide the reader in supporting his or her patients in their quest for optimal oral health.

Acknowledgments: The author is grateful to Ms. A. Brodie, Mr. H. Bright, and Mr. V. Tedeschi, librarians at A.T. Still University of Health Sciences in Mesa, Arizona, USA, for their assistance in retrieving documents; and Ms. B.J. LeBaron for her assistance in preparing the manuscript.

Appendix 1: Chairside Checklist

1. Interpersonal Communication
- What is the provider's tone of voice?
- Is it warm, expressing empathy and concern?
- Is the manner of speaking authoritarian or collaborative?
- Are messages framed to motivate the patient by emphasizing the benefits of disease prevention, rather than evoking fear of disease?
- Does the provider seek to promote the patient's self-efficacy by offering encouragement and identifying role models, and building upon past successes?

2. Expectations for Treatment
- What are the provider's expectations for treatment, and how might these differ from those of the patient?
- What is the patient's perception of his or her oral health quality of life, and does this need to be reconciled with the expectations of the care provider?

3. Defining Goals and Identifying Resources Needed to Reach and Maintain Them
- What are the desired preventive goals, and are they clearly defined?
- What are the subgoals (i.e., steps along the way that must be reached on the way to achieving the main goal)?
- What resources and skills are needed to reach the goals?
- What are potential barriers to achieving the goals and how might the patient plan ways to address these barriers?
- Is the patient aware that repetition of the desired behavior will lead to mastery and support the long-term maintenance of the goals?
- How will the patient monitor his or her progress toward the goals?
- How can the patient connect with the internal rewards of success, such as feeling pride in one's accomplishment?
- How can the goals be integrated into the patient's lifestyle so they become automatic?

4. Lifespan Considerations
- Are the goals and recommendations age appropriate and realistic in terms of the patient's level of comprehension and motor skills?
- Is there a caregiver in addition to the patient?
- Is this caregiver included in important conversations?

5. Environmental Factors that Influence the Patient's Behavior
- What kinds of cultural norms might be influencing the patient's behavior?
- Are there economic constraints that impose limitations on the patient's ability to care for him- or herself, or purchase health necessities such as toothbrush and toothpaste?
- Who are the important people in the patient's life who can be sources of support and encouragement?
- Might there be people in the patient's life who can potentially sabotage the patient's efforts for behavior change? If so, how might the patient make a plan for dealing with this situation?

6. Barriers to Preventive Care
- What are potential barriers to self-care, and how can the patient cope or overcome the barriers? Has the patient anticipated barriers and identified strategies to overcome the barriers?
- Are there unsupportive people who detract

from the desired goals? How can the patient be assertive and navigate around these people?
- If finances are a barrier, are there alternate paths to the goals? Can the patient and provider brainstorm and arrive at creative solutions?
- If the patient is experiencing stress, which people in the patient's life can assist with both emotion-focused coping and action-focused coping?

7. Basic Literacy
- Can the person read and write and, if so, at what level of literacy? How might the clinician adapt communication to optimize patient engagement in the conversation?
- Do the consent forms, educational materials, and appointment reminders need to be adapted to the patient's literacy level?
- Is the patient being treated respectfully, even if his or her literacy level is low?
- Might the teach-back method enhance patient understanding of his or her situation?

8. Health Literacy
- Is communication with the patient respectful, free of jargon, and clearly understood?
- Has the patient been asked to "teach back" to demonstrate his or her level of understanding of critical concepts?

9. Resources to Support the Patient in Self-Care
- Which person or people in the patient's life can be a source of encouragement, support, and stress reduction?
- Which resources, such as Internet sites and educational materials and guides, might be of use to the patient?
- Are there smartphone applications (apps) or other technologies that the patient can use to set up reminders and to track progress toward a goal?

10. Stressors and Coping Resources
- What are the demands that the patient (or parent of child patient) is experiencing that interfere with carrying out health behavior?
- What kinds of emotional support might help the patient to achieve his or her goals?
- What kinds of practical support might help the patient to achieve his or her goals?
- Are there individuals in the patient's life who might be recruited to support the patient in the pursuit of his or her health behavior?

11. Patient's Self-Dialogue
- Is the patient speaking in a manner that connotes hopelessness or helplessness? If so, how might the clinician increase the patient's self-efficacy?
- How might the clinician respectfully counter the patient's negative self-talk?
- Does the patient need additional help if he or she is expressing a degree of helplessness or hopelessness that prevents achievement of the goal?
- Are there family members and friends who can be recruited to encourage and support the patient?

12. Medical Referral
- Does the patient have unhealthy habits that have implications for poor oral health, and is there a need for medical consultation?
- Does the patient present with medical conditions that impede self-care?
- Might the patient have a systemic condition such as diabetes that interferes with achieving good oral health?
- If the patient's medication is exerting a negative side effect on the oral cavity, are there alternatives that have fewer side effects?

13. Referral to a Behavioral Health Provider
- Does the patient engage in unhealthy behaviors, such as unhealthy diet, tobacco use, and alcohol misuse, and might he or she benefit from a referral for counseling?
- Does the patient present with signs of depression, anxiety, substance use, or other psychological problems? If so, might the patient benefit from a psychological referral?

- If the patient is having trouble establishing healthy habits, would a psychological referral be beneficial?

14. Structures and Resources to Help the Patient Maintain Lasting Habits
- What kinds of stressors might be occurring in the patient's life that prevent him or her from maintaining a healthy behavior?
- What kinds of environmental barriers might be influencing the patient's behavior?
- What are ways to promote the patient's self-efficacy—especially if the patient is expressing loss of hope?
- Is the patient adequately connected with the rewards and benefits of the healthy behavior, rather than focused on the efforts to achieve the goal?
- What kinds of internal rewards might boost the patient's motivation?

REFERENCES

1. Engel GL. The need for a new medical model: a challenge for biomedicine. *Science*. 1977;196:129–136.
2. Schroeder SA. We can do better—improving the health of the American people. *N Engl J Med*. 2007;357:1221–1228.
3. Glanz K, Bishop DB. The role of behavioral science theory in development and implementation of public health interventions. *Annu Rev Public Health*. 2010;31:399–418.
4. Braverman P, Gottleib L. The social determinants of health: it's time to consider the causes of the causes. *Public Health Rep*. 2014;129(suppl 2):19–31.
5. Kawachi I, Subramanian SV, Almeida-Filho N. A glossary for health inequalities. *J Epidemiol Community Health*. 2002;56:647–652.
6. World Health Organization. *Dying for Change: Poor People's Experience of Health and Ill Health*. Report no. 33125. Geneva, Switzerland: World Health Organization; 2005.
7. Haushofer J, Fehr E. On the psychology of poverty. *Science*. 2014;344(6186):862–867.
8. Goldman AS, Yee R, Holmgren CJ, Benzian H. Global affordability of fluoride toothpaste. *Global Health*. 2008;4:7.
9. WHOQOL Group. The World Health Organization Quality of Life Assessment (WHOQOL). Development and psychometric properties. *Soc Sci Med*. 1998;46:1569–1585.
10. Bennadi D, Reddy CVK. Oral health related quality of life. *J Int Soc Prev Community Dent*. 2013;3:1–6.
11. Vettore MV, Aqeeli A. The roles of contextual and individual social determinants of oral health-related quality of life in Brazilian adults. *Qual Life Res*. 2015; Sep 5. [Epub ahead of print.]
12. Yiengprugsawan V, Somkotra T, Seubsman SA, Sleigh AC; Thai Cohort Study Team. Oral health-related quality of life among a large national cohort of 87,134 Thai adults. *Health Qual Life Outcomes*. 2011;9:42.
13. Enoki K, Ikebe K, Matsuda KI, Yoshida M, Maeda Y, Thomson WM. Determinants of change in oral health-related quality of life over 7 years among older Japanese. *J Oral Rehabil*. 2013;40:252–257.
14. Brennan DS, Spencer JA. Life events and oral-health-related quality of life among young adults. *Qual Life Res*. 2009;18:557–565.
15. Khatri SG, Acharya S, Srinivasan SR. Mother's sense of coherence and oral health related quality of life of preschool children in Udupi Taluk. *Comm Dental Health*. 2014;31:32–36.
16. Almozino G, Aframian DJ, Sharav Y, Sheftel Y, Mzabaev A, Zini A. Lifestyle and dental attendance as predictors of oral health-related quality of life. *Oral Dis*. 2015;21:659–666.
17. World Health Organization. *Health Promotion Glossary*. Geneva, Switzerland: World Health Organization; 1998.
18. Nouri S, Rudd RE. Health literacy in the "oral exchange": an important element of patient-provider communication. *Patient Educ Couns*. 2015;98:565–571.
19. Kickbusch I, Pelikan JM, Apfel F, Tsouros AD, eds. *Health Literacy: The Solid Facts*. Geneva, Switzerland: World Health Organization; 2012.
20. Watt RG, Sheiham A. Integrating the common risk factor approach into a social determinants framework. *Comm Dent Oral Epidemiol*. 2012;40:289–296.
21. Heilmann A, Sheiham A, Watt RG, Jordan RA. The common risk factor approach—an integrated population- and evidence-based approach for reducing social inequalities in health [in German]. *Gesundheitswesen*. 2015; Sep 3. [Epub ahead of print.]
22. Bandura A. *Social Foundations of Thought and Action: A Social Cognitive Theory*. Englewood Cliffs, NJ: Prentice-Hall; 1986.
23. Prochaska JO, DiClemente CC, Norcross JC. In search of how people change. Applications to addictive behaviors. *Am Psychol*. 1992;47:1102–1114.
24. Lazarus RS, Folkman S. *Stress, Appraisal and Coping*. New York, NY: Springer Publishing; 1984.
25. Miller WR, Rose GS. Toward a theory of motivational interviewing. *Am Psychol*. 2009;64(6):527-37
26. Askelson AM, Chi DL, Momany ET, et al. The importance of efficacy: Using the extended parallel process model to examine factors related to preschool-age children enrolled in Medicaid receiving preventive dental visits. *Health Educ Behav*. 2015;42:805–813.

27. Gholami M, Knoll N, Schwarzer R. A brief self-regulatory intervention increases dental flossing in adolescent girls. *Int J Behav Med.* 2015;22:645–651.
28. Thoits PA. Stress and health: major findings and policy implications. *J Health Soc Behav.* 2010;51(suppl):S41–S53.
29. Folkman S, Lazarus RS, Dunkel-Schetter C, DeLongis A, Gruen RJ. Dynamics of a stressful encounter: cognitive appraisal, coping, and encounter outcomes. *J Pers Soc Psychol.* 1986;50:992–1003.
30. DeLongis A, Folkman S, Lazarus RS. The impact of daily stress on health and mood: psychological and social resources as mediators. *J Pers Soc Psychol.* 1988;54:486–495.
31. Cahill K, Lancaster T, Green N. Stage-based interventions for smoking cessation. *Cochrane Database Syst Rev.* 2010;(11):CD004492.
32. Gao, X, Lo EC, Chan KC. Motivational interviewing in improving oral health: a systematic review of randomized clinical trials. *J Periodontol.* 2014;85:426–437.
33. Borrelli B, Tooley EM, Scott-Sheldon LA. Motivational interviewing for parent-child health interventions: a systematic review and meta-analysis. *Pediatr Dent.* 2015;37:254–265.
34. Foxcroft DF, Coombes L, Wood S, Allen D, Almeida Santimano NM. Motivational interviewing for alcohol misuse in young adults. *Cochrane Database Syst Review.* 2014;(8):CD007025.
35. Lindson-Hawley N, Thompson TP, Begh R. Motivational interviewing for smoking cessation. *Cochrane Database Syst Rev.* 2015;(3):CD006936.
36. Miller WR, Rollnick S. Ten things that motivational interviewing is not. *Behav Cogn Psychother.* 2009;37:129–140.
37. Collett BR, Huebner CE, Seminario AL, Wallace E, Gray KE, Speltz ML. Observed child and parent toothbrushing behaviors and child oral health. *Int J Paediatr Dent.* 2015; Jul 4. [Epub ahead of print.]
38. Tiwari T, Albino J, Batliner TS. Challenges faced in engaging American Indian mothers in an early childhood caries preventive trial. *Int J Dent.* 2015;2015:179189.
39. Wang TF, Huang CM, Chou C, Yu S. Effect of oral health education programs for caregivers on oral hygiene of the elderly: a systematic review and meta-analysis. *Int J Nurs Studies.* 2015;52:1090–1096.
40. Brennan L, Strauss J. Cognitive impairment in older adults and oral health considerations: treatment and management. *Dent Clin North Am.* 2014;58:815–828.
41. Lally P, Gardner B. Promoting habit formation. *Health Psychol Rev.* 2013;7(suppl):S137–S158.
42. Ambady N, LaPlante D, Nguyen MA, Rosenthal R, Chaumeton N, Levinson W. Surgeon's tone of voice: a clue to malpractice history. *Surgery.* 2002;132:5–9.
43. Kessler RC, Bromet EJ. The epidemiology of depression across cultures. *Annu Rev Public Health.* 2013;34:119–138.
44. Chan HL, Lin CK, Chau YL, Chang CM. The impact of depression on self-care activities and health care utilization among people with diabetes in Taiwan. *Diabetes Res Clin Pract.* 2012;98:e4–7.
45. Baxter AJ, Scott KM, Vos T, Whiteford HA. Global prevalence of anxiety disorders: a systematic review and meta-regression. *Psychol Med.* 2013;43:897–910.

Chapter 3
Risk Assessment

JoAnn R. Gurenlian

As each patient completes a comprehensive oral evaluation or assessment, the data collected must be reviewed to determine whether the patient can participate in the planned dental or dental hygiene treatment. This process, referred to as a *risk assessment*, is used to determine if treatment outweighs the potential risks to the patient.

Risk assessment has been defined in various ways. Little and colleagues[1] described risk assessment as involving the following four components: (1) the nature, severity, control, and stability of the patient's medical condition; (2) functional capacity of the patient; (3) emotional status of the patient; and (4) type and magnitude of the planned procedure. In *Standards for Clinical Dental Hygiene Practice* of the American Dental Hygienists' Association, risk assessment is described as the "qualitative and quantitative evaluation gathered from the assessment process to identify any risks to general and oral health."[2] These data "provide the clinician with the information to develop and design strategies for preventing or limiting disease and promoting health."[2] Within this standard, risk is classified as high, moderate, or low. Examples include fluoride exposure, smoking, systemic diseases, xerostomia, age, gender, family history, physical disability, and psychological and social considerations.

This chapter discusses risk assessment for both systemic health and oral health conditions. Risk assessment tools to support clinical practice are addressed to aid dental professionals in creating accurate risk profiles for their patients as a means of preventing medical complications and oral diseases to the extent possible.

RISK ASSESSMENT FOR SYSTEMIC HEALTH

Dental professionals assess the general health status of their patients as part of the comprehensive health history obtained during an initial appointment. This health history should be updated routinely at subsequent patient appointments. One purpose of completing a health history is to identify risk factors that may be present, placing the patient at risk for a potential medical emergency during the dental or dental hygiene appointment. Another purpose is to identify possible risks for health conditions not yet identified. In this section, risk assessment is demonstrated through discussion of the systemic conditions of cardiovascular disease and stroke, diabetes mellitus, and sleep-related breathing disorders.

Cardiovascular Disease and Stroke
Key Considerations

Each year, the American Heart Association (AHA), the Centers for Disease Control and Prevention (CDC), the National Institutes of Health (NIH), and other government agencies join together to identify current statistics related to cardiovascular, cerebrovascular, and metabolic diseases, and present them as a statistical update.[3] The AHA statistical update titled "Heart Disease and Stroke Statistics—2015 Update: A Report from the American Heart Association" appears in the journal *Circulation* (downloadable from http://circ.ahajournals.org) and serves as the basis for a fact sheet that appears on the joint website of the AHA and the American Stoke Association (ASA).[3] From this resource, it is apparent that cardiovascular disease (CVD) remains the leading cause of death globally and in the United States, and among both men and women. Approximately 787,000 Americans died from heart disease, stroke, and other CVD in 2011, accounting for one of every three deaths in the United States (see Figure 1). Considered another way, one person dies from CVD every 40 seconds. CVD is also the leading cause of death worldwide, representing 31% of all global deaths in 2012. Of these deaths, approximately 7.4 million were due to coronary heart disease.[4] Although the death rate from heart disease continues to fall, the burden and risk factors remain alarmingly high. In particular, almost 735,000 Americans have myocardial infarctions each year, and approximately 120,000 die.[3]

Stroke is the fifth leading cause of death in the United States, killing someone once every 4 minutes, and is the leading preventable cause of disability.[3] Approximately 795,000 people have a stroke every year, equating to one every 40 seconds.

Figure 1. Percentage Breakdown of Deaths Attributable to Cardiovascular Disease in the United States

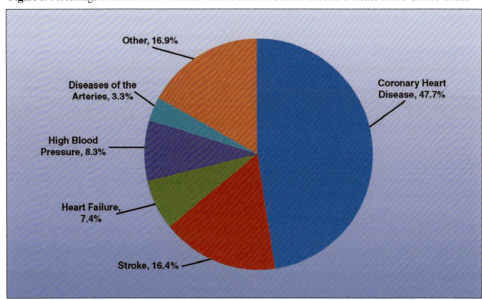

Source: Circulation. 2015;131:e29–e322. © American Heart Association. All rights reserved. Reprinted with permission.

Worldwide, there were 6.7 million deaths due to stroke in 2012.[4]

Risk factors, prevention, and lifestyle interventions have been studied extensively to improve cardiovascular health. Current evidence supports a multidimensional strategy that encompasses individual-focused approaches, healthcare system approaches, and population-based approaches. Each facet targets lifestyle, treatment, health behavior, and health factor changes—in the home, school, workplace, local community, state, and nation—and involves healthcare providers, families, and support teams to improve health. The AHA and ASA have established the goal *to improve the cardiovascular health of **all** Americans by 20%, and reduce deaths from cardiovascular diseases and stroke by 20%, by the year 2020.*[3] To measure progress toward that goal, the AHA and ASA have defined cardiovascular health as the absence of disease and the presence of seven key health factors and behaviors referred to as Life's Simple 7. These seven factors and behaviors are:

- Not smoking
- Physical activity
- Healthy diet
- Healthy body weight
- Control of cholesterol
- Control of blood pressure
- Control of blood glucose

Table 1 presents the measurements used by the AHA and ASA to determine whether someone is in ideal, intermediate, or poor cardiovascular health. Figure 2 demonstrates the prevalence of cardiovascular health metrics and 2020 projections, while Figure 3 provides age-standardized prevalence estimates of US adults meeting different numbers of criteria for ideal cardiovascular health.

Influencing the determination of Life's Simple 7 were the following statistics[3]:

- Worldwide, tobacco smoking (including secondhand smoke) was one of the top three leading risk factors for disease and contributed to an estimated 6.2 million deaths in 2010.
- In 2012 there were approximately 6,300 new cigarette smokers every day.
- About one in every three US adults—31%—reports participating in no leisure-time physical activity.
- Less than 1% of US adults meet the AHA's definition for "ideal healthy diet." Essentially

Table 1. American Heart Association Definition of Cardiovascular Health

Life's Simple 7	Poor	Intermediate	Ideal
Blood pressure			
Adults > 20 years of age	SBP ≥ 140 or DBP ≥ 90 mm Hg	SBP 120–139 or DBP 80–89 mm Hg or treated to goal	< 120/< 80 mm Hg
Children 8–19 years of age	> 95th percentile	90th–95th percentile or SBP ≥ 120 or DBP ≥ 80 mm Hg	< 90th percentile
Physical activity			
Adults > 20 years of age	None	1–149 min/wk mod or 1–74 min/wk vig or 1–149 min/wk mod+vig	≥ 150 min/wk mod or ≥75 min/wk vig or ≥ 150 min/wk mod+vig
Children 12–19	None	> 0 and < 60 min of or vig every day	≥ 60+ min of mod or vig every day
Cholesterol			
Adults > 20 years of age	≥ 240 mg/dL	200–239 mg/dL or treated to goal	< 170 mg/dL
Children 6–19 years of age	≥ 240 mg/dL	170–199 mg/dL	
Healthy diet			
Adults > 20 years of age	0–1 components	2–3 components	4–5 components
Children 5–19	0–1 components	2–3 components	4–5 components
Healthy weight			
Adults > 20 years of age	≥ 30 kg/m^2	25–29.9 kg/m^2	< 25 kg/m^2
Children 2–19 years of age	> 95th percentile	85th–95th percentile	< 85th percentile
Smoking status			
Adults > 20 years of age Children 12–19 years of age	Current smoker Tried prior 30 days	Former smoker	Never/quit ≥ 12 mo
Blood glucose			
Adults > 20 years of age	≥ 126 mg/dL	100–125 mg/dL or treated to goal	< 100 mg/dL
Children 12–19 years of age	≥ 126 mg/dL	100–125 mg/dL	< 100 mg/dL

DBP, diastolic blood pressure; mod, moderate; SBP. systolic blood pressure; vig, vigorous.
Source: Circulation. 2010;121:586–613.

no children meet the definition.
- Eating patterns have changed dramatically in recent decades. Women consumed an average of 22% more calories in 2004 than in 1971, and men consumed an average of 10% more in that span.
- Most Americans older than 20 years of age—more than 159 million US adults, or about 69%—are overweight or obese.
- About 32% of US children—nearly one in three—are overweight or obese. About 24 million are overweight, and about 13 million (17%) are obese.
- About 43% of Americans have total cholesterol higher than 200 mg/dL, and 13% have total cholesterol over 240 mg/dL.
- Nearly one in every three Americans has high levels of low-density lipoprotein (LDL)

Figure 2. Prevalence of Health Metrics Developed by the American Heart Association

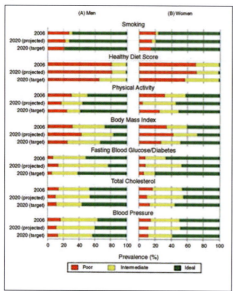

Source: Circulation. 2015;131:e29–e322. © American Heart Association. All rights reserved. Reprinted with permission.

cholesterol, and 20% of Americans have low levels of high-density lipoprotein (HDL) cholesterol.

- About 80 million US adults (33%) have hypertension. Although 77% of these adults use antihypertensive medication, in only 54% is the condition controlled.
- The number of Americans with hypertension is projected to increase by about 8% between 2013 and 2030.
- The total number of people with diabetes mellitus worldwide is projected to rise from 285 million in 2010 to 439 million in 2030.

Since the AHA and ASA initiated the Life's Simple 7 campaign, some progress has been noted. With the exception of diet and physical activity, children are making progress toward ideal levels of health behaviors and health factors—in contrast to adults. The age-standardized death rate attributed to CVD decreased by 11.5% and the stroke death rate decreased by 12.9% for all individuals. These are signs of improvement; however, to meet the

Figure 3. Age-Standardized Prevalence Estimates of US Adults Meeting Criteria for Ideal Cardiovascular Health (NHANES, 2009–2010).

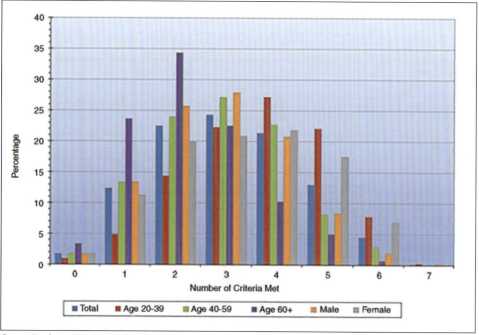

Source: Circulation. 2015;131:e29–e322. © American Heart Association. All rights reserved. Reprinted with permission.

target goal, diet quality, physical activity, and body weight metrics will need to change significantly, and all metrics will continue to require a major focus. The AHA and ASA emphasize the need for treatment of acute cardiovascular events as well as secondary prevention through management of risk factors and health behaviors.

Application to Clinical Practice
To reduce the risk of medical emergencies in the dental office setting, it is recommended that dental professionals obtain vital signs for all patients at each appointment, including blood pressure, respirations, temperature, and pulse.[5] If patients present with obvious signs of medical emergency (chest pain, shortness of breath, significantly elevated pulse or hypertension, unilateral numbness, speech disturbance, etc.), oral treatment should be deferred and immediate medical care sought, using emergency medical services (EMS) as needed. Height and weight are additional forms of vital signs that should be measured, and cardiovascular health assessment should be clearly addressed. Smoking should also be assessed as part of the health history. If these factors raise concern, the next step in assessment is to perform the AHA/ASA My Life Check™–Life's Simple 7 risk assessment with the patient. The assessment, which evaluates the risk factors and health behaviors discussed earlier, takes approximately 5 minutes to complete. The patient receives a score from 1 to 10, with 10 representing an ideal heart score. The assessment can be performed in English or Spanish. Recommendations are then made concerning next steps and goals for the future, and patients are encouraged to repeat the assessment to see if progress is made over time. The My Life Check™–Life's Simple 7 assessment can be found online at www.heart.org/mylifecheck.

Another assessment model, advocated in the European Guidelines on Cardiovascular Disease Prevention in Clinical Practice (version 2012), is the HeartScore® electronic risk assessment system.[6] This system evolved from the earlier Systemic Coronary Risk Evaluation (SCORE) project used to predict and manage risk of heart attack and stroke in Europe.[7] The tool is based on the 2007 European Guidelines on CVD Prevention and offers two European versions based on low-risk and high-risk models and risk charts. It is designed to provide a graphic picture of absolute CVD risk to help address the benefits of preventive interventions. The clinician can then discuss the impact of modifiable risk factors and tailor health advice based on the individual risk profile of the patient. HeartScore® can be accessed at www.heartscore.org.

The dental professional can complete the Life's Simple 7 assessment or HeartScore® with the patient and provide education about oral health, particularly periodontal health and its relationship with cardiovascular health. For example, a systematic review conducted by the AHA Committee on Rheumatic Fever, Endocarditis, and Kawasaki Disease found that observational studies support a consistent association between periodontal disease and atheromatous diseases independent of known confounders.[8] Meta-analyses have been conducted pertaining to the association between atherosclerosis and periodontal disease. Meurman and colleagues found a 20% increase in the risk for CVD among patients with periodontal disease (95% confidence interval [CI]: 1.08–1.32) and a higher risk ratio for stroke, varying from 2.85 (95% CI: 1.78–4.56) to 1.75 (95% CI: 1.08–2.81).[9] Khader and associates[10] reported relative risk estimates of 1.19 (95% CI: 1.08–1.32) whereas Vettore[11] noted 1.15 (95% CI: 1.06–1.25). Helping patients appreciate that a connection exits between cardiovascular and stroke health and oral health, particularly periodontal health, is an important step in empowering them to take charge of their lifestyle behaviors and home efforts to improve their general and oral health.

Diabetes Mellitus
Key Considerations
The *National Diabetes Statistics Report, 2014* estimate of diabetes prevalence in the United States noted that 29.1 million people have diabetes, and 8.1 million of these individuals do not know they have the disease.[12] Figure 4 illustrates the percentages of individuals diagnosed and undiagnosed with diabetes and those whose condition is well managed versus uncontrolled. Further demonstrating the

magnitude of this disease, 86 million individuals have prediabetes.[12] Diabetes is the seventh leading cause of death in the United States.[12] Worldwide, it is estimated to affect 347 million people and is predicted to become the seventh leading cause of death by the year 2030.[13] The global epidemic of diabetes is linked to rapid increases in overweight and physical inactivity.[13] This serious disease leads to complications and coexisting conditions, including hypoglycemia and hyperglycemic crisis, hypertension, high blood LDL cholesterol, cardiovascular disease and stroke, blindness and other eye problems, kidney disease and end-stage renal failure, amputations, nerve disease, nonalcoholic fatty liver disease, hearing loss, erectile dysfunction, depression, and complications of pregnancy. In addition to systemic complications, there are oral effects of diabetes, including caries, periodontal disease, and abscesses; dry, burning mouth; gingival proliferation; abnormal wound healing; candida infection; acetone breath; increased salivary viscosity; and asymptomatic parotid gland swelling.

It is estimated that one in three people is at risk of developing type 2 diabetes in his or her lifetime. Risk factors for type 2 diabetes include[14]

- Age 45 years or older
- Overweight or obese—body mass index (BMI) of 25 kg/m² or greater (≥ 23 kg/m² for Asian Americans) or waist circumference in men greater than 40 inches (102 cm) or in women greater than 35 inches (88 cm)
- Family history of diabetes (i.e., parent or sibling)
- Member of a high-risk population (i.e., African American, Hispanic/Latino, American Indian, Alaska Native, Asian American, Pacific Islander)
- History of gestational diabetes mellitus (GDM) or giving birth to a baby weighing 9 pounds (4 kg) or more
- Physical inactivity
- Hypertension
- High-density lipoprotein cholesterol (HDL-C) level ≤ 35 mg/dL (0.90 mmol/L)
- Fasting triglyceride (TG) level ≥ 250 mg/dL (2.82 mmol/L)
- Acanthosis nigricans, nonalcoholic steatohepatitis, polycystic ovary syndrome, and other conditions associated with insulin resistance
- Atherosclerotic cardiovascular disease
- Depression
- Treatment with atypical antipsychotics or glucocorticoids
- Obstructive sleep apnea and chronic sleep deprivation (< 6 hours per day)—identified as emerging risk factors

Figure 4. Diabetes Mellitus Awareness, Treatment, and Control in Adults Aged 20 Years and Older (NHANES, 2009–2012).

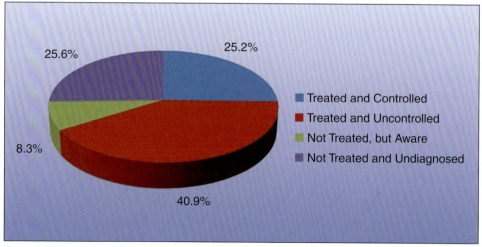

Source: Circulation. 2015;131:e29–e322. © American Heart Association. All rights reserved. Reprinted with permission.

To address and reverse the high incidence and prevalence of type 2 diabetes, the National Diabetes Education Program (NDEP) created "Guiding Principles for the Care of People With or at Risk for Diabetes" for healthcare professionals, key stakeholders, and patients. These principles are briefly presented in Table 2, and can be reviewed in detail at http://ndep.nih.gov/hcp-businesses-and-schools/guiding-principles.[15] These principles demonstrate that all healthcare providers, including dentists and dental hygienists, can have a more active role in the detection and management of patients with diabetes, particularly type 2 diabetes mellitus.

Further, the American Medical Association (AMA) and the CDC partnered to create a toolkit titled "Prevent Diabetes STAT" (Screen, Test, Act-Today) as an immediate action because people with prediabetes who are overweight are at risk for developing type 2 diabetes within 5 years unless they lose weight. This toolkit is a guide for physicians and other healthcare providers as to the best methods to screen and refer high-risk patients to diabetes prevention programs in their communities. Dentists and dental hygienists interested in adopting this program for patients with prediabetes can access the toolkit at www.cdc.gov/diabetes/prevention/pdf/STAT_toolkit.pdf. Online screening tools are also available at www.preventdiabetesstat.org (patient screening) and www.cdc.gov/diabetes (prediabetes screening), the latter as part of the CDC's National Diabetes Prevention Program.

Other risk-scoring algorithms have been developed for estimating diabetes risk and are summarized in the toolkit titled "Take Action to Prevent Diabetes: A Toolkit for the Prevention of Type 2 Diabetes in Europe." This document is available at www.idh.org. One of the featured risk assessments in this document—and highlighted in the "Guidelines on Diabetes, Prediabetes, and Cardiovascular Diseases: Executive Summary"[16]—is the Finnish Diabetes Risk Score (FINDRISC). This screening device examines predictive variables such as age; BMI; waist circumference; use of antihypertensive therapy; history of high blood glucose; physical activity; consumption of fruits, vegetables, and berries; and family history of diabetes. The tool predicts a 10-year risk of type 2 diabetes with 85% accuracy and detects current asymptomatic diabetes and abnormal glucose tolerance.[17-19] Individuals screened and identified to be at high risk should have subsequent glucose testing.

Application to Clinical Practice

To reduce the risk of hypoglycemia or a hyperglycemic crisis in the dental office, appointments for patients with a known history of diabetes mellitus should begin with a glucometer reading. Levels less than 70 mg/dL indicate hypoglycemia; common signs and symptoms include perspiration, confusion, anxiety, mood changes, tachycardia, hunger, and nausea. If the patient is conscious, a sugar source such as candy, 4 ounces of fruit juice, or a glucose tablet can be offered. If the patient loses consciousness, the dental provider should call EMS, provide basic life support, and administer intravenous 50% dextrose or intramuscular glucagon (1 mg). The best way to prevent hypoglycemia is to remind patients to eat after taking their diabetes medication and to monitor their glucose before their appointment. If the patient is taking insulin, it is important to inquire when the peak effect of the specific insulin being used is likely to occur and avoid scheduling appointments around that time. For patients presenting with a glucometer reading of 300 mg/dL or greater, representing dangerous hyperglycemia, the dental provider is advised to defer treatment, contact EMS, provide basic life support, and allow the EMS personnel to give necessary medication and treatment. Treatment can be resumed when the patient's blood glucose is better controlled.

Because diabetes and CVD are closely associated, a risk factor assessment is recommended for adult patients. The risk factors described earlier can be generated into a screening form and used to identify level of risk for type 2 diabetes. Patients can be counseled to seek further evaluation with a medical specialist if multiple risk factors are identified. In addition, for patients unaware of their prediabetes or diabetes status, a screening test can be implemented while the patient is in the reception

Table 2. Guiding Principles for the Care of People With or at Risk for Diabetes

Guiding Principle	Topics Covered
Principle 1— Identify people with undiagnosed diabetes and prediabetes	Why test for diabetes and prediabetes Whom to test for diabetes and prediabetes, and how often Risk factors for type 2 diabetes How to test for diabetes and prediabetes How to test for gestational diabetes Test criteria for prediabetes, diabetes, and gestational diabetes
Principle 2— Manage prediabetes to prevent or delay the onset of type 2 diabetes	Weight loss and physical activity for prevention of type 2 diabetes Medication for type 2 diabetes prevention Cardiovascular disease risk management
Principle 3— Provide ongoing self-management education and support for people with or at risk for diabetes and its complications	Definition and purpose of diabetes self-management education and diabetes self-management support What is self-management How to provide self-management and support Community-based and other resources
Principle 4— Provide individualized nutrition therapy for people with or at risk for diabetes	Nutrition therapy providers Macronutrient intake for people with or at risk for diabetes Weight management for overweight and obese individuals Helpful behaviors and practices for weight management Amount and frequency of medical nutrition therapy for diabetes
Principle 5— Encourage regular physical activity for people with or at risk for diabetes	Encourage physical activity Aerobic physical activity Muscle-strengthening activity Goal setting Appropriate precautions
Principle 6— Control blood glucose to prevent or delay the onset of diabetes complications and avert symptoms of hyperglycemia and hypoglycemia	Risks of blood glucose control Hemoglobin A1C treatment goals Blood glucose management Blood glucose assessment Bariatric surgery
Principle 7— Provide blood pressure and cholesterol screening and control, smoking cessation, and other therapies to reduce cardiovascular disease	Evidence for blood pressure control Blood pressure management Therapy considerations Evidence for statin therapy Cholesterol management Multiple risk factor management Antiplatelet therapy Tobacco use cessation
Principle 8— Provide regular assessments to detect and monitor diabetes microvascular complications and treatment to slow their progression	Nephropathy assessment Nephropathy management Neuropathy assessment Foot assessment Neuropathy management Retinopathy assessment Retinopathy management
Principle 9— Consider the needs of special populations: children, women of childbearing age, older adults, and high-risk racial and ethnic groups	Children and adolescents Women of childbearing age Older adults High-risk racial and ethnic groups
Principle 10— Provide patient-centered diabetes care	Considerations of health literacy and numeracy Comorbid conditions that involve team care coordination Patient-centered care of common morbidities

Source: Adapted from National Diabetes Education Program. *Guiding Principles for the Care of People With or at Risk for Diabetes.* Available at: http://ndep.nih.gov/hcp-businesses-and-schools/guiding-principles. Accessed November 29, 2015.

area waiting for his or her appointment. These tests can be downloaded from the previously listed websites (sample forms appear as Figures 5 and 6). When the patient is present in the operatory, the dental provider can offer the patient the option of a screening hemoglobin A1C test. The NDEP recommends screenings be performed for people who are asymptomatic and older than age 45 years, or for adults of any age who are overweight or obese and have one or more of the previously listed risk

Figure 5. Diabetes Risk Assessment Tool

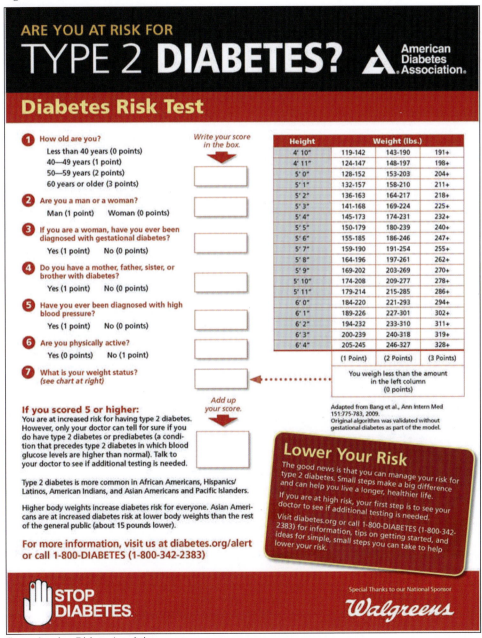

Source: American Diabetes Association.

factors. The A1C test does not require fasting and can be performed chairside. The patient should be advised that the testing performed in the dental office will not be diagnostic of diabetes and that findings will need to be confirmed after further laboratory analysis. However, this screening may help the patient become more aware of a diabetic condition and begin a treatment program. Studies of dental

Figure 6. Finnish Diabetes Risk Score Assessment Tool

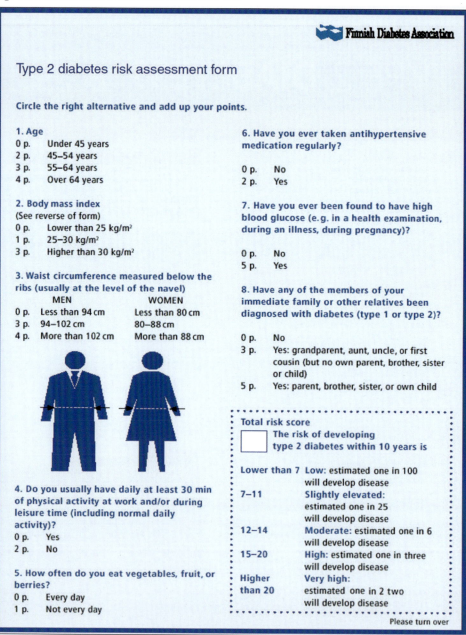

Source: Lars Rydén et al. *Eur Heart J.* 2007;28:88–136. © 2007 The European Society of Cardiology and European Association for the Study of Diabetes (EASD). All rights reserved. Reprinted with permission.

patients have demonstrated that A1C testing can be performed safely in a dental office setting, and further, that it is beneficial in identifying patients with unrecognized prediabetes and diabetes.[20-22]

In addition, patients should be counseled that diabetes is a risk factor for periodontal disease,[23-27] and that the impact of successful routine nonsurgical periodontal treatment on blood glucose is similar in magnitude to adding a second oral antidiabetes medication.[28] This concept is of clinical importance in managing type 2 diabetes. Patients should appreciate the importance of improving periodontal and oral health while improving glycemic control and their systemic health.

Sleep-Related Breathing Disorders
Key Considerations
According to the National Sleep Foundation, more than 18 million American adults have a sleep-related breathing disorder or obstructive sleep apnea (OSA).[29] OSA is a medical disorder in which breathing is briefly and repeatedly interrupted during sleep. The "apnea" refers to a breathing pause that lasts at least 10 seconds. In addition, the muscles in the posterior portion of the throat fail to keep the airway open. Another form of sleep apnea is central sleep apnea, defined as a decrease in proper brain control of breathing during sleep. The end result is ineffective and shallow breaths. Complex sleep apnea is a combination of OSA and central sleep apnea.

Symptoms of OSA generally begin slowly and may be present for years before the patient is referred for or seeks treatment. Nocturnal and daytime symptoms are noteworthy. Nocturnal symptoms include snoring, witnessed apneas, gasping and choking sensations that arouse the patient from sleep, nocturia, insomnia, and restless sleep. Daytime symptoms include nonrestorative sleep or waking up as tired as when going to bed, morning headache, dry or sore throat, excessive daytime sleepiness (EDS), daytime fatigue or tiredness, chronic deficits (memory and intellectual impairments), decreased vigilance, personality and mood changes, sexual dysfunction, gastroesophageal reflux, hypertension, and depression.[30]

Multiple risk factors exist for OSA. These include obesity (BMI > 30 kg/m^2), large neck circumference (> 17 inches [43 cm] in men and 15 inches [38 cm] in women), abnormal Mallampati score (see Figure 7), narrowing of the lateral airway walls, enlarged tonsils, retrognathia or micrognathia, large degree of overjet, high-arched hard palate, systemic

Figure 7. Mallampati Classification[34]

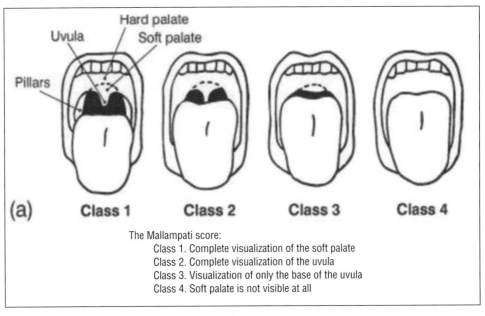

The Mallampati score:
Class 1. Complete visualization of the soft palate
Class 2. Complete visualization of the uvula
Class 3. Visualization of only the base of the uvula
Class 4. Soft palate is not visible at all

arterial hypertension (in approximately 50% of patients), congestive heart failure, pulmonary hypertension, stroke, metabolic syndrome, type 2 diabetes mellitus, alcohol consumption, smoking, and nasal congestion.[30-32] Further, due to increased risk for EDS, individuals with OSA are at increased risk for motor vehicle accidents.[33]

In their review of the literature on OSA, Kornegay and Brame report that OSA is linked to multiple systemic diseases, most notably cardiovascular conditions such as hypertension, stroke, congestive heart failure, cardiac arrhythmias, and myocardial infarction.[34] Further, OSA is associated with diabetes mellitus, and with diminished quality of life and neurocognitive function.[34] Recent research suggests that the blood-brain barrier becomes more permeable in OSA, which could contribute to brain injury and enhance or accelerate damage affecting memory, mood, and cardiovascular risk, likely due to reduction in oxygen from repeated breathing interruptions. Although this study was conducted on a small sample, it suggests that treatment needs to focus on improving breathing in patients with OSA as well as repairing and improving blood-brain barrier function.[35]

Application to Clinical Practice
Several screening tools exist to assess patients for OSA. The STOP questionnaire[36] is a brief tool that can easily be administered in the dental office setting (see Table 3). Patients who answer "yes" to two or more questions are considered to be at high risk. Analysis of this screening tool revealed a moderately high sensitivity and specificity.[36] Another screening tool is the STOP-Bang questionnaire, an eight-item instrument (see Table 4) that has a high probability of OSA detection. If a patient answers "yes" to three or more items, he or she is considered at high risk for OSA.[37]

As patients are evaluated for risk factors and either of the above screening tools is completed, they should be counseled that research demonstrates an association between OSA and periodontitis[37-39]; therefore, a thorough periodontal evaluation is warranted. In light of the oral health concerns and systemic health risks, patients should give serious consideration to seeking treatment for OSA and improving their quality of life.

RISK ASSESSMENT FOR ORAL HEALTH

Once the comprehensive health history is completed, the oral professional continues with a dental history and evaluates the patient for oral disease risks. This section focuses on risks for oral health diseases, including oral cancer, caries, periodontal disease, and xerostomia. Many of these problems share risk factors. Available screening tools are presented so that oral professionals can utilize measures to help their patients become aware of the risk for serious oral conditions that impact their health and quality of life, as well as ways to prevent or minimize risk.

Oral Cancer
Key Considerations
According to the American Cancer Society, an estimated 48,330 new cases of oral and pharyngeal

Table 3. STOP Questionnaire[36]

Snoring	Do you snore loudly?
Tired	Do you often feel tired, fatigued, or sleepy during the daytime?
Observed	Has anyone observed you stop breathing during your sleep?
Blood Pressure	Do you have or are you being treated for high blood pressure?

Table 4. STOP-Bang Questionnaire[37]

Snoring	Do you snore loudly?
Tired	Do you often feel tired, fatigued, or sleepy during the daytime?
Observed	Has anyone observed you stop breathing during your sleep?
Blood Pressure	Do you have or are you being treated for high blood pressure?
Basal Metabolic Index (BMI)	Is your BMI > 35 kg/m2?
Age	Are you older than 50 years?
Neck circumference	Is your neck circumference > 40 cm?
Gender	Are you male?

cancer (OPC) will occur in the United States in 2016, resulting in 9,570 deaths.[40] Unfortunately, OPC diagnoses are predicted to rise significantly over the next 15 years.[41] Survival rates are significantly higher when OPC is diagnosed early. However, less than one third of new cases are diagnosed at the localized stage compared with over half that are diagnosed in advanced stages. These data suggest the impact that regular oral examination and risk factor assessment in patients could have on OPC morbidity.

Signs and symptoms of OPC include red or white lesions of the soft tissue of the oral cavity, an ulcer or sore that does not heal within 14 days, a lump or thickening in the oral soft tissues, soreness or a feeling that something is caught in the throat, difficulty chewing or swallowing, ear pain, difficulty moving the jaw or tongue, hoarseness, numbness of the tongue or other areas of the mouth, or swelling of the jaw that causes dentures to fit poorly or become uncomfortable.

Numerous risk factors exist for OPC. Tobacco and alcohol consumption remain the major chemical risk factors for oral cancer development. The role of oncogenic viruses has been an emerging area of research interest with attention paid to the human papillomavirus (HPV), particularly HPV-16, HPV-18, HPV-31, and HPV-33. Other viruses associated with oral squamous cell carcinoma include herpes simplex virus, human immunodeficiency virus, Epstein Barr virus, and cytomegalovirus. Genetic susceptibility, genetic alterations, genetic syndromes (i.e., Fanconi's anemia, dyskeratosis congenital), and tumor suppressor genes are examples of molecular pathological changes that affect oral carcinogenesis. Other risk factors include gender, age, exposure to ultraviolet light, weakened immune system, graft-versus-host disease, and lichen planus.[40,42,43]

Application to Clinical Practice

Currently no validated scales assess risk for OPC. However, several risk assessment tools can be used to increase patients' awareness of their risk, and to begin discussion about early detection measures for OPC.

Health Canada provides an online eight-item Oral Cancer Self-Assessment Quiz[44] (see Table 5) that patients can use to assess their personal risk for developing oral cancer. The more items checked "yes," the higher the patient's risk will be. Individuals are advised to conduct self-examination for signs and symptoms associated with oral cancer, and to speak with a dental provider or healthcare provider and ask for an oral cancer screening.

Another tool is the Oral Cancer Risk Assessment from PreViser™, available at www.previser.com. It considers risk based on the parameters of patient and family history of cancer, race, smoking history, alcohol consumption, and lesions noted during the oral examination. A risk profile for oral cancer is

Table 5. Health Canada Oral Cancer Self-Assessment Quiz

Indicate "yes" or "no" to each of the following questions.
Are you over the age of 40? ☐ Yes ☐ No
Are you male? ☐ Yes ☐ No
Do you have human papillomavirus (HPV)? ☐ Yes ☐ No
Are you sexually active and not regularly tested for sexually transmitted infections (STIs)? ☐ Yes ☐ No
Do you use tobacco products? ☐ Yes ☐ No
Do you drink a lot of alcohol and have done so consistently for a long period of time? ☐ Yes ☐ No
Are your lips exposed to the sun on a regular basis? ☐ Yes ☐ No
Is your diet low in fruits and vegetables? ☐ Yes ☐ No

Source: Health Canada. Available at: http://www.hc-sc.gc.ca/hi-vs/oral-bucco/disease-maladie/cancer-eng/php.

created based on a scale of 1 to 5 (less risk to more risk), and preventive treatment options the patient should consider—pertaining to visits to the dentist, oral cancer screening examinations, alcohol use, and family cancer history—are provided. Additional online cancer resources are included as part of the risk assessment for patients seeking more information.

Philips has created the CARE (Customizable Assessment and Risk Evaluator) Tools to help dental professionals identify patients at risk for oral diseases and develop plans for preventing and managing oral conditions across the lifespan. Among these is the six-step Oral Pathology CARE Tool. Step 1 is a patient interview that includes a section related to disease indicators, a section focusing on risk factors, and a section on protective factors. Step 2 is an assessment of risk, which ranges from low to moderate, high, or extreme. Step 3 involves review of clinical guidelines based on the identified risk category. In step 4, the clinician selects a protocol based on the risk profile of the patient. A customized protocol is created and downloaded for the patient in step 5. Topics to be discussed may include biopsy, HPV susceptibility testing, routine screenings, additional follow-up, other instructions, counseling, and lifestyle habits. Step 6 encompasses any other product recommendations, questions, and answers. Additional information about the Oral Pathology CARE Tool can be found at www.philipsoralhealthcare.com.

Caries

Key Considerations

Dental caries remains one of the most serious chronic oral health conditions across the lifespan. At epidemic proportions, caries is the most chronic infection of children.[45] The National Institute of Dental and Craniofacial Research provides summaries of the National Health and Nutrition Examination Survey (NHANES) data collected between 1999 and 2004. Key findings for dental caries follow.[46]

- Among children 2 to 11 years of age, 42% have had dental caries in their primary teeth, and 23% have untreated dental caries.
- Among children 6 to 11 years of age, 21% have had dental caries in their permanent teeth, and 8% have untreated dental caries.
- Among adolescents 12 to 19 years of age, 59% have had dental caries in their permanent teeth, and 20% have untreated caries.
- Among adults 20 to 64 years of age, 92% have had dental caries in their permanent teeth, and 26% have untreated caries.
- Among seniors 65 years of age and older, 93% have had dental caries in their permanent teeth, and 15% have untreated caries.
- Black and Hispanic subgroups and those with lower incomes and less education have had more caries and more untreated primary and permanent teeth.

Signs and symptoms of dental caries include pain, sensitivity, visible pits in tooth surfaces, and brown or white lesions on tooth surfaces. Risk factors for dental caries have been studied in developed and developing countries. A systematic review of the literature and pediatric clinical practice guidelines have identified the following risk factors for dental caries in children and adolescents: diet, fluoride exposure, microflora (*Streptococcus mutans, Lactobacillus*), level of education, a susceptible host, oral hygiene, parental oral health, enamel hypoplasia, and social, cultural, and behavioral factors.[47,48]

Applications to Clinical Practice

The American Academy of Pediatric Dentistry's Clinical Practice Guidelines include risk assessment tools for children from birth to 3 years of age for physicians and other nondental healthcare providers, a caries-risk assessment tool for those from birth through 5 years of age for dental providers (see Table 6), and a caries risk assessment form for children 6 years of age and older for dental professionals (see Table 7).[48] These forms were developed based on available evidence and incorporate biological risk factors, protective factors, and clinical findings from examination. Risk is classified as low, moderate, and high. Caries management protocols are provided within the Clinical Practice Guidelines for each risk category pertaining to diagnostics, preventive interventions, and restorative care. These forms are available at www.aapd.org.

Another evidence-based approach to preventing or treating dental caries at an early stage is Caries Management by Risk Assessment (CAMBRA).[49] Disease indicators highlighted in CAMBRA include visible cavities or radiographic penetration of the dentin, radiographic approximal enamel lesions (not in the dentin), white spots on smooth surfaces, and restorations within the past 3 years. Risk factors or biological predisposing factors evaluated are mutans streptococci (MS) and lactobacilli (LB), both median or high (by culture); visible heavy plaque on teeth; frequent snacks (more than three times daily between meals); deep pits and fissures; recreational drug use; inadequate saliva flow by observation or measurement; saliva-reducing factors; exposed roots; and orthodontic appliances. Protective factors are also evaluated. These factors include fluoride experience, chlorhexidine use, xylitol use, calcium and phosphate paste during the past 6 months, and adequate saliva flow.[49] The form assesses caries risk as low, moderate, high, and extreme. To learn more about CAMBRA, and prevention and treatment interventions for each risk level, visit the CDA Foundation at www.cdafoundation.org.

The American Dental Association has a Caries Risk Assessment Form for children from birth through 6 years of age, and another for children older than age 6. These forms are divided into risks based on contributing conditions (fluoride exposure; sugary foods and drinks; caries experience of mother, caregiver, or siblings; and dental home); general health conditions (special health care needs, chemotherapy or radiation therapy, eating disorders, medications that reduce salivary flow, and drug or alcohol abuse); and clinical conditions. Risk is categorized as low, moderate, or high. These forms are available at www.ada.org.

Periodontal Disease
Key Considerations
Periodontal disease is a chronic inflammatory disease that has become an important public health problem in the United States. In a recent study that monitored the extent of this oral health condition

Table 6. Caries-Risk Assessment Form for Children from Birth to 5 Years of Age[48]

Factors	High Risk	Moderate Risk	Low Risk
Biological			
Mother/primary caregiver has active carries	Yes		
Patient/caregiver has low socioeconomic status	Yes		
Child has > 3 between-meal sugar-containing snacks or beverages per day	Yes		
Child is put to bed with a bottle containing natural or added sugar	Yes		
Child has special healthcare needs		Yes	
Child is a recent immigrant		Yes	
Protective			
Child receives optimally fluoridated drinking water or fluoride supplements			Yes
Child has teeth brushed daily with fluoridated toothpaste			Yes
Child receives topical fluoride from health professional			Yes
Child has dental home/regular dental care			Yes
Clinical Findings			
Child has > 1 decayed/missing/filled surfaces	Yes		
Child has active white spot lesions or enamel defects	Yes		
Child has elevated mutans streptococci levels	Yes		
Child has plaque on teeth		Yes	

Circling those conditions that apply to a specific patient helps the practitioner and parent understand the factors that contribute to or protect from caries. Risk assessment categorization of low, moderate, or high is based on preponderance of factors for the individual. However, clinical judgement may justify the use of one factor (e.g., frequent exposure to sugar-containing snacks or beverages, more than one decayed/missing/filled surfaces) in determining overall risk.
Overall assessment of the child's dental caries risk: High Moderate Low

using a full mouth periodontal examination protocol, 47.2% of adults aged 30 years and older had some form of periodontal disease, and 70.1% of those 65 years and older had periodontitis.[50]

Varied risk factors influence the clinical presentation and rate of periodontal disease progression. They include smoking, poorly controlled diabetes, pathogenic bacteria and poorly controlled oral hygiene, genetic factors, extent and severity of alveolar bone loss, gingival bleeding, gender, and stress.[51-55] While some authors suggest that age is a risk factor for periodontal disease, age alone is not a risk factor. Studies have shown minimal loss of attachment in aging subjects enrolled in preventive programs throughout their lives. Periodontal disease is not an inevitable fate of the aging process, and aging does not increase disease susceptibility.[56,57]

Application to Clinical Practice

In its *Guidelines for the Management of Patients with Periodontal Diseases*,[58] the American Academy of Periodontology (AAP) promotes risk assessment for periodontal disease as an important part of comprehensive periodontal evaluation. A comprehensive periodontal evaluation checklist available at www.aap.org includes components related to teeth, dental implants and subgingival areas, plaque or biofilm, dentition, occlusion, diagnostic-quality radiographs, and discussion of patient risk factors. The AAP states "Utilizing risk assessment helps dental professionals predict the potential for developing periodontal diseases and allows them to focus on early identification and to provide proactive, targeted treatment for patients who are at risk for progressive/aggressive diseases."[51]

In 2015, Lang, Suvan, and Tonetti[59] published results of their systematic review of periodontal disease risk factor assessment tools. Prospective and retrospective cohort studies were evaluated as no randomized controlled clinical trials were available to review. Five risk assessment tools were examined: DenPlan Excel/PreVisor® Patient Assessment (DEP-PA) and its modifications, the Health Improvement in Dental Practice (HIDEP) model, Risk Assessment-Based Individualized Treatment (RABIT), the Dentition Risk System (DRS) at both the patient and tooth level, and the Periodontal Risk Assessment (PRA)

Table 7. Caries-Risk Assessment Form for Children 6 Years of Age and Older[48]

Factors	High Risk	Moderate Risk	Low Risk
Biological			
Patient is of low socioeconomic status	Yes		
Patient has > 3 between-meal sugar-containing snacks or beverages per day	Yes		
Patient has special healthcare needs		Yes	
Patient is a recent immigrant		Yes	
Protective			
Patient receives optimally fluoridated drinking water			Yes
Patient brushes teeth daily with fluoridated toothpaste			Yes
Patient receives topical fluoride from health professional			Yes
Additional home measures (e.g., xylitol, MI Paste™, antimicrobial)			Yes
Patient has dental home/regular dental care			Yes
Clinical Findings			
Patient has ≥ 1 interproximal lesions	Yes		
Patient has active white spot lesions or enamel defects	Yes		
Patient has low salivary flow	Yes		
Patient has defective restorations		Yes	
Patient wearing an intraoral appliance		Yes	

Circling those conditions that apply to a specific patient helps the practitioner and patient/parent understand the factors that contribute to or protect from caries. Risk assessment categorization of low, moderate, or high is based on preponderance of factors for the individual. However, clinical judgement may justify the use of one factor (e.g., ≥ 1 interproximal lesions, low salivary flow) in determining overall risk.

Overall assessment of the child's dental caries risk: High Moderate Low and its modifications. The authors noted that the majority of these tools are variations of the Periodontal Risk Calculator (PRC) and the PRA. Findings showed that periodontitis progression and tooth loss might be predicted based on risk using these tools; however, no data were available on the impact of risk assessment and patient management. The authors reported that the PRA and its modifications have been validated on multiple occasions and that this tool has applicability for clinical practice.

Lang and Tonetti[60] introduced the PRA in 2003. It uses six vectors weighted equally to evaluate the patient's risk for susceptibility and progression of periodontal disease. These parameters are percentage of bleeding on probing, prevalence of pockets greater than 4 mm, loss of teeth from a total of 28 teeth, loss of periodontal support in relation to the patient's age, systemic and genetic conditions, and environmental factors such as smoking. Each parameter has its own scale for minor-, moderate-, and high-risk profiles. The diagram is shaped like a spider web and the shape of the web changes as specific areas of risk increase. The PRA can be accessed at www.perio-tools.com.

The Periodontal Assessment Tool, part of the Oral Health Information Suite from www.previser.com, is an online tool designed to create a periodontal diagnosis and risk score for future disease. A report is prepared for the clinician's documentation and for the patient. Parameters reviewed include history of smoking, diabetes status, prior periodontal treatment, probing depth and bleeding in each quadrant, and estimate of bone loss. Risk scores range from 1 (lowest risk) to 5 (highest risk). The disease state score ranges from 1 (health) to 100 (severe periodontitis).[61] Studies have validated that the risk scores calculated by the Periodontal Assessment Tool predicted future periodontal status with a high level of accuracy.[62,63]

Xerostomia
Key Considerations
Saliva plays an important role in oral health. It serves as a lubricant for the oral cavity and offers protective functions, providing antimicrobial activity, control of pH, and remineralization, and maintaining the integrity of the oral mucosa. In addition, saliva has a mechanical cleansing action. Without these actions, individuals would be at an increased risk for developing oral diseases such as caries, periodontal disease, and fungal infections.

Hyposalivation is the decreased flow of saliva that may result in xerostomia (dry mouth). Xerostomia is often referred to as a subjective sensation.[64] Current estimates of xerostomia and hyposalivation based on epidemiological studies are unavailable, but older studies emphasize widespread complaints of oral dryness among the general population with increases among the elderly.[65] Negative consequences of hyposalivation with xerostomia, in addition to increased risk for oral diseases, include difficulty eating, swallowing, speaking, sleeping, and wearing prostheses; impaired social function; and decreased quality of life.[65]

Multiple risk factors are associated with hyposalivation with xerostomia. The primary risk factor is the use of prescription and nonprescription medications. Other risk factors include sex (more common in women versus men), smoking, diabetes, autoimmune disorders (Sjögren's syndrome), radioactive iodine treatment for thyroid malignancy, and anxiety.[43]

Application to Clinical Practice
There are currently no validated risk assessment tools for xerostomia. However, the ADHA has created a Screening Tool for Hyposalivation with Xerostomia[66] (see Figure 8) designed to help detect the presence of disease and its nature. The screening tool comprises a questionnaire and clinical examination by which the practitioner identifies a risk level of low, moderate, or high. Planning and implementation options are provided for each level of risk.[66] Further evaluation of this instrument is warranted to establish its validity and utility as a screening tool.

SUMMARY

Risk assessment provides dental professionals an opportunity to strengthen their understanding of the patient's health profile prior to providing planned interventions. As this chapter emphasizes, multiple tools are available that can be used to assess systemic and oral health. Some of these instruments can be completed before the appointment while others are best conducted directly with the patient to maximize discussion, awareness, and education, and to coordinate treatment between dental and other healthcare providers. Risk factors overlap between systemic and oral health, and they may vary as the patient's health changes. Therefore, continuous evaluation of risk is imperative.

REFERENCES

1. Little JW, Falace DA, Miller CS, et al. *Little and Falace's Dental Management of the Medically Compromised Patient.* 8th ed. St. Louis, MO: Elsevier; 2013.

Figure 8. Hyposalivation with Xerostomia Screening Tool

Name				/ /
HYPOSALIVATION with XEROSTOMIA SCREENING TOOL				**Points**
SOURCE BY DENTAL HYGIENE ASSESSMENT				
CONTRIBUTORY HISTORY	☐ None	☐ Present (10 pts each); indicate related history below		
DIRECT RELATIONSHIP ☐ Autoimmune Disorder: Sjögren's Syndrome or Other ☐ Cancer Therapy: Recent Chemo and/or H&N Radiation ☐ Diabetes (either type) ☐ Dialysis ☐ _____		☐ Diet Disorder: Anorexia, Bulimia, and/or Dehydration ☐ Infection: Hepatitis, HIV, Tuberculosis, or Other ☐ Mental Condition or Dementia ☐ Thyroid Disease: Hypo/Hyperthyroidism ☐ _____		*DIRECT RELATIONSHIP*
LONG-TERM DAILY INTAKE	☐ None	☐ One (5 pts); check type below	☐ Two or more (10 pts total); check type below	
MORE THAN ONE MONTH ☐ Alcohol (any form) ☐ Antidepressant ☐ Antidiarrheal ☐ Antihistamine or Decongestant ☐ _____		☐ Antihypertensive ☐ Antipsychotic ☐ Bronchodilator ☐ Caffeine (any form) ☐ Diuretic	☐ Garlic, Gingko, or Other ☐ Non-Steroidal Antiinflammatory ☐ Painkiller, Sedative, or Tranquilizer ☐ Tobacco (any form) ☐ _____	*MORE THAN ONE MONTH*
SYMPTOM QUESTIONS BY DENTAL HYGIENE ASSESSMENT				
Feeling Constantly Thirsty?	☐ None	☐ Slight (1 pt)	☐ Moderate (2 pts)	☐ Severe (3 pts)
Difficulty Chewing Food?	☐ None	☐ Slight (1 pt)	☐ Moderate (2 pts)	☐ Severe (3 pts)
Difficult Swallowing Food?	☐ None	☐ Slight (1 pt)	☐ Moderate (2 pts)	☐ Severe (3 pts)
Saliva Amount?	☐ Regular	☐ Low (1 pt)		☐ Very Low (2 pts)
Dryness Amount?	☐ Regular	☐ High (1 pt)		☐ Very High (2 pts)
Dryness Frequency?	☐ None	☐ Occasional (1 pt)	☐ Constant (2 pts)	
Dryness Duration?	☐ None	☐ Short-term (1 pt)	☐ Long-term (2 pts)	
Mouth Changes? Select below	☐ None	☐ One (1 pt)	☐ Two (2 pts)	☐ Three or More (3 pts)
ASK ☐ Bad or Stale Breath? ☐ Burning Mouth?		☐ Denture Poor Hold? ☐ Spicy Food Sensitivity?	☐ Soreness in Mouth? ☐ Stickiness of Tongue?	☐ Taste Sensation Loss? ☐ Tooth Sensitivity? *ASK*
Additional Eye, Nose, Throat, Skin, Genital Dryness?			☐ None	☐ Yes (1 pt)
ORAL SIGNS BY DENTAL HYGIENE DIAGNOSIS				
Tissue Changes? If noted, circle specific signs (1 pt each group)	☐ None	☐ Atrophy/ Redness	☐ Cheilitis/ Fissured	☐ Glossitis/ Stickiness	☐ Ulcers/ Debris
Oral Diseases? (1 pt each)	☐ None	☐ Caries	☐ Fungal	☐ Halitosis	☐ Periodontal
Saliva/Gland Changes? (1 pt each)	☐ None	☐ Enlarged	☐ No Pooling	☐ Stone(s)	☐ Thick/White
Failure To Express? Indicate gland(s) (1 pt each)	☐ None	☐ Parotid	☐ Sublingual/Submandibular		
RISK LEVEL BY DENTAL HYGIENE ASSESSMENT (tally points and circle level)				**TOTAL**
LOW RISK		**MODERATE RISK**		**HIGH RISK**
From 1 to 10 points		From 11 to 20 points		Greater than 20 points
DENTAL HYGIENE PLANNING AND IMPLEMENTATION				
☐ Document in patient record; ☐ Correlate with other oral disease risk tools; ☐ Recommend palliative management; ☐ Monitor by evaluation over next 6-month period		☐ Document in patient record; ☐ Correlate with other oral disease risk tools; ☐ Recommend palliative management; ☐ Perform diagnostic salivary tests to evaluate for high risk ☐ If negative, monitor by evaluation over next 3-month period; ☐ If positive, consider high risk and proceed with planning		☐ Document in patient record; ☐ Correlate with other oral disease risk tools; ☐ Recommend palliative management; ☐ Perform diagnostic salivary tests for baseline ☐ Refer to oral surgeon and/or physician for further testing if from unknown source or for prescribing medication(s), and follow-up evaluation/treatment

Source: ADHA © 2010. ADHA *Standards for Clinical Dental Hygiene*; Fehrenbach MJ. American Dental Hygienists' Association hyposalivation with xerostomia screening tool. *Access*, December, 2010.

2. American Dental Hygienists' Association. *Standards for Clinical Dental Hygiene Practice*. Chicago, IL: American Dental Hygienists' Association; 2008.
3. Mozaffarian D, Benjamin EJ, Go AS, et al. on behalf of the American Heart Association Statistics Committee and Stroke Statistics Committee. Heart disease and stroke statistics—2015 update: a report from the American Heart Association. *Circulation*. 2015;131:e29–e322.
4. World Health Organization. Cardiovascular disease (CVDs). Fact sheet No. 317. Available at: http://www.who.int/mediacentre/factsheets/fs317/en/. Accessed February 27, 2016.
5. Pickett FA, Gurenlian JR. *Preventing Medical Emergencies: Use of the Medical History in Dental Practice*. 3rd ed. Baltimore, MD: Wolters Kluwer Health; 2015.
6. Perk J, Backer GD, Gohike H, et al. European Guidelines on cardiovascular disease prevention in clinical practice (version 2012). *Eur Heart J*. 2012;33:1635–1701.
7. Conroy RM, Pyörälä K, Fitzgerald AP, et al. Estimation of a ten-year risk of fatal cardiovascular disease in Europe: The SCORE project. *Eur Heart J*. 2003;24:987–1003.
8. Lockhart PB, Bolger AF, Papapanou PN, et al. American Heart Association Rheumatic Fever, Endocarditis, and Kawasaki Disease Committee of the Council on Cardiovascular Disease in the Young, Council on Epidemiology and Prevention, Council on Peripheral Vascular Disease, and Council on Clinical Cardiology. Periodontal disease and atherosclerotic vascular disease: does the evidence support an independent association? A scientific statement from the American Heart Association. *Circulation*. 2012;125:2520–2544.
9. Meurman JF, Sanz M, Janket SJ. Oral health, atherosclerosis and cardiovascular disease. *Crit Rev Oral Biol Med*. 2004;15:403–413.
10. Khader YS, Albashaiereh ZS, Alomari MA. Periodontal diseases and the risk of coronary heart and cerebrovascular diseases: a meta-analysis. *J Periodontol*. 2004;75:1046–1053.
11. Vettore MS. Periodontal disease and cardiovascular disease. *Evid Based Dent*. 2004;5:69.
12. Centers for Disease Control and Prevention. *National Diabetes Statistics Report: Estimates of Diabetes and Its Burden in the United States, 2014*. Atlanta, GA: U.S. Department of Health and Human Services; 2014.
13. World Health Organization. 10 facts about diabetes. Available at: http://ww.who.int/features/factfiles/diabetes/facts/en/. Accessed February 27, 2016.
14. National Diabetes Education Program. Risk factors for type 2 diabetes. Available at: http://ndep.nih.gov/hcp-businesses-and-schools/guiding-principles/principles-01-idenify-undiagnosed-diabetes-and-prediabetes-aspx. Accessed November 29, 2015.
15. National Diabetes Education Program. Guiding principles for the care of people with or at risk for diabetes. Available at: http://ndep.nih.gov/hcp-businesses-and-schools/guiding-principles. Accessed November 29, 2015.
16. Rydén L, Standl E, Bartnik M, et al. Guidelines on diabetes, prediabetes, and cardiovascular diseases: executive summary. *Eur Heart J*. 2007;28:88–136.
17. Lindstrom J, Tuomilehto J. The diabetes risk score: a practical tool to predict type 2 diabetes risk. *Diabetes Care*. 2003;26:725–731.
18. Saaristo T, Peltonen M, Lindstrom J, et al. Cross-sectional evaluation of the Finnish Diabetes Risk Score: a tool to identify undetected type 2 diabetes, abnormal glucose tolerance and metabolic syndrome. *Diab Vasc Dis Res*. 2005;2:67–72.
19. De Berardis G, Pellegrini F, Franciosi M, et al. Longitudinal assessment of quality of life in patients with type 2 diabetes and self-reported erectile dysfunction. *Diabetes Care*. 2005;28:2637–2643.
20. Lalla E, Kunzel C, Burkett S, et al. Identification of unrecognized diabetes and prediabetes in a dental setting. *J Dent Res*. 2011;29;90:855–860.
21. Genco R, Schifferle R, Dunford R, et al. Screening for diabetes mellitus in dental practices: a field trial. *J Am Dent Assoc*. 2014;145:57–64.
22. Wolff R, Wolff L, Michalowicz B. A pilot study of glycosylated hemoglobin levels in periodontitis cases and healthy controls. *J Clin Periodontol*. 2009:80:1057–1061.
23. Bossart M, Calley KH, Gurenlian JR, et al. HBA1C chairside screening for diabetes in patients with chronic periodontitis. *Int J Dent Hyg*. Mar 2015; Mar 23. [Epub ahead of print.]
24. Mealey BL, Ocampo GL. Diabetes mellitus and periodontal disease. *Periodontol 2000*. 2007;44:127–153.
25. Lamster IB, Lalla E, Borgnakke WS, et al. The relationship between oral health and diabetes mellitus. *J Am Dent Assoc*. 2008;139(suppl):19S–24S.
26. Taylor GW, Borgnakke WS. Periodontal disease associations with diabetes, glycemic control and complications. *Oral Dis*. 2008;14:191–203.
27. Taylor GW, Manz MC, Borgnakke WS. Diabetes, periodontal diseases, dental caries, and tooth loss: a review of the literature. *Compend Contin Educ Dent*. 2004;24:179–184, 186–178, 190.
28. Bornakke WS. Hyperglycemia/diabetes mellitus and periodontal infection adversely affect each other. In: Genco RJ, Williams RC, eds. *Periodontal Disease and Overall Health: A Clinician's Guide*. 2nd ed. Yardley, PA: Professional Audience Communication, Inc; 2014:99–122.
29. National Sleep Foundation. Sleep apnea. Available at: http://sleepfoundation.org/sleepdosrders-problems/sleep-apnea. Accessed December 5, 2015.
30. Downey R. Obstructive sleep apnea. Available at: http://emedicine.medscape.com/article295807. Accessed December 5, 2015.
31. Lee W, Nagubadi S, Kryger MD, et al. Epidemiology of obstructive sleep apnea: a population-based perspective. *Expert Rev Respir Med*. 2008;2:349–364.
32. Seo WH, Cho ER, Thomas RJ, et al. The association between periodontitis and obstructive sleep apnea: a pre-

liminary study. *J Periodontal Res.* 2012;48:500–506.
33. Levendowski DJ, Olmstead R, Popovic D, et al. Assessment of obstructive sleep apnea risk and severity in truck drivers: validation of a screening questionnaire. *Sleep Diagnosis Ther.* 2007;2(2):20–26.
34. Kornegay EC, Brame JL. Obstructive sleep apnea and the role of dental hygienists. *J Dent Hyg.* 2015;89:286–292.
35. Palomares JS, Tummala S, Wang D, et al. Water exchange across the blood-brain barrier in obstructive sleep apnea: an MRI diffusion-weighted pseudo-continuous arterial spin labeling study. *J Neuroimaging.* 2015;25:900–905.
36. Chung F, Yegneswaran B, Lia P, et al. STOP questionnaire: a tool to screen patients for obstructive sleep apnea. *Anesthesiology.* 2008;108:812–821.
37. Ahmad NE, Sanders AE, Sheats R, et al. Obstructive sleep apnea in association with periodontitis: a case-control study. *J Dent Hyg.* 2013;87:188–199.
38. Gunaratnam K, Taylor B, Curtis B, et al. Obstructive sleep apnea and periodontitis: a novel association? *Sleep Breath.* 2009;13:233–239.
39. Seo W, Cho ER, Thomas RJ, et al. The association between periodontitis and obstructive sleep apnea: a preliminary study. *J Periodont Res.* 2012;48:500–506.
40. American Cancer Society. *Cancer Facts & Figures 2016.* Atlanta, GA: American Cancer Society; 2016.
41. Laronde DM. Oral cancer and the dental hygienist: making a difference and saving lives. *Can J Dent Hyg.* 2014;48:5–6.
42. Ram H, Sarkar J, Kumar H, et al. Oral cancer: risk factors and molecular pathogenesis. *J Maxillofac Oral Surg.* 2011;10:132–137.
43. Regezi JA, Sciubba JJ, Jordan RCK. *Oral Pathology: Clinical Pathologic Correlations.* 5th ed. St. Louis, MO: Saunders; 2008.
44. Health Canada. Healthy living. Oral health. Oral diseases. Available at: http://www.hc-sc.gc.ca/hi-vs/oral-bucco/disease-maladie/cancer-eng/php. Accessed December 6, 2015.
45. Colak H, Dülgergil CT, Dalli M, Hamidi MM. Early childhood caries update: A review of causes, diagnoses, and treatments. *J Nat Sci Biol Med.* 2013;4:29–38.
46. National Institute of Dental and Craniofacial Research. Dental caries. Available at http://www.nidc.nih.gov/DataStatistics/FindDataByTopic/DentalCaries/htm. Accessed December 9, 2015.
47. Harris R, Nicoll AD, Adair PM, et al. Risk factors for dental caries in young children: a systematic review. *Community Dental Health.* 2004;21(suppl):71–85.
48. American Academy of Pediatric Dentistry, Council on Clinical Affairs. Guidelines on caries-risk assessment and management for infants, children, and adolescents. *Pediatr Dent.* 2014;37(6):132–139.
49. Featherstone JD, Domejean-Orliaguet S, Jenson L, et al. Caries risk assessment in practice for age 6 through adult. *J Calif Dent Assoc.* 2007;35:703–713.
50. Eke PI, Dye BA, Wei L, et al. Prevalence of periodontitis in adults in the United States: 2009 and 2010. *J Dent Res.* 2012;91:914–920.
51. American Academy of Periodontology. American Academy of Periodontology statement on risk assessment. Available at: http://www.aap.org. Accessed December 9, 2015.
52. van Winkelhoff AJ, Bosch-Tijhof CJ, Winkel EG, et al. Smoking affects the subgingival microflora in periodontitis. *J Periodontol.* 2001;72:666–671.
53. Demmer RT, Jacobs DR Jr, Desvarieux M. Periodontal disease and incident type 2 diabetes: results from the first National Health and Nutrition Examination Survey and its epidemiologic follow-up survey. *Diabetes Care.* 2008;31:1371–1379.
54. Michalowicz BS, Diehl SR, Gonsolley JC, et al. Evidence of a substantial genetic basis for risk of adult periodontitis. *J Periodontol.* 2000;71;1699–1707.
55. Linden GJ, Mullally BH, Freeman R. Stress and the progression of periodontal disease. *J Clin Periodontol.* 1996;23:675–680.
56. Brown LJ, Oliver RC, Loe H. Evaluating periodontal status of US employed adults. *J Am Dent Assoc.* 1990;121:226–232.
57. Novak KF, Novak MJ. Clinical risk assessment. In: Newman MG, Takei HN, Klokkevold PE, et al. *Carranza's Clinical Periodontology.* 12th ed. St. Louis, MO: Elsevier; 2015.
58. American Academy of Periodontology. Guidelines for the management of patients with periodontal diseases. *J Periodontol.* 2006;77:1607–1611.
59. Lang NP, Suvan JE, Tonetti MS. Risk factor assessment tools for the prevention of periodontitis progression a systematic review. *J Clin Periodontol.* 2015:42(suppl 16):S59–S70.
60. Lang NP, Tonetti MS. Periodontal risk assessment (PRA) for patients in supportive periodontal therapy (SPT). *Oral Health Prev Dent.* 2003;1:7–16.
61. Page RC, Martin JA, Loeb CF. The Oral Health Information Suite (OHIS): its use in the management of periodontal disease. *J Dent Ed.* 2005:69:509–520.
62. Page RC, Krall EA, Martin JA, et al. Validity and accuracy of a risk calculator in predicting periodontal disease. *J Am Dent Assoc.* 2002;133:569–576.
63. Page RC, Martin JA, Krall EA, et al. Longitudinal validation of a risk calculator for periodontal disease. *J Clin Periodontol.* 2003;30:819–827.
64. Fehrenbach MJ, Phelan JA, Ibsen OAC. Immunity and immunologic oral lesions. In: Ibsen OAC, Phelan JA. *Oral Pathology for the Dental Hygienist.* 6th ed. St. Louis, MO: Elsevier; 2014:78–113.
65. Turner MD, Ship JA. Dry mouth and its effects on the oral health of elderly people. *J Am Dent Assoc.* 2007;138(suppl):15S–20S.
66. Fehrenbach MJ. American Dental Hygienists' Association hyposalivation with xerostomia screening tool. *Access.* December 22–25, 2010.

Chapter 4
Dental Caries

J.M. ("Bob") ten Cate and Erik R. Roskam

Dental caries has an interesting association with wealth. Human skulls from various periods in history show tooth decay when the subject could afford luxury foods. More specifically, diets with a high intake of refined sugars were associated with tooth decay. Today, this pattern is noticed in emerging economies. Improving economics may lead to a shift in dietary patterns and allow opportunities to consume a healthier diet, but often the diet is also more cariogenic. Additionally, the necessary improvement in attention to oral health often lags behind. This may result in a dramatic increase in dental caries in youngsters. (See Box 1.) However, increasing wealth also enables people to afford proper dental care, and gradually this drives the desire to keep a dentition that is "worth being seen." Generally speaking, a society and its role models set the norms that dictate the behavior of individuals.

Without question this applies to choices in dentistry, such as the choice of orthodontics based on aesthetics rather than functionality, a wish to bleach teeth, and a preference for white fillings and porcelain-coated crowns and bridges.

Several decades ago, a full denture was the treatment option preferred by many patients, as keeping one's own teeth was considered neither feasible nor affordable. In a population where most individuals over a particular age were edentulous, having a denture was not a stigma, as it probably is today. The expectation of keeping one's teeth in a functional and aesthetically acceptable state spread gradually among the population. This development was important in setting the research priorities for preventive dentistry. It meant that prevention became an issue for all age groups, expanding beyond children and young adults to include the elderly.

A pivotal question still concerns the preferred scheme for caries prevention in patients older than 30 years of age. Toothbrushing—more specifically toothbrushing with a fluoridated toothpaste—developed as the norm over the past 50 years. However, few data evaluating successful additional tools for caries prevention in middle-aged and older adults are available as most efficacy studies involved schoolchildren. Although it is tempting to generalize these findings to older patients, it should be noted that oral physiology changes with age. This applies in particular to elderly patients, who generally take multiple forms of medication or suffer from

Box 1. Dental Caries: Still a Worldwide Problem

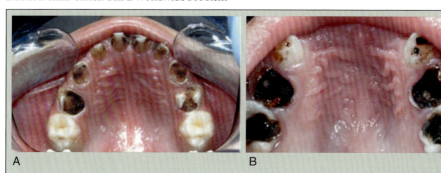

A   B

Figures 1A and B show two examples of extreme tooth decay in the primary dentition: one from South America, the other from Europe. One is from an area with high living standards and easily accessible, properly funded dental care. The other is from an area with poor dietary habits and adequate dental care only for the happy few. Can you see a difference?

other conditions (e.g., dementia, loss of dexterity) that limit their ability to follow an effective oral hygiene routine. Dental health for the elderly is now prominent on the agenda in many countries such as Japan, where the 80/20 program (20 teeth at the age of 80 years) is highly esteemed.

The wish to keep teeth for extended periods also changed the focus of research. Epidemiological data convincingly showed that keeping one's own teeth is preferable for maintaining a functional dentition. Research therefore has focused on improving our understanding of the pathogenesis and etiology of dental caries, with the objective of developing science-based schemes for prevention. These efforts have generated many new insights and have dramatically changed our understanding of the processes leading to dental caries and its prevention.

This chapter aims to provide the reader with some insights into the various developments and achievements in understanding the pathophysiology of the oral cavity. Present-day medical, and therefore dental, care requires a solid scientific foundation. Findings in science precede the development of new treatment modalities. It is thus important for dental practitioners to be aware of major developments in dental science so they will be prepared to make well-founded decisions when considering novel treatments for patients in their clinics.

CARIES PREVENTION
Trends and Challenges

Dental caries and their prevention is an issue that requires lifelong attention. In a unique study in Dunedin, New Zealand, all babies born in 1973 have been followed with periodic assessments of their dental health in relation to other parameters.[1] This project has provided an extremely valuable database on the fate of the dentition over a more than 40-year period. Studies of this type of "natural history" of a disease should ideally be performed periodically and in various countries, as epidemiological data are the basis for decision making in dental public health and necessary to optimize prevention schemes. (See Box 2.)

The Dunedin data reveal that the population split into three groups comprising high (15%),

Box 2. The Famous Case of the British Colony Tristan da Cunha

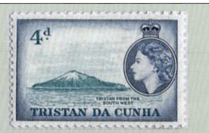

Tristan da Cunha, primarily known for its stamps, is documented as one of the most convincing examples showing the effect of dental deterioration due to an adjustment of standard of living (i.e., the consumption of refined carbohydrates). Until World War II, the inhabitants of this volcanic island in the South Atlantic had a diet based on fish and potatoes, their only harvest. Despite a lack of dental care and poor hygiene, most of the population was free of caries. Studies in the late 1930s indicated that the prevalence of caries in the first permanent molars of 6 to 19 year olds was zero.

When war began, military stations and new factories came to the island, leading to an increased standard of living that, in turn, enabled a change in the diet. The islanders' traditional diet, in which refined fermentable carbohydrates were largely absent, changed to a diet high in these constituents. A volcanic eruption in 1961 led to temporary evacuation of the whole population to England, where their teeth were checked again. By then, the prevalence of caries in the first permanent molars of 6 to 19 year olds had increased to 50%. By 1966, 3 years after their return to the island, caries had increased to 80%. The most prominent change in the islanders' life conditions involved diet, with a decrease in the consumption of potatoes and a compensatory increase in consumption of sugar. It is estimated that the daily consumption of sugar rose from 1.8 g in 1938 to 150 g in 1966.

moderate (45%), and low (40%) rates of incidence of disease. Irrespective of this discrimination in levels of caries progression, it was found that for all subjects the number of surfaces and teeth affected by or treated for caries increased with time. This rate of increase was obviously lowest in the low caries subgroup. These data also prove that caries is not a disease limited to childhood or adolescence. On this point it should be noted that with progressing age many surfaces received new restorations, which presumably were larger (i.e., included additional surfaces) than the original restorations. In the high caries group, by the age of 38 years, the average value on the Decayed, Missing, Filled Surfaces (DMFS) Index was 50, compared with 8 in the low caries group.[1]

For various reasons it is of interest to further consider these findings. The studied population grew up in a period when fluoride toothpastes had just become widely available and were, in fact, widely used. However, the prevailing procedures in dental practice were largely still oriented to early restoration. It is interesting to speculate what the data would have shown if a more restrictive surgical treatment policy had been followed.

From clinical trials on fluoride efficacy, such as the Tiel-Culemborg drinking water fluoride study performed in the 1960s and 1970s, we know that lesions are arrested or even reversed as a result of using fluoride.[2] The fact that early lesions may remineralize or be arrested requires that practitioners maintain a policy of "watchful waiting" and be very restrictive in placing restorations. This "modern" type of operative dentistry focusing on nonoperative interventions (often referred to as a nonoperative caries treatment program [NOCTP]) is still not common practice throughout the world. A large-scale clinical study was very successfully performed at the Danish municipality of Nexo; since then this method is often referred to as the Nexo approach.[3] The NOCTP approach evaluated at Nexo is based on four pillars: (1) dental education of children and caretakers; (2) intensive training of these individuals in maintaining oral hygiene, with a focus on the quality of hygienic practice; (3) early nonrestorative interventions based on early detection of signs of disease; and (4) individually determined recall schemes based on caries risk assessment. This approach has many similarities with minimally invasive dentistry.

Dental caries is more than just cavities. Numerous studies have identified the stages that precede the formation of a cavity. In particular, when fluoride is available it takes several years before a sound surface is cavitated. During this period both patient and dentist should be made aware of surfaces in the dentition that appear to be at particular risk. The study of the pathogenesis of dental caries has demonstrated that the early stages of caries are characterized by a preferential dissolution of tooth mineral from weak spots in the tissue, at both the microscopic and macroscopic level. During an average day, when a patient consumes sugars, several periods of dissolution of the teeth occur. When, at the end of such a specific episode, all sugars are fermented and acids are neutralized by saliva, the physiology returns to a stable situation with calcium phosphates being redeposited from saliva into the damaged areas. This remineralization process is enhanced in the presence of fluoride. However, it should be noted that this remineralization is typically up to 10 times slower than the preceding demineralization. Practically, this implies that about 5 hours of remineralization are needed to repair a 30-minute demineralization episode. It is also clear that a pattern of continuous consumption of cariogenic food will impair the possibility for a fluoride-enhanced "natural" repair. Simply stated, there is a limit to fluoride efficacy in caries prevention. This is important to remember as patients (and dentists) often think that brushing with a fluoride toothpaste makes the teeth strong and able to withstand cariogenic snacking.

A focus on early caries prevention and reversal is also reflected in novel methods of early detection of caries, both to assess the state of disease in the hard tissue (level of demineralization of enamel and dentin) and characteristics of the dental plaque that might result in caries. Using such methods, caries can be detected long before it has progressed into a cavity, or can even be identified in the average dental practice. Firstly, it is possible to see early caries as white spot lesions after removal of plaque, drying the surface, and proper illumination of the sites at risk. Secondly, more advanced techniques involving a change in the optical properties of enamel have been developed. One of these optical properties is its intrinsic fluorescence, which results from the mineral hydroxyapatite and is lost when the mineral is dissolved. Thus, when demineralized enamel is illuminated with visible light, a change in fluorescence can be observed and quantified. This technique, known as quantitative light fluorescence (QLF), is used in epidemiological surveys and in randomized controlled trials (RCTs) to assess the effects of caries preventive treatments. The rationale for both methods is that assessing the early stages of caries is important to quantify the level of new disease, particularly at a point when the damage is still reversible. For RCTs, the added benefit of QLF and similar techniques is that it is possible to evaluate efficacy of new preventive agents in a shorter time period and, more specifically, to determine what the effects of a novel preventive treatment are on the onset and possibly the natural, saliva-induced, repair of decay. (See Box 3.)

Better than screening for early signs of loss of hard tissue are methods that have become available to quantify dental plaque and the cariogenic potential of plaque. Again optical properties based on fluorescence have shown the potential to better visualize potential problems, in this case of the dental plaque biofilm. This method is an improvement over the traditional red disclosing tablets, as it does not leave the patient with an awkwardly red mouth afterward (see Box 3, Figures 3A and B). Moreover, it seems more predictive of caries-inductive

Box 3. Modern Diagnostic Methods: Fluorescence

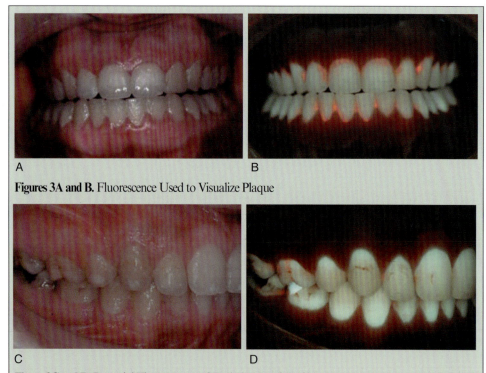

Figures 3A and B. Fluorescence Used to Visualize Plaque

Figure 3C and D. Bacterial Fluorescence of Early Stages of Caries

New optical methods are promising tools for the detection of plaque (see Figures 3A and B) and caries (see Figure 3C and D) and are used in minimally invasive treatment regimens. Newly developed equipment can assist by performing a rapid and complete assessment of the patient's oral health without the need for disclosing solutions. Fluorescence (panels B and D) is not only an accurate diagnostic method for use by the general practitioner but is also an efficient motivational tool for patients.

plaque. It is foreseeable that this optical phenomenon can be employed in smart tools to be used by dentists, and patients, as motivation for better oral hygiene.[4]

The Dunedin study, a new classic in oral epidemiology, is very informative about changes in oral health in an age cohort as it passes through stages in life. Other interesting data are obtained from cohorts at a given age in time. The World Health Organization has chosen particular age groups for this purpose. Using this database, countries may be compared and their respective success in implementing oral care improvement programs can be evaluated. The past 40 years have, by and large, shown a significant improvement in oral health: average levels of disease decreased, and the number of individuals without disease increased. Despite the overall success of reduced caries levels, there are indications that improvements in oral health have halted and may have been somewhat reversed.[5] This trend has been reported for countries that initially showed the largest reductions in caries. It is unknown whether this pattern will continue or spread to other countries. Additional data are needed to further our understanding of what contributed to slowing of improvement in the caries rate.

Paradigm Shifts in Etiology

Oral bacteria have been the subject of study for almost four centuries. In 1674, Antony van Leeuwenhoek used one of the first microscopes to observe dental plaque. Some later findings were already hinted at in his early correspondence with the Royal Society of Medicine, such as the acid susceptibility of the small "creatures" he was observing. The role of acids produced by bacteria was also the basis for the theories on dental caries that were described by W.D. Miller in the last decade of the nineteenth century. Still, the study of bacteriology and oral microbiology remained very similar in terms of the methods used to identify bacteria: bacteria were cultured on various types of agar media that enabled a phenotypic discrimination between species. The discovery of antibiotics obviously led to a major improvement in health, as infectious diseases were no longer the most common cause of death early in life.

A major breakthrough in microbiology took place a few decades ago with the introduction of various methods enabling manipulation of DNA, and the development of techniques to analyze and characterize the genomes of species. Around the time that the human genome was decoded, the first DNA sequences of bacteria were reported. This made it possible to link specific genes to physiological properties, and allowed a more comprehensive approach to understanding the bacterial world. A striking finding was that numerous bacteria identified by their DNA had never been isolated using the traditional culturing method. A practical consequence was that bacteria could be assessed "dead or alive." Even in prehistoric samples it became possible to search for traces of life, including bacteria. As a result of these DNA methods, the taxonomy ("name giving") of bacteria changed: bacteria that were previously considered to be related were repositioned in the phylogenic tree of life. As it was now possible to study specific genes, the research of structure and function of bacterial communities could go to a higher, "supra-species," level.

Bacteria provide vital components of the human physiology. It takes courage to accept that 90% of the cells in our body are bacterial cells. We would never survive without bacteria living in a symbiotic relationship with us and inside us. The pivotal survival strategy for humans is without question to encourage and cherish the beneficial bacteria and to fight the pathogenic ones! Still, the most prevalent diseases in the oral cavity are caused by bacteria. These diseases could be classified as infectious diseases—although typically infectious diseases are caused by pathogenic bacteria that are not part of the normal, commensal bacterial flora.

Various hypotheses have been proposed over time to explain the etiology of dental caries. In the 1970s, the intellectual fight was between groups of scientists who supported the specific versus the nonspecific plaque hypothesis. Briefly, they asked: Is it the volume of plaque or the presence of certain bacteria in the plaque that is responsible for the dissolution of the dental hard tissues? A decade later,

Marsh and Bradshaw (reviewed in 1993) formulated a compromise in the now widely accepted ecological plaque hypothesis.[6] The essence of this theory is that ecological changes, in particular the consumption of large amounts of fermentable carbohydrates (sugars), lead to an intense acidification of dental plaque. This, in turn, results in a shift in microbial composition of dental plaque with an increase of those bacteria that survive periods of high acidity (i.e., low pH). These so-called aciduric bacteria usually also form high amounts of acid. Collectively this implies that changes in bacterial composition shift the natural balance between demineralization (dissolution) and remineralization (repair) to an overall loss of tooth tissue, eventually leading to cavitation. A similar reasoning can be made to explain the enrichment of plaque with bacteria that are associated with infections of the gingival tissues.

Although the ecological plaque hypothesis focused research efforts to better understand the causes of oral disease, several points merit mention and remain the topics of current investigations. It was found that species other than the "arch-criminal of caries," *Streptococcus mutans*, were able to form large amounts of acids and, more importantly, survive in the acidic environment they create. With DNA-based methods, the oral cavity was studied in great detail and thousands of different bacterial species were identified in a group of about 100 people.[7] A separate study showed that various sites in the mouth differ in bacterial composition, with notable differences seen among saliva, soft tissues of the tongue and gingiva, and tooth surfaces. A quick analysis of saliva, therefore, is not a good indicator of the bacterial load at various sites that are at risk for caries or periodontal disease. The microbial variability is far greater than the classically reported difference between supra- and subgingival plaque.

The oral cavity also provided nine sites that were sampled in the large Human Microbiome Project, in which an inventory was made of the bacterial flora of the total human body.[8] A consequence of this generic approach to study bacteria and biofilms was that the oral cavity as habitat for bacterial communities was chosen to address fundamental research issues by colleagues from outside the traditional oral/dental research field. The oral biofilms of dental plaque are very similar in structure and function when compared with other biofilms. This finding holds promise because discoveries derived from biofilms in nature may have applicability to the prevention of oral diseases.

Our deepened understanding of the living microscopic world in our mouths has already resulted in paradigm shifts in caries etiology that have implications for practical prevention. For instance, it is now accepted that, beyond the use of chemotherapeutic agents, preventive efforts should consider routes to attain a healthy microbiome. Research groups that study the microbiome from a more foundational perspective should be able to devise creative approaches that hit "bad" bacteria at their weakest spots and encourage "good" bacteria that help to foster health. Another insight concerns the interplay between bacteria and other microscopic species, such as fungi and viruses, as well as interactions with the host. This microworld, which is now slowly being disclosed, is governed by complex signaling systems between the various components. As described later in this chapter, this information has translational potential.

Evidence for Efficacy: Focus on Fluoride

For the past 40 years, prevention of dental caries has centered around fluoride, in various forms of application. The discovery of fluoride was a classic example of serendipity. Dentist Frederick McKay, a careful observer, noticed that although the teeth of his patients were stained, they also had lower levels of tooth decay when compared with patients in similar communities elsewhere in the country. It took several decades before the cause of this "fluorosis" and the associated reduced levels of dental caries was unravelled and effective caries prevention agents were formulated. In the early 1970s, fluoride toothpastes became available, marking the onset of significant reductions in tooth decay.

Numerous RCTs were completed to quantify the effects of various preventive products. These studies focused on the type of fluoride in a paste or rinse, the fluoride level, and the effects of other additives. As is generally done, the results of these studies were combined in meta-analyses in which data from individual studies were critically reconsidered and combined. This procedure is followed to overcome the risk of accidentally positive or negative outcomes. The conclusions are then often documented in the Cochrane Collaboration Library. This comprehensive evaluation confirmed that fluoride toothpastes are highly effective in caries prevention. Additional benefits were found from using fluoride gels and rinses.[9] Theoretical considerations led to a consensus that fluoride is mainly active though a localized effect in the oral cavity. This implied that fluoride, brought into the mouth during toothbrushing, is most effective when given with "high" frequency—that is, preferably at least twice daily. This mode of action speaks against the use of fluoride tablets and other forms of fluoride administration in which fluoride is present only transiently in the oral cavity. Understanding how a treatment works is essential, given the current emphasis on evidence-based treatments or, in general, evidence-based medicine. For any type of medical, and thus dental, treatment, rigorous and scrutinized data should be available before it is used in patients.

CARIES RISK ASSESSMENT AND NON-FLUORIDE INTERVENTIONS

In recent years there has been increasing support for a more restrictive, truly conserving, approach in restorative dentistry. The rationale is that placing a filling is the irreversible start of a series of re-restorations that, in time, increase the risk of losing the whole tooth. A decision to place a restoration means having "lost the battle" as a result of inadequate prevention to safeguard the respective tooth against decay. The Dunedin study cited earlier in this chapter provides irrefutable data that invasive treatment gradually leads to more surfaces being restored or teeth being lost. With this in mind, research has focused on evaluating nonoperative anticaries approaches in conjunction with a caries risk assessment. One of the promising approaches has been the Caries Management by Risk Assessment (CAMBRA) initiative. Based on this principle, several clinical studies have now been reported. In high-risk adults, Chaffee and colleagues studied three types of anticaries agents.[10] The study design encompassed separate groups in which the protocol followed a single or repeated delivery of agents, and a no-additions control group. The three treatments chosen were 0.12% chlorhexidine gluconate, 5,000 ppm fluoride toothpaste or varnish, and xylitol products. The study revealed that the one-time delivery group had similar caries scores as the control group that followed the basic dental care. However, the group that received the repeated, spaced delivery showed a significantly higher anticaries benefit, with on average one additional restoration being prevented in every three subjects during the 18 months of the study.

Encouraged by the success of fluoride, considerable efforts were taken to find other agents that could positively influence the demineralization–remineralization balance. Remineralization is enhanced by low levels of fluoride in the oral fluids. However, calcium and phosphate also are required to form new hydroxyapatite. Calcium and phosphate additions have been researched in several chemical forms, notably tricalcium phosphate, calcium glycerophosphate, and nanoparticulate hydroxyapatite. Currently, information is limited and none of these additions has reached the level of a thorough Cochrane review with a positive recommendation. Of particular interest have been products based on casein phosphopeptide–amorphous calcium phosphate (CPP-ACP). The rationale for developing this compound was that the milk-derived CPP binds high levels of calcium and phosphate in an amorphous form. Accumulation of CPP-ACP in dental plaque increases the calcium and phosphate levels, which may then be expected to increase mineral deposition as a remineralization of enamel. Numerous papers have focused on elucidating the mode of action of CPP-ACP and, more recently, determining the clinical efficacy of CPP-ACP–based products. In spite of this extensive research, a review recently concluded that there is a lack of evidence to support the use of products based on this technology at this time.[11] The authors suggest that further, well-designed RCTs are needed before there is widespread recommendation of these products for the prevention and treatment of early dental caries in the general population.

NOVEL APPROACHES: A FOCUS ON THE PLAQUE BIOFILM

The stagnation in the improvement of oral health, mentioned earlier, has intensified efforts in cariology research to find new antimicrobial agents. Such compounds should have an effect additive to fluoride. The rationale is that fluoride is primarily effective in enhancing the remineralization of early caries lesions and, in general, the mineral–tissue reactions. For patients with a cariogenic lifestyle (i.e., too-frequent snacking), the deleterious effect of numerous acid attacks on the teeth cannot be counteracted by remineralization. Various studies have confirmed that no more than about six cariogenic meals or snacks can still be repaired by (fluoride-enhanced) remineralization from saliva.[12]

The new information about the dental plaque biofilm, and bacteria in general, has led to promising new approaches for interfering with the bacterial etiology of caries.[13] In general, these encompass the new insights of biofilm properties. Some of these routes are described in the next paragraphs. One of the perplexing questions in understanding life in a biofilm has been how it is possible for so many different bacteria to live together in a crowded environment. From studies on individual species it is evident that bacteria are very different in terms of optimal growth conditions and growth rates. Why, then, is dental plaque not dominated by a particular species that outgrows all the others? One explanation is that bacteria possess smart signaling systems. Among these, the quorum sensing system is vital to enable bacteria to sense neighboring species. When a colony begins to exceed a particular density, the bacteria adjust their physiology in a way that allows all to survive—a very intelligent approach that humans can only dream about! With our knowledge of the quorum sensing system, and more specifically the tools to control (shut off) this system, we could upset the balanced bacterial life in a biofilm. Initial experiments have shown that this will result in reduced overall bacterial growth in the treated biofilms. Bacteria also share advanced metabolic networks. The metabolic waste of one species is food for another. Again, if reactions in this network are impaired, it will lead to a buildup of intermediate products and a metabolic congestion with effects similar to overloaded highways on Friday afternoon!

Another possible approach centers on the question, can we modify the bacterial composition of our biofilms? In principle this is difficult as the biofilm composition is the result of a long historic evolution. Fortunately, a bacterial invader, often a pathogen, is not easily accepted in a bacterial community. This so-called colonization resistance serves an important purpose for the host (us, in this case): Without it, we would be more often struck by pathogens and the resultant bacterial infections. Despite this protective mechanism, selected bacteria may be taken up in biofilms and assume a role in the overall physiology. (See Box 4.)

The role of probiotics in affecting the bacterial flora in the gut is a classic example. Probiotics are microorganisms that are believed to provide health benefits when consumed. Commonly claimed benefits include a decrease in potentially harmful gastrointestinal microorganisms, reduction of gastrointestinal discomfort, and strengthening of the immune system. There is anecdotal evidence that individuals who regularly take probiotics have a higher life expectancy. With respect to oral diseases, some studies have shown a limited benefit when schoolchildren drank milk with added probiotics, or used probiotics in another form. As there have also been negative study outcomes, the final verdict for probiotics in oral health is still pending. Of historic interest is the related Replacement Theory, which was first proposed in the 1970s. Hillman and colleagues modified *Streptococcus mutans* to reduce its acidogenic potential and added other features to the genome to give it an ecological advantage.[14] Eventually this approach was abandoned as the many legal

Box 4. Nature versus Nurture

> When we examine members of the same family, we often observe the same health trends in different generations. For example, when parents present with multiple decayed teeth, most likely, their children will present with the same problem. Conversely, parents with excellent oral health often have children with healthy mouths as well. This prompts an important question: What role does nature play in caries risk, and which part is nurture?
>
> Genetics has an impact on several oral risk factors: the composition and quantity of saliva, the shape of the teeth, and whether the enamel is in "good shape." The position of the teeth, crowding, and bite issues are also important variables when considering a predisposition to caries. Good dental hygiene and careful maintenance may help overcome these negative factors. However, patients with more risk factors will have to be more committed to performing their best oral hygiene.
>
> What are the "nurture" factors that require extra vigilance on the part of dental professionals? Bacteria that cause caries and periodontal disease were not present in the oral cavity at birth. Unfavorable bacterial flora are acquired, passed from person to person, and thrive with an unhealthy diet. Sharing utensils, drinks, and even kissing can result in the sharing of "bad" bacteria among all members of the family.
>
> Encourage adult patients to set the right example for their children. The numbers of sugary drinks and in-between snacks ingested each day are crucial determinants in the caries debate. Drinking plain water, maintaining thorough brushing and flossing habits, and seeing a dental professional regularly are helpful in reducing caries risk. As a practitioner, keep a keen eye on arising problems. Use of current oral care products, methods, and technologies—such as dental sealants and interceptive orthodontics—can help patients keep their smiles healthy and beautiful.

restrictions for this type of genetic modification made it too difficult to pursue. Other investigators have studied bacteria that selectively eliminate pathogens, which might be called "predator bacteria." The discovery that bacteria can now be manufactured by introducing selected genes has undoubtedly great potential but is, in terms of its applications, still in the realm of science fiction.

A potentially more promising approach involves prebiotics. Prebiotics are chemicals that induce the growth or activity of bacteria and fungi that contribute to the well-being of their host. Stated more simply, these are not bacteria but rather food for bacteria. Dental caries is caused by acids formed in the dental plaque; therefore, if bacteria could either break down or neutralize these acids it would be advantageous. In the search for such bacteria, arginolytic bacteria were found: Various streptococci (e.g., *Streptococcus gordonii* and *sanguinis*) catabolise arginine or urea to form ammonium, and thereby elevate the pH of the medium. Although a first patent to include arginine in oral care products dates from 1978, it took almost 30 years before a toothpaste with fluoride and arginine was introduced.[15] The first studies with arginine in toothpastes and confectionary have shown the great potential of this approach, with outcomes similar to fluoride control groups. Recent clinical trials in Thailand and China confirmed that the addition of arginine provided an additional anticaries benefit of about 25% compared with a fluoride control paste.[16] This is a significant development as the search for other active substances that would significantly boost fluoride has so far not been successful.

In the search for chemical formulations that have antimicrobial properties, researchers have investigated many types of compounds. The rationale for this comprehensive research is the need to also search for a medication that might be a next-generation antibotic agent. Avenues that have been researched include both active compounds and vehicles that would specifically target pathogens with antimicrobial agents. If the medicament could be made to actively search for pathogens, a reduced dose would probably suffice to kill the pathogen. Such selective targeted antimicrobial peptides (STAMPs) have shown promise, although for dental caries it is now clear that the disease does not result from a mono-infection. In general, developments in nanotechnology and nanoparticulate materials offer numerous opportunities. For instance, nano-sized calcium phosphate particles can penetrate deeply into biofilms, serving as sources of calcium and phosphate, and in addition can carry a "load" of an antimicrobial to be released at the site where it is most needed.[17]

SUMMARY

Major paradigm shifts in all issues related to dental caries have occurred in recent decades. First and foremost is probably the changed perception regarding the importance of oral health in relation to general health. The following editorial plea in *The Lancet* is a clear and important message to a wide readership, from general medical practitioners to insurance companies and policy makers: "Politically, commitment is needed to integrate oral disease prevention into programmes to prevent chronic diseases and into public-health systems. Good oral health should be everyone's business."[18]

Secondly, the notion has spread that it is doable to keep one's teeth for a lifetime, but that it is not an easy task to achieve. As part of the collaboration between patient and dental professional, prevention-oriented schemes should be set and followed. Maintaining a functional dentition is primarily the patient's responsibility, and this should be acknowledged. However, dental practitioners should start or continue to change their focus from a restorative approach to a prevention-oriented one. The decision to place a restoration should only be made when all other options have failed. Although today's dental restorations are acceptable from both aesthetic and functional perspectives, they are inferior to the original tooth. Similarly, it should be stressed that dentures are not really an acceptable alternative to one's natural dentition.

In terms of dental public health, the search should continue for the most effective and cost-effective programs for caries prevention. This discussion and outcome will depend on the economic conditions of the groups under study. The finding that caries is still highly prevalent among economically deprived individuals demands a reconsideration of available schemes. This requires not only evaluating products for oral care, but also numerous food types that are components of the causative diets. Overweight, obesity, and dental caries often go hand in hand; therefore, we should join forces with colleagues working in food research or as dietary consultants. A dietary evaluation is the task of dental practitioners during the dental visit.

Numerous agents and products are on the drawing board and it is conceivable that promising new products will become available in the next decade. It is the task of the dental community, including manufacturers of oral care products, to make these products available to and affordable for the consumer at large.

The argument that good oral health is vital for general health should help to remove the borders between the respective disciplines. The most prevalent human diseases are, or originate from, infectious diseases. Our improved understanding of the importance of bacteria in the body and insights regarding their functions should induce a more rational approach to controlling them. Undoubtedly this is the most appealing, challenging, and potentially most rewarding facet of the dental care agenda for the future.

CASE 1: Caries in Adolescent Patients

Despite careful instructions regarding dental hygiene, the absence of responsibility often seen among adolescents may lead to a lack of dental hygiene for extended periods of time. As seen in Figures 4A and 4B, a stable, caries-free dentition may deteriorate if the patient does not follow instructions. This case depicts the need for enhanced oral attention during orthodontic treatment. Observations such as these are, unfortunately, rather common in general practice and could result in heated discussions with parents or caretakers about responsibility,

Figures 4A and B. Deterioration of Dentition in an Adolescent Patient

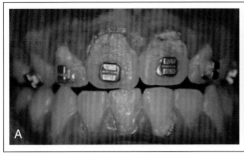
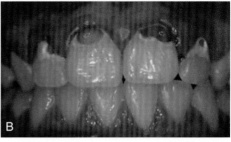

and even attempts to assign liability.

The same applies to dietary intake among members of this age group. A high consumption of carbonated drinks, often with high sugar intake, can lead to extensive erosive lesions. Sometimes these lesions are so deep that the patient complains of irreversible hypersensitivity. In the case shown in Figures 4C and 4D, the adolescent patient required root canal treatment in the mandibular first molar.

In contrast, the patient shown in Figures 4E through 4H has excellent dental hygiene: Her mother is dental nurse in our office! Nevertheless, note the loss of enamel in the first molars within a span of only 4 years (contrast Figures 4E–F with Figures 4G–4H).

CASE 2: Caries in Elderly Patients

Dental care for the elderly is challenging. Improvements in access to dental care and caries pre-vention over the past five decades have resulted in a large group of elderly patients who have kept their teeth; however, difficulties with maintenance of good oral hygiene often increase with age.

Mrs O. is almost 94 years old. Her health is consistent with what is to be expected of a person of this age: a minor heart condition, trouble with walking, and blindness. However, she is cognitively intact. She is still able to take care of her teeth by herself at home and comes to the office for her regular visits (see Figures 5A–5D).

Another large group of elderly patients resides in nursing homes and long-term care facilities. Many of these patients also still have their own dentition, but due to physical and cognitive impairments, they are either personally unable or their caretakers have a lack of interest in maintaining good oral hygiene. Thus, their oral condition rapidly deteriorates.

A recent article from the American Dental

Figures 4C and D. Female Patient, Aged 19 Years

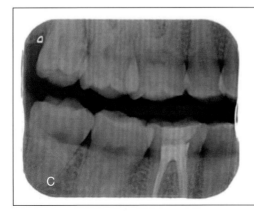
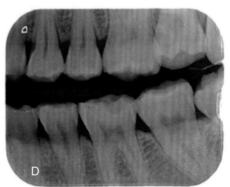

Figures 4E and F. Female Patient, Aged 15 Years (*compare with Figures 4G and H*)

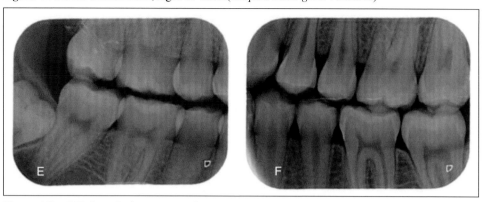

Figures 4G and H. Same Patient as 4E and F, Now Aged 19 Years

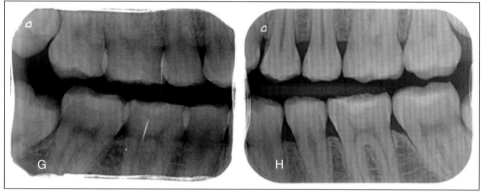

Association[19] describes needed actions for managing this growing population group:

Legislation currently before the US Congress would provide grants to organizations that help expand access to care for the elderly in nursing homes. In the United States, approximately 1.3 million nursing home residents face the greatest barriers to access dental care of any population group. Federal law requires nursing home facilities to provide dental care to residents, including routine and emergency care. But delivering dental care to these patients has been problematic. Currently, dentists across the United States are adopting nursing homes in their communities using the existing public health safety net. This is an immediate and affordable solution to coordinate free dental care to poor and disabled adults, including senior citizens.

Similar schemes are being set up in other countries as well. Schemes to provide dental education for caregivers are getting more and more common. But most of all, those responsible for the care of these elderly patients should feel it is primarily their obligation to take care of their dental needs.

CASE 3: Oral Health and General Health

PATIENT OVERVIEW

Medical history: H.B is a 43-year-old male with diabetes mellitus type 1—2006; four bypasses—2014. After his first appointment more than 10 years ago, the dental team was hardly able to improve the dental condition of this patient. After being diagnosed with diabetes and being put on medication in 2006, his dental condition did improve but even with

Figures 5A–D. Elderly Female Patient, Aged 94 Years

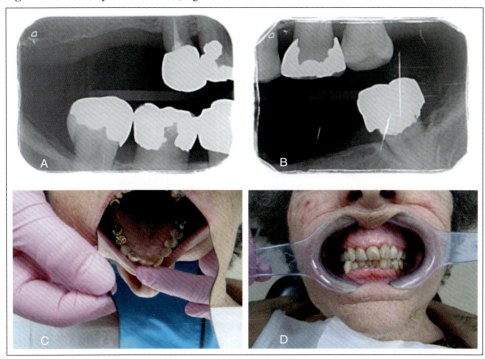

Figures 6A–D. Male Patient with Complications of Diabetes Mellitus Type 1

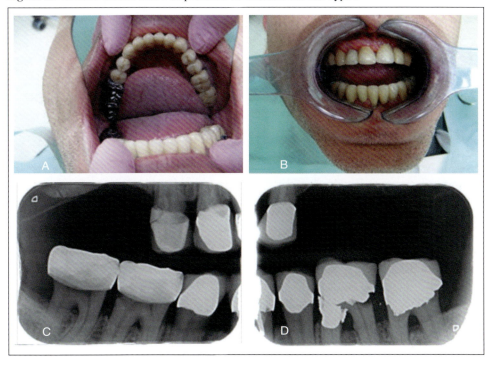

maximal support from the dental hygienist still stayed at a rather poor level. But after coronary surgery in 2014 his overall condition as well as his dental condition improved markedly.

Risk Assessment/Risk Factors: As dental practitioners we know it all too well. On the intake examination we see poor dentition, poorly maintained oral hygiene, and a long history of dental work (see Figures 6A–D). For the medical anamneses, we then typically expect the same: a highly compromised history with many medical issues.

It was previously known that poor oral hygiene substantially increases the risk for cardiovascular disease. But recently, poor dentition and poor oral hygiene have been suspected of having links to numerous systemic diseases, such as diabetes, osteoporosis, rheumatoid arthritis, pneumonia, and chronic obstructive pulmonary disease. Studies have also linked obesity to gum disease. Researchers are investigating the possible role of oral health during pregnancy. Infection and inflammation in general seem to interfere with the development of a fetus in the womb. General and dental health are possibly already affected by the development of immune responses at that stage (see Chapter 12).

Acknowledgments

The authors are indebted to Drs. Catherine Chaussain, Rita Villena, Monique van der Veen, and Janneke Krikken for allowing the use of case information as illustrations for this chapter.

REFERENCES

1. Broadbent JM, Foster Page LA, Thomson WM, Poulton R. Permanent dentition caries through the first half of life. *Br Dent J*. 2013;215:E12.
2. Groeneveld A. Longitudinal study of prevalence of enamel lesions in a fluoridated and non-fluoridated area. *Community Dent Oral Epidemiol*. 1985;13:159–163.
3. Ekstrand KR, Christiansen ME. Outcomes of a non-operative caries treatment programme for children and adolescents. *Caries Res*. 2005;39:455–467.
4. van der Veen MH. Detecting short-term changes in the activity of caries lesions with the aid of new technologies. *Curr Oral Health Rep*. 2015;2:102–109.
5. Bagramian RA, Garcia-Godoy F, Volpe AR. The global increase in dental caries. A pending public health crisis. *Am J Dent*. 2009;22:3–8.
6. Marsh PD, Bradshaw DJ. Microbiological effects of new agents in dentifrices for plaque control. *Int Dent J*. 1993;43(4 suppl 1):399–406.
7. Keijser BJ, Zaura E, Huse SM, et al. Pyrosequencing analysis of the oral microflora of healthy adults. *J Dent Res*. 2008;87:1016–1020.
8. Human Microbiome Project Consortium. Structure, function and diversity of the healthy human microbiome. *Nature*. 2012;486:207–214.
9. Marinho VC. Cochrane reviews of randomized trials of fluoride therapies for preventing dental caries. *Eur Arch Paediatr Dent*. 2009;10:183–191.
10. Chaffee BW, Cheng J, Featherstone JD. Non-operative anti-caries agents and dental caries increment among adults at high caries risk: a retrospective cohort study. *BMC Oral Health*. 2015;15:111.
11. Raphael S, Blinkhorn A. Is there a place for Tooth Mousse® in the prevention and treatment of early dental caries? A systematic review. *BMC Oral Health*. 2015;15:113.
12. Duggal MS, Toumba KJ, Amaechi BT, Kowash MB, Higham SM. Enamel demineralization in situ with various frequencies of carbohydrate consumption with and without fluoride toothpaste. *J Dent Res*. 2001;80:1721–1724.
13. ten Cate JM, Zaura E. The numerous microbial species in oral biofilms: how could antibacterial therapy be effective? *Adv Dent Res*. 2012;24:108–111.
14. Hillman JD, Brooks TA, Michalek SM, Harmon CC, Snoep JL, van Der Weijden CC. Construction and characterization of an effector strain of *Streptococcus mutans* for replacement therapy of dental caries. *Infect Immun*. 2000;68:543–549.
15. Kleinberg I. A mixed-bacteria ecological approach to understanding the role of the oral bacteria in dental caries causation: an alternative to *Streptococcus mutans* and the specific-plaque hypothesis. *Crit Rev Oral Biol Med*. 2002;13:108–125.
16. Li X, Zhong Y, Jiang X, et al. Randomized clinical trial of the efficacy of dentifrices containing 1.5% arginine, an insoluble calcium compound and 1450 ppm fluoride over two years. *J Clin Dent*. 2015;26:7–12.
17. Zhou C, Weir MD, Zhang K, Deng D, Cheng L, Xu HH. Synthesis of new antibacterial quaternary ammonium monomer for incorporation into CaP nanocomposite. *Dent Mater*. 2013;29:859–870.
18. Editorial. Oral health: prevention is key. *Lancet*. 2009;373(9657):1.doi: http://dx.doi.org/10.1016/S0140-6736(08)61933-9.
19. American Dental Association. *Action for Dental Health. Provide Care Now to People Suffering with Untreated Dental Disease*. Chicago, IL: ADA; 2015. Available at: http://www.ada.org/en/public-programs/action-for-dental-health. Accessed May 4, 2016.

Chapter 5
Gingival Diseases

Rebecca Wilder and Antonio Moretti

PART 1: OVERVIEW OF THE CONDITION
This chapter focuses on gingivitis and chronic periodontitis associated with dental plaque, which are the most common forms of periodontal diseases. Topics covered are classification, epidemiology, etiology and pathogenesis, risk assessment, and interventional and preventative measures. In addition, the chapter reports on the emerging evidence of similar inflammatory conditions affecting peri-implant tissues.

PERIODONTAL DISEASES: DEFINITIONS AND CLASSIFICATION

Gingivitis is inflammation of the gingiva (gums) surrounding the teeth, with no radiographic evidence of bone loss. Periodontitis is inflammation of the supporting tissues of the teeth. Periodontitis is usually a progressively destructive process leading to the loss of the surrounding structures of the teeth. It is, in fact, an extension of inflammation from the gingiva into the adjacent structures (i.e., alveolar bone and periodontal ligament).[1] Periodontitis is clinically characterized by gingival pocket formation or gingival recession, or both. One can normally observe the presence of biofilm (bacterial plaque) and calculus. Radiographically, one can notice alveolar bone loss, especially in moderate to severe cases.

The last comprehensive Classification System for Periodontal Diseases and Conditions was published in 1999 by the American Academy of Periodontology (AAP).[2] This was based on the knowledge and consensus report of approximately 60 periodontist clinicians and researchers from around the world who participated in the International Workshop for a Classification of Periodontal Diseases and Conditions.[2] Table 1 summarizes the main conditions discussed and presented to the dental profession approximately 17 years ago.

More recently, the AAP published a Task Force Report on the update to the 1999 Classification of Periodontal Disease and Conditions.[3] The Academy also announced that a comprehensive update to the 1999 Classification would commence in 2017. Meanwhile, minor modifications have been introduced, which are discussed below.

Formulation of a diagnosis of periodontitis is based on multiple clinical and radiographic parameters, all of which may not be required. In general, a patient has periodontitis when one or more sites have inflammation exhibiting bleeding on probing (BOP), radiographic alveolar bone loss, and increased probing pocket depth (PPD) or clinical attachment loss (CAL).[3] Table 2 summarizes the most recent guidelines for determining the severity of periodontitis in patients.

Chronic and Aggressive Periodontitis

Chronic periodontitis is the most common form of periodontitis seen in the adult population. It has been recommended as a descriptor to denote the slowly progressive nature of the condition. However, there are, in some patients, short periods of rapid destruction of the periodontal structures.[3] Aggressive periodontitis is a rare condition that occurs in patients who otherwise are clinically healthy (except for periodontal disease). Common features include rapid attachment and alveolar loss; familial aggregation is also common. Normally, the amounts of microbial deposits (biofilm) and calculus are inconsistent with the severity of the disease. Phagocyte abnormalities are observed, as well as elevated proportions of *Aggregatibacter actinomycetemcomitans* and, in some populations, *Porphyromonas gingivalis.*[1] The recent AAP Task Force Report has recommended that patient age younger than 25 years at the time of the disease onset be used, along with other signs or criteria, to support the diagnosis of aggressive periodontitis.[3] Currently, there are no definitive biomarkers that can differentiate between aggressive and chronic periodontitis or between generalized and localized forms of aggressive periodontitis. The clinician must base diagnostic decisions on the patient history and clinical and radiographic signs.[3] Additional information on classification of

Table 1. AAP 1999 Classification of Periodontal Diseases and Conditions

1	Gingival diseases	Dental plaque-Induced	Dental plaque only Modified by systemic factors Modified by medications Modified by malnutrition
		Non–plaque-induced gingival lesions	Specific bacterial origin Viral origin Fungal origin Genetic origin Manifestation of systemic conditions Traumatic lesions Foreign body reactions
2	Chronic periodontitis		Localized or generalized
3	Aggressive periodontitis		Localized or generalized
4	Periodontitis as a manifestation of periodontal diseases		Associated with hematologic disorders Associated with genetic disorders
5	Necrotizing periodontal diseases		Necrotizing ulcerative gingivitis Necrotizing ulcerative periodontitis
6	Abscesses of the periodontium		Gingival abscess Periodontal abscess Pericoronal abscess
7	Periodontitis associated with endodontic lesions		
8	Developmental or acquired deformities and conditions		Localized tooth-related factors that modify or predispose to plaque-induced gingival diseases/periodontitis Mucogingival deformities and conditions around teeth Mucogingival deformities and conditions on edentulous ridges Occlusal trauma

Source: Ann Periodontol. 1999;4:1–6.[2]

Table 2. Guidelines for Determining Severity of Periodontitis

	Slight (Mild)	Moderate	Severe (Advanced)
Probing depths	> 3 and < 5 mm	≥ 5 and < 7 mm	≥ 7 mm
Bleeding on probing	Yes	Yes	Yes
Radiographic bone loss	Up to 15% of root length or ≥ 2 mm and ≤ 3 mm	16% to 30% or > 3 mm and ≤ 5 mm	>30% or > 5 mm
Clinical attachment loss	1–2 mm	3–4 mm	≥ 5 mm

Source: J Periodontol. 2015;7:835-838.[3]

periodontitis as localized or generalized can be found in the same AAP Task Force Report.[3]

Epidemiology of Gingivitis and Chronic Periodontitis
Gingivitis
The recent update on prevalence of periodontitis in adults in the United States (National Health and Nutrition Examination Survey [NHANES] 2009 to 2012) did not include all forms of periodontal diseases. BOP (indicative of active inflammation) was not part of the data collection.[4] Albandar and Kingman, in 1999, found that 50% of adults had gingival bleeding in one or more sites.[5] More recently, Li and colleagues investigated the prevalence and severity of gingivitis in a representative cohort of American adults.[6] The authors found that only 6.1% of the individuals showed low levels of gingival inflammation. Estimates of the general prevalence of gingivitis vary from 50% to 100% of the adult population.[7] Regarding age, gingivitis typically starts in early childhood, increases in both prevalence and severity during

adolescence, and remains stable in the second decade of life.[7] There is a small increase in the *prevalence* of gingival bleeding with age, but with a more marked increase in the *extent* of gingival bleeding. In addition, the prevalence and extent of gingival bleeding have been reported to be significantly higher in males than in females.[5]

Chronic Periodontitis

Periodontitis affects almost 50% of the US adult population aged 30 years and older. The prevalence is higher in Hispanics followed by non-Hispanic blacks. Non-Hispanic Asians are the third most affected group followed by non-Hispanic whites. Other important factors that can negatively affect the prevalence of periodontitis are (1) being a current smoker, (2) sex (males are more affected than females), and (3) lower socioeconomic status (including either poverty or education).[4] Eke and associates noted that US estimates appear to be much lower than those reported for certain European populations.[4] Around the world, epidemiological studies show a large variation when defining and classifying periodontal diseases. More importantly, the great disparity among populations makes it difficult to compile data from the various sources. Nevertheless, chronic periodontitis is a very significant healthcare problem. Severe periodontitis is the sixth most prevalent disease in humans.[8]

Etiology and Pathogenesis of Periodontal Diseases

Gingivitis and periodontitis are best viewed as a continuum of a chronic inflammatory disease entity, with periodontitis representing a perturbation of host–microbial homeostasis in susceptible individuals that leads to irreversible destruction of tissues.[9] Bacterial plaque or biofilm has long been recognized as a major factor contributing to the initiation and persistence of gingival inflammation.[10] The bacterial challenge elicits the innate immune system with the production of cytokines and chemokines in the gingival tissues, leading to the expression of adhesion molecules, increased permeability of gingival capillaries, and chemotaxis of polymorphonuclear neutrophils and macrophages. As the process continues, the adaptive immune system brings other critical participants such as T and B lymphocytes and plasma cells. These have both protective and nonprotective features. A great number of proinflammatory mediators (e.g., prostaglandin E_2, interleukin-1β [IL-1β], tumor necrosis factor- , and matrix metalloproteinases), microorganisms other than bacteria (i.e., viruses and fungi), and additional events and conditions are involved in this very complex process. The poor and imbalanced interaction between the host and the microbial challenge leads to irreversible pathological alveolar bone resorption, mostly of slow progression, that eventually, if untreated, may lead to tooth loss.

Diagnostic Testing of Periodontal Diseases

Over the past two to three decades, both clinicians and scientists have been focused on the important goals of early diagnosis and treatment of periodontal diseases, preventing the irreversible loss of structures. The destructive nature of chronic periodontitis makes early detection and intervention particularly important. There is still much to be learned in this field. Despite tremendous development in both basic and clinical sciences, clinicians continue to rely primarily on clinical and radiographic findings to diagnose, prevent, and treat periodontal diseases.

Several diagnostic biomarkers exist that might help the clinician. These molecular markers of tissue destruction can be present in the gingival crevicular fluid, saliva, and serum. However, Buduneli and Kinane concluded that there is no single or combination of biomarkers than can disclose periodontal tissue destruction adequately.[11] Microbial sampling has also been considered of limited value. In a systematic review, Listgarten and Loomer concluded that for chronic periodontitis, there is lack of strong evidence that microbial identification is a valuable adjunct to its management.[12] Another more recent systematic review that explored the association of susceptible genotypes to periodontal disease concluded that IL-1–positive genotypes increase the risk for tooth loss.[13] Regarding imaging, Aljehani reviewed the diagnostic application of cone-beam computed tomography (CBCT) in the field of periodontology.[14] It was concluded that bony defects, craters, and furcation involvement seem to be better depicted on CBCT, whereas bone quality and periodontal ligament space scored better on conventional intraoral radiography. The author concluded that CBCT does not offer a significant advantage over conventional radiography for assessing periodontal bone levels.

Periodontal Prognosis and Risk Assessment
It is well-known that periodontal diseases have a complex and multifactorial etiology. For the clinician, it is important to determine the relative risk for disease progression in a once-treated patient.[15] Although periodontal prognosis relates to treatment outcome for the tooth or dentition, or both, risk assessment is more global and involves a more thorough understanding of the patient and his or her future oral health. Both prognosis and risk assessment are integral parts of practice. However, according to Kwok and Caton, there is limited direct evidence in the literature regarding the assignment of periodontal prognosis.[16] It thus remains a nonscientific aspect of the professional routine. Conversely, a recent systematic review by Lang and coworkers identified five available periodontal risk assessment tools in the literature.[15] The various assessment tools and multiple publications associated with their methods support the possibility that periodontitis progression and tooth loss can be predicted in a treated population based on risk segmentation. The authors also stated that there are no data yet to determine the impact that risk assessments may have on patient management.

The frequency of periodontal maintenance recalls has been discussed, along with the idea that it may help in treatment planning; however, the suggestion remains unsubstantiated. One risk assessment tool in the public domain was introduced by Lang and Tonetti in 2003.[17] The tool may be accessed from the website at the University of Bern School of Dental Medicine, Switzerland (www.perio-tools.com/pra/en/). (Chapter 3, Risk Assessment, includes additional information about periodontal risk assessment.)

PERI-IMPLANT DISEASES

Peri-implant diseases can be divided into peri-implant mucositis and peri-implantitis. Very similar to the bacterial plaque–induced inflammatory process that occurs surrounding natural teeth, peri-implant mucositis affects the mucosal tissues adjacent to the implants without loss of the supporting alveolar bone. Conversely, peri-implantitis involves both inflammation of the mucosa and the irreversible loss of alveolar bone. From a clinical and radiographic standpoint, when tracing a parallel between natural teeth and dental implants, peri-implant mucositis is the equivalent of gingivitis and peri-implantitis is the equivalent of periodontitis.

According to the 2013 paper published by the AAP Task Force on Peri-Implantitis, peri-implant mucositis includes BOP or suppuration, or both, which is usually associated with probing depths of 4 mm or greater and no evidence of radiographic loss of bone beyond bone remodeling.[18] When the same parameters are present with any degree of detectable bone loss following initial bone remodeling after implant placement, a diagnosis of peri-implantitis is made.[18] This diagnostic threshold can only be applied in cases in which a baseline radiograph has been taken at the time of placement of the prosthesis. Sanz and Chapple have recommended use of a threshold vertical distance of 2 mm from the expected marginal bone level following remodeling post-implant placement as the threshold for the diagnosis of peri-implantitis in cases where a baseline radiograph is absent.[19]

Epidemiology
The frequency of peri-implant diseases has been studied.[20,21] Both scientists and clinicians still have arduous work ahead to understand the etiology, pathogenesis, and especially the magnitude of these conditions affecting the global population. In a systematic review, the estimated frequency of peri-implant mucositis has been reported in approximately 64% of individuals and 31% of implants.[21] In addition, peri-implantitis frequency has been estimated to affect approximately 19% of

individuals and 10% of implants.[21] Atieh and colleagues concluded that high-risk groups should receive planned long-term maintenance care to reduce risk of peri-implantitis. They also strongly suggested that informed consent is needed, including the commitment to long-term maintenance therapy, when planning for implant therapy.[21]

Pathogenesis
In 2014, Belibasakis described how peri-implant mucositis and peri-implantitis involve a sequence of inflammatory events and qualitative composition of the immune cells similar to gingivitis and periodontitis but of greater magnitude.[22] The author also stated that the molecular events that govern these processes are not yet fully characterized. No specific genotype or systemic inflammatory marker exists that can reliably indicate peri-implant disease progression or susceptibility. When analyzing the differences in peri-implant microbiota between fully and partially edentulous patients, it was concluded that partially edentulous patients harbor a potentially more pathogenic peri-implant microflora than fully edentulous patients.[23]

Risk Assessment
When assessing risk for dental implant patients, the literature includes levels of oral hygiene, cigarette smoking, history of periodontitis, and diabetes as potentially relevant factors. In addition, other considerations include genetic traits, osteoporosis, type of implant design or surface, and occlusion. To date, there have been numerous prospective studies to guide the clinician in addressing this matter with accuracy. Nevertheless, the clinician is expected to advise patients who need tooth replacement therapy. A meta-analysis revealed that smoking led to a rate of implant bone loss of 0.164 mm per year. Exposure to smoking had a negative impact on implant alveolar bone loss.[24] The correlation between implant failure and marginal bone loss due to a history of periodontitis has been reported to be of moderate level of evidence in at least two systematic reviews and meta-analyses.[25,26] Finally, the effect of occlusal overload and bone implant loss was systematically reviewed by Naert and coworkers in 2012.[27]

The authors concluded that there is little or no evidence to support a cause-and-effect relationship.

PART 2: PATIENT MANAGEMENT AND INTERVENTIONS

Maintaining low levels of biofilm is essential to the prevention of most gingival and periodontal diseases, including natural teeth and implants.[28] Fifty years of experimental research and clinical trials have confirmed the importance of effective plaque removal to periodontal health.[10] Methods investigated to remove or prevent oral biofilm production have included those rendered in an oral healthcare setting by clinicians, as well as those performed by patients at home. Following is a review of evidence-based strategies to prevent disease or disease progression of the gingival diseases.

IN-OFFICE PREVENTIVE TREATMENTS AND STRATEGIES FOR THE PREVENTION OF GINGIVAL DISEASES

Although the evidence supports care by a clinician for reduction or prevention of gingival diseases, there is little evidence for the traditional 6-month recare appointment typically recommended to patients.[29-31] More importantly, it is the quality of biofilm removal along with other indicators of oral–systemic health or risk for disease that should be considered when determining recare appointment intervals.

In-office preventive strategies should be performed based on the evidence available. Preventive and therapeutic methods should include mechanical and adjunctive treatments to reduce biofilm and its byproducts for the prevention of periodontal diseases, including gingivitis, chronic periodontitis, peri-implant mucositis, and peri-implantitis.

Mechanical Therapy
Scaling and root planing (SRP) is considered the mainstay of periodontal therapy, reversing microbial shifts associated with disease and reestablishing microbiota seen in periodontal health.[32] Mechanical therapy using SRP is an essential component in the removal of plaque biofilm and calculus deposits.[33,34] Considered the gold standard

of periodontal therapy, its efficacy is well documented in the literature.[33-36] SRP has been shown to result in gains in clinical attachment loss (CAL) between 0.55 mm and 1.29 mm, reductions in probing pocket depth (PPD) between 1.29 mm and 2.16 mm, and reduction of BOP.[34] While clinicians should try to remove as much of the deposits as possible, investigators have shown that as PPD depth increases it becomes difficult for clinicians to thoroughly remove deposits.[37-40] In addition, success in deposit removal is highly dependent on the skill of the clinician and his/her attention to detail.[41,42]

Hand instruments and powered instrumentation have been shown to be equally effective in the removal of deposits and disruption of the biofilm, although power-driven instruments remove calculus at a faster rate.[33,34,43,44] Influencing factors in the success of mechanical therapy include the pocket depth, furcations, and bony lesions, as well as patient habits, such as use of tobacco and adherence to home care instructions for biofilm reduction.[34]

New therapies have been proposed and investigated for prevention and reduction of plaque biofilm, and, in some cases, calculus removal. These include laser technologies, full-mouth disinfection, subgingival air abrasive systems with glycine powder air polishing (GPAP), dental endoscopy, and others.

Laser Technology

Lasers have been used as an adjunctive treatment to SRP. Potential therapeutic benefits include reduction in inflammation and enhancement of the healing process.[45] Lasers are categorized according to the wavelength of emitted light. In 2012, Sanz and coworkers reported on the current evidence for nonsurgical treatment of periodontitis. The authors concluded that soft tissue lasers are not indicated in periodontal therapy as they do not remove dental biofilm or calculus.[34] In addition, they reported that although the Er:YAG (erbium–yttrium aluminium garnet) laser has shown efficacy as a monotherapy, it does not demonstrate superiority when used as an adjunct to conventional periodontal instrumentation.[34] Additional clinical research is needed in this field.

In 2015, Smiley and colleagues reported on evidence-based treatments for chronic periodontitis by means of SRP with and without adjuncts.[46] The group of expert reviewers, convened by the ADA Council on Scientific Affairs, conducted a systematic review of randomized controlled trials that were at least 6 months in duration. They also selected CAL as the sole measure to assess treatment effectiveness as it is routinely reported in the scientific literature as a valid measurement of disease progression and is considered the most important outcome in arresting or reversing periodontal disease onset and progression. The use of lasers was reviewed as an adjunctive treatment to SRP. Compared with SRP alone, the Nd:YAG (neodymium–yttrium aluminium garnet) laser resulted in a 0.41-mm mean gain in CAL (95% confidence interval [CI], −0.12 to 0.94). The Er:YAG, resulted in a 0.18-mm mean gain in CAL (95% CI, −0.63 to 0.98). Both were judged to have an overall *low* level of certainty in the evidence on the basis of the evidence profile. Based on the review, a clinical practice guideline was developed by the ADA that provides treatment recommendations to clinicians using a scale of *strong, in favor, weak, expert opinion for, expert opinion against,* and *against*.[47,48] Expert opinion *against* is the recommendation for use of lasers for patients with moderate to severe chronic periodontitis because the "current evidence shows no net benefit when used as an adjunct to SRP."[46] The authors noted that lasers have no defined and accepted protocol for standard usage and that larger clinical trials are needed to properly evaluate the benefits of utilizing lasers as an adjunct to SRP. The photodynamic therapy diode (PDT) laser was the only laser that the reviewers noted as having a "moderate" level of certainty as an adjunctive treatment to SRP. The PDT has shown a 0.53-mm CAL (95% CI, 0.06 to 1.00) gain over SRP alone.[46]

Full-Mouth Disinfection

Full-mouth scaling and root planing (FMSRP) is a mode of periodontal therapy that consists of

SRP (with hand or ultrasonic instrumentation) of all pockets within a 24-hour time frame. Full-mouth disinfection (FMD) is SRP of all pockets in combination with topical application of chlorhexidine within 24 hours. The rationale for this therapy is that it avoids bacterial transmission to other parts of the oral cavity, such as the tongue, mucosa, and untreated periodontal pockets.[34] Although early studies showed significant improvements in clinical outcomes, other studies have shown no benefits as compared with conventional staged debridement (CSD), or SRP over several weeks. Eberhard and coworkers, in a systematic review, reported that FMD resulted in higher PPD reductions in 5- to 6-mm pockets as compared with CSD. However, they concluded that all three interventions (FMD, FMSRP, CSD) could result in improvements in clinical outcomes.[49] Recently two papers have reported on the clinical and microbiological effects of FMSRP compared with CSD. Zijnge and associates reported no differences in PPD or BOP after 3 months.[50] Similarly, after a 12-month randomized controlled trial, Knöfler and colleagues reported that FMSRP and CSD were similar in targeting periodontal pathogens.[51] Fang and colleagues published a systematic review and meta-analysis comparing FMD, FMSRP, and quadrant scaling and root planing (Q-SRP). FMD showed an additional effect in PPD reduction (0.25 mm) and CAL gain (0.33 mm) versus Q-SRP in studies longer than 3 months. The authors reported no differences in patient discomfort post-treatment, and less time was needed to complete treatment with FMD. However, the authors concluded that FMD, FMSRP, and Q-SRP are all effective in the treatment of chronic periodontitis.[52] Since conventional treatment, FMD, and FMSRP are all clinically effective, clinicians should make treatment decisions based on their judgment and clinician and patient preferences.

Dental Endoscopy

A fiber-optic endoscopic system was introduced to dentistry in the late 1990s to assist clinicians in viewing the subgingival area. Used as an adjunct to SRP, the technology produces a real-time video showing the subgingival environment, thus allowing the clinician to see the tooth structure, gingival attachment, and sulcus wall, as well as residual calculus remaining on the root surface at a magnification of 24 to 48 times their actual size.[53] A randomized controlled trial conducted by Geisinger and coworkers reported significantly less residual calculus in deeper probing depths when clinicians used the dental endoscope for detection but no difference in shallower probing depths. In addition, differences in PPD at treated sites were significant only at deeper sites greater than 4 mm for buccal and lingual surfaces and greater than 6 mm for interproximal surfaces.[54] In a subsequent study, the same investigators reported that the endoscope showed no significant improvement in calculus removal in multirooted molar teeth.[55] A smaller but more recent study reported that clinicians were able to detect more calculus when using the dental endoscope versus a dental explorer in patients with moderate periodontitis.[56] More studies are needed to determine how using the periodontal endoscope results in improved clinical parameters.

Subgingival Air Polishing

Air polishing devices were first introduced in the 1940s for tooth restorative preparation.[57] Using an abrasive slurry of particles, the powder inside the chamber is stirred up by pressurized air allowing air and water to be transported to the top of the device. Plaque and stain can be removed while the device tip is held 3 to 4 mm from the enamel surface and moved in a circular motion. Although air polishing with sodium bicarbonate (mean particle size up to 250 μm) has been utilized since the 1980s as a treatment for removal of oral biofilms and stains, safety concerns regarding damage to exposed root surfaces, gingival tissues, and restorative materials have limited its use.[32] Recently, fine-grain glycine powder has been investigated for subgingival removal of biofilm. Glycine is 80% lower in abrasiveness (45- to 60-μm particle size) when compared with air polishing using sodium bicarbonate powder.[58] Many studies have been conducted to investigate the efficacy, safety, and patient perceptions of glycine powder air polishing (GPAP) as compared with traditional methods of SRP.[57-61]

A nozzle is available for supra- and subgingival GPAP, depending on the pocket depth. Subgingival GPAP has been shown to reach pocket depths up to 9 mm. In one study by Flemmig and coworkers, subgingival GPAP was more efficacious in removing subgingival biofilm in 4- to 9-mm pockets than SRP.[59] In addition, time for biofilm removal was shown to be less with subgingival GPAP (10 seconds per site) than with ultrasonic debridement (30 seconds per site). The time did not include calculus removal as subgingival GPAP does not remove hard deposits.[60,61]

In 2012, a consensus conference on mechanical biofilm management was conducted during the Europerio 7 Congress in Vienna. Specifically, the conference experts were charged with reviewing the current evidence from the peer-reviewed literature on the clinical relevance of subgingival use of air polishing and to make practical recommendations for clinicians.[62] The consensus was that air polishing devices are efficient in removing both sub- and supragingival biofilm and stains. The subgingival nozzles provide better access to subgingival and interdental areas, and when compared with hand curettes, air polishing removes significantly more biofilm in shallow and deeper pockets. GPAP is faster than hand or ultrasonic instrumentation and is perceived by patients as being more comfortable.[62]

Subgingival GPAP has been investigated in patients presenting with peri-implantitis.[57] A recent study reported on the biofilm removal and surface roughness of 10 instruments on implant surfaces. Biofilm on titanium disks was cleaned using nine mechanical implant cleaning instruments or an erbium laser. Cleaning methods included plastic instruments, carbon curettes, traditional prophylaxis, powered instrumentation, and an air polishing device using glycine powder particles of less than 63 μm. The best cleaning with the least amount of damage resulted with the GPAP method and the sonic-driven polyether ether ketone (PEEK) plastic tip.[63]

Protocol for use of subgingival GPAP includes using the glycine air polishing prior to using powered or hand instruments for stain and calculus removal. High-volume evacuation should be used with air polishing. Although a traditional air polishing device should never be directed into the gingival sulcus, subgingival GPAP uses an application tip designed for subgingival tissue and is required to reach depths of up to 10 mm in a pocket (see Figure 1). Although the risk is low, facial emphysema can occur. Flemmig and coworkers estimated the probability of this condition occurring from subgingival GPAP as 1 in 666,666.[59]

Figure 1. Glycine Powder Air Polishing

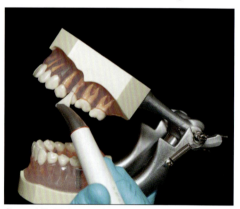

Source: AIR-FLOW® Perio, used with permission from Hu-Friedy, Chicago, IL, USA).

Given the available evidence, subgingival GPAP is safe and effective for biofilm removal and may reduce clinician time.

Supra- and Subgingival Irrigation

Several devices have been used by clinicians to irrigate periodontal pockets. These include syringes, a jet irrigator with a cannula, and an ultrasonic unit. Many studies have been conducted to determine the efficacy of in-office subgingival irrigation to improve the parameters of gingivitis and periodontitis.[64] Currently there are limited data to support the benefits of a single episode of subgingival irrigation while the patient is receiving professional treatment.[64] Although data are very limited, the exception may be with multiple irrigations in-office using antimicrobials to treat sites that do not respond to traditional therapies. The lack of efficacy for a one-time irrigation treatment may be related to the quick elimination of subgingivally placed fluids.[64] However, at-home irrigation by patients has been shown to be beneficial for the reduction of gingivitis and is discussed later in this chapter.

Local and Systemic Therapies, Including Antimicrobials and Antibiotics

In-office treatments for gingivitis control typically consist of debridement and scaling or debridement of the biofilm and calculus. For chronic periodontitis, other therapies, adjunctive to SRP, have been developed and proposed in recent years. Although patients with chronic periodontitis should see improved results from SRP, some sites and patients may not respond adequately. SRP of deep pockets has its limitations, such as clinician inability to reach the depth of the pocket and difficulty with SRP of furcations. Certain pathogens are resistant to SRP, oral niches make SRP very difficult, and clinicians may be limited due to time, patient sensitivity, and other factors. In addition, recolonization of subgingival biofilm is a concern and dependent to some degree on good daily oral hygiene by the patient. With poor supragingival plaque control, bacteria may reestablish themselves in a short period following SRP. For example, Sbordone and coworkers reported that after a single episode of SRP and in the absence of oral hygiene, recolonization of subgingival sites with periodontal pathogens may occur at 3 weeks. They also reported that at 60 days, there was no significant variation in any clinical and microbiological parameters as compared with pretreatment levels. Conclusions were that for patients without good oral hygiene who are at risk for periodontal disease, more frequent recare visits may be necessary.[65] For all of these reasons, adjunctive treatments may be necessary for the control and treatment of chronic periodontitis and to prevent further destruction.

Adjunctive treatments to SRP, such as systemic antibiotics and locally delivered antimicrobials and antibiotics, have been used in recent years by clinicians. As the focus of this chapter is on the *prevention* of gingivitis and periodontitis, we provide only a brief discussion of the treatments.

Locally Delivered Antimicrobials and Antibiotics

Site-specific, locally delivered, controlled-release antimicrobials and antibiotics have been available in dentistry since the 1980s. These agents, used as adjuncts to SRP, deliver an antimicrobial or antibiotic to the base of the periodontal pocket with the goals of improving PPD and CAL gains, and reducing BOP. One benefit of using a locally delivered antimicrobial is substantivity, or the ability of an agent to remain in an area or site without becoming diluted or washed away by gingival crevicular fluid or salivary action.[66] Agents delivered in this way slowly release active ingredients at a high minimal inhibitory concentration (MIC) level required to inhibit growth of a planktonic bacterial population. The premise for use of site-specific locally delivered agents is that due to higher and longer substantivity, the MIC is maintained at a level needed to significantly reduce the level of pathogens over what can be achieved by SRP alone, with the intended outcome being improvements in periodontal parameters. Substantivity varies from approximately 7 days for the chlorhexidine chip and doxycycline hyclate gel to about 14 to 21 days for minocycline microspheres.[67–70]

As mentioned earlier, the ADA Council on Scientific Affairs conducted a systematic review and meta-analysis of nonsurgical treatments of chronic periodontitis utilizing SRP with or without adjuncts.[46] Using CAL as the outcome measure, the authors assessed the overall level of certainly in the body of evidence as high, moderate, or low. SRP alone resulted in a 0.49-mm gain in CAL and was judged to be moderate on the basis of the evidence profile. When compared with SRP alone, the chlorhexidine chip plus SRP resulted in a 0.40-mm mean gain in CAL (95% CI, 0.24 to 0.56) and was judged *moderate* based on the evidence profile. Doxycycline hyclate gel resulted in a 0.64-mm gain in CAL (95% CI, 0.00 to 1.28), and minocycline microspheres resulted in a 0.24-mm gain in CAL (95% CI, −0.06 to 0.55), and both were judged to be *low* based on the evidence profile. A clinical practice guideline was developed by the ADA based on the review and provided recommendations for these treatments based on a scale of *strong, in favor, weak, expert opinion for, expert opinion against,* and *against*.[47] Regarding locally delivered antimicrobials and antibiotics, the chlorhexidine chip was rated *weak*, and doxycycline hyclate gel and minocycline microspheres received *expert opinion for.* Experts emphasized that *"expert opinion for"* does not imply endorsement but signifies that evidence is lacking and the level of certainty in the evidence is low. Clinicians should determine use based on their professional judgment and the patient's needs and preferences. A chairside guide is available for clinicians on the ADA Center for Evidence-Based Dentistry website (http://ebd.ada.org/en/).[48]

Systemic Antibiotics
Systemic antibiotics have been utilized for the treatment of chronic periodontitis as adjunctive therapy to SRP. The rationale is that they can affect periodontal pathogens in saliva and gingival crevicular fluid. They can also reduce the microbial load in multiple subgingival areas and at extracrevicular sites that have been insufficiently treated by SRP.[71] Frequently used antibiotics are amoxicillin, metronidazole, erythromycin, tetracycline, doxycycline, and others. Sgolastra and colleagues reported on a systematic review and meta-analysis of combination amoxicillin (AMX) and metronidazole (MET) as an adjunctive treatment to SRP.[71] The selection process included four randomized clinical trials. They concluded that there was overall effectiveness of AMX/MET as an adjunct to SRP compared with SRP alone in the treatment of chronic periodontitis. Six major groups of antibiotics were reported in the systematic review and meta-analysis conducted by Smiley and others at the ADA.[46] Compared with SRP alone, SRP plus systemic antimicrobials resulted in a 0.35-mm mean gain in CAL (95% CI, 0.20 to 0.51). Experts judged the overall level of certainty in the evidence to be *moderate* on the basis of the evidence profile.

Another systemic antibiotic has been used for the adjunctive treatment of chronic periodontitis since the late 1990s and is considered a host modulating agent. Systemic subantimicrobial dose doxycycline (SDD) is provided at low doses (20 mg), which may be taken twice a day up to 9 months. It is sold in the United States as generic 20 mg doxycycline tablets. Systemic levels do not reach inhibitory concentrations against bacteria. The drug inhibits collagenase activity in vitro and may prevent further breakdown of connective tissue and alveolar bone. Compared with SRP alone, Smiley and colleagues reported that SDD resulted in a 0.35-mm gain in CAL (95% CI, 0.15 to 0.56). The overall level of certainty in the evidence is *moderate* based on the evidence profile. The experts concluded that for patients with moderate to severe chronic periodontitis, clinicians may consider SSD (20 mg twice daily) for 3 to 9 months as an adjunct to SRP, with a small net benefit expected. The strength is *in favor*.[46,47]

Maintenance and Recall
Most clinicians would agree that a combination of professional care and oversight coupled with excellent home care by the patient is ideal to prevent or control most forms of gingivitis and chronic periodontitis.[29] However, patient recall and periodontal maintenance intervals have been debated for many years. Traditionally, a 6-month recall system has been advocated by dentistry, but other intervals have been recommended, including 2 weeks, 2 to 3 months, 3 months, 3 to 4 months, 3 to 6 months, and 12 to 18 months.[72] A systematic review published by Beirne and coworkers in 2007 revealed that there is insufficient evidence from randomized controlled trials to make any evidence-based recommendations on the benefits or harm of altering the recall interval between dental checkups.[30] Farooqi and associates published a systematic review on appropriate recall intervals for periodontal maintenance. Eight cohort studies met the inclusion criteria. The authors concluded that there is weak evidence for a specific recall interval for patients following periodontal therapy. They also

suggested that the merits of a risk-based recommendation over fixed recall interval regimens should be investigated.[72]

Worthington and others conducted a systematic review to determine the level of evidence for routine SRP for periodontal health in adults.[73] They concluded that some statistically significant evidence favored SRP at more frequent intervals, particularly between 3- and 12-month visits for gingivitis reduction (evaluated at 24 months). There was also some evidence for reduced calculus with more frequent recalls. Needleman and coworkers reported that more frequent professional mechanical plaque control can improve plaque, bleeding, and attachment loss; however, the strength of the evidence is low.[74] Both reviews stressed the lack of high-quality clinical trials in this area of prevention. As there is little evidence to guide the frequency of mechanical plaque control, clinicians are advised to make professional judgments based on a needs and risk assessment for each patient, including the patient's adherence to oral hygiene biofilm removal.[75]

A recent study conducted by Giannobile and colleagues investigated how risk for periodontal disease and number of preventive visits per year impacted tooth loss.[76] The retrospective study involved more than 5,000 patients over a 16-year period. The authors investigated how smoking, diabetes, and the IL-1 genotype influenced tooth loss in patients who had preventive visits either once or twice per year. Patients were deemed high risk if they had one or more of the conditions. Patients at low risk did not experience a significant difference in tooth loss rates whether they had one or two visits a year. High-risk patients had better periodontal outcomes if they attended two preventive visits a year. These results support the use of risk-based assessment as one method of determining maintenance intervals.[76]

The prevention of gingivitis and chronic periodontitis is of concern in fixed prosthodontics as well as implant-borne restorations. Recently, the American College of Prosthodontists (ACP) convened a panel of experts to critically evaluate and debate recently published findings from two systematic reviews. After consensus, the panel published "Clinical Practice Guidelines for Recall and Maintenance of Patients with Tooth-Borne and Implant-Borne Dental Restorations."[77] The ACP experts noted that to their knowledge, these are the first clinical practice guidelines addressing patient recall regimen, professional maintenance regimen, and at-home maintenance regimen for these patients (see Tables 3 and 4). Although the recommendations are intended for healthy adult patients and not those with peri-implant disease or periodontal disease, the authors noted that the recall and maintenance regimen guidelines may be helpful to patients with these diseases.[77]

AT-HOME PREVENTIVE TREATMENTS AND STRATEGIES

Previous studies have reported that patients retain more teeth over time if they brush more than once a day, perform interdental cleaning, and obtain professional dental care.[29,78] A 2015 systematic review found that there is likely little value in providing professional mechanical plaque control (PMPC) without oral hygiene instruction.[79] PMPC consists of supragingival and subgingival plaque and calculus removal using hand or powered instruments. PMPC plus oral hygiene instruction results in the greatest benefit. In fact, the authors emphasized that oral hygiene instruction is as influential as PMPC for periodontal health.[79] Since most individuals are unable to accomplish complete disruption and removal of biofilm at and below the gingival margin, professional intervention is required.[9] Tonetti and coworkers reported on expert consensus regarding effective prevention of periodontal and peri-implant diseases. Opinions and recommendations from the group included[9]

- repeated and individually tailored oral hygiene instruction is the key element in achieving gingival health;
- patients should have professional supervision for PMPC and have appropriate oral hygiene instruction tailored to their needs and monitored for efficacy; and

Table 3. Clinical Practice Guidelines for Recall and Maintenance of Patients with Tooth-Borne Dental Restorations

Number	Topic	Guideline	Strength of Evidence*
1.	Patient recall	Patients with tooth-borne restorations (fixed or removable) should be advised to obtain a dental professional examination at least every 6 months as a lifelong regimen.	D
		Patients categorized by the dentist as higher risk based on age, ability to perform oral self care, biological or mechanical complications of natural teeth or tooth-borne restorations should be advised to obtain a dental professional examination more often than every 6 months, depending upon the clinical situation.	D
2A.	Professional maintenance: Tooth-borne removable restorations (partial removable dental prostheses)	Professional maintenance for patients with tooth-borne removable restorations should include an extra- and intraoral health and dental examination, oral hygiene instructions for existing natural teeth and any restorations, oral hygiene intervention (cleaning of natural teeth and restorations), and use of oral topical agents as deemed clinically necessary.	A, C, D
		Professional maintenance of the partial removable dental prostheses should include hygiene instructions, detailed examination of the prosthesis, prosthetic components, and patient education about any foreseeable problems that impair optimal function with the restoration. The partial removable dental prosthesis should be professionally cleaned extraorally using professionally accepted mechanical and chemical methods.	D
		Professionals should recommend and/or prescribe appropriate oral topical agents and oral hygiene aids suitable for the patient's at-home maintenance needs.	D
2B.	Professional maintenance: Tooth-borne fixed restorations (intracoronal restorations, extracoronal restorations, veneers, single crowns, and partial fixed dental prostheses)	Professional maintenance for patients with tooth-borne fixed restorations should include an extra- and intraoral health and dental examination, oral hygiene instructions for natural teeth and the fixed restorations, oral hygiene intervention (cleaning of natural teeth and restorations), and use of oral topical agents as deemed clinically necessary.	A, C, D
		Professionals should recommend and/or prescribe appropriate oral topical agents and oral hygiene aids suitable for the patient's at-home maintenance needs.	D
		When clinical signs indicate the need for an occlusal device, professionals should educate the patient and fabricate an occlusal device to protect the tooth-borne fixed restorations.	D
		Professional maintenance of the occlusal device should include hygiene instructions, detailed examination of the occlusal device, and patient education about any foreseeable problems that impair optimal function with the occlusal device. The occlusal device should be professionally cleaned extraorally, using professionally accepted mechanical and chemical methods.	D
3A.	At-home maintenance: Tooth-borne removable restorations (partial removable dental prostheses)	Patients with tooth-borne removable restorations should be educated about brushing existing natural teeth and restorations twice daily, and the use of oral hygiene aids such as dental floss, water flossers, air flossers, interdental cleaners, and electric toothbrushes.	C, D
		Patients with tooth-borne removable restorations should be educated about cleaning their prosthesis at least twice daily using a soft brush and the professional recommended denture-cleaning agent.	D
		(Continued on next page)	

Table 3. Clinical Practice Guidelines for Recall and Maintenance of Patients with Tooth-Borne Dental Restorations (cont'd)

Number	Topic	Guideline	Strength of Evidence*
		Patients with multiple and complex restorations on existing teeth supporting or surrounding the removable restoration should be advised to use oral topical agents such as toothpaste containing 5,000-ppm fluoride, toothpaste with 0.3% triclosan, and supplemental short-term use of chlorhexidine gluconate when indicated.	A, C, D
		Patients with tooth-borne removable restorations should remove the restoration out of the mouth during sleep. The removed prosthesis should be stored in a prescribed cleaning solution.	D
3B	At-home maintenance:	Patients with tooth-borne fixed restorations should be educated about brushing twice daily, and the use of oral hygiene aids such as dental floss, water flossers, air flossers, interdental cleaners, and electric toothbrushes.	A, D
	Tooth-borne fixed restorations (intracoronal restorations, extracoronal restorations, veneers, single crowns, and partial fixed dental prostheses)	Patients with multiple and complex restorations on existing teeth should be advised to use oral topical agents such as toothpaste containing 5,000-ppm fluoride, toothpaste with 0.3% triclosan, and supplemental short-term use of chlorhexidine gluconate when indicated.	A, C, D
		Patients prescribed with occlusal devices should be advised to wear the occlusal device during sleep.	D
		Patients prescribed with occlusal devices should be educated about cleaning their occlusal device before and after use, with a soft brush and the prescribed cleaning agent. Patients should also be educated about proper methods for storage of the occlusal device when not in use.	D

ppm, parts per million.
*Strength of evidence to support the guideline.
Source: *J Prosthodont.* 2016;25(suppl 1):S32–S40.[77]

research is needed to determine if there is a threshold of gingival inflammation (in terms of severity and duration) that is compatible with long-term periodontal health.

Following is a review of effective oral hygiene instruction strategies and the evidence for their use.

Manual Oral Care

Toothbrushes

Toothbrushes are utilized by 80% to 90% of the population once or twice a day.[28] More frequent brushing is recommended, as reports indicate patients use a manual toothbrush on average between 30 and 60 seconds and only remove 60% of overall plaque per brushing session.[80] Chapple and coworkers reported that a single exercise of manual toothbrushing leads to a reduction in plaque scores of approximately 42% from pre-brushing scores when manual brushes are used and 46% with powered brushing.[81] General consensus from individual studies (not systematic reviews) is that effective manual brushing reduces gingival inflammation.[81] To date, there are no meta-analyses reporting the impact of manual toothbrush design on gingival inflammation. However, Chapple and coworkers reported a 24% to 47% reduction in plaque scores for flat-trim bristle designs, 33% to 54% for multilevel bristles, and 39% to 61% for criss-cross designs.[81] Manual toothbrush design continues to change and improve, but efficacy of biofilm removal is still dependent on the skill and motivation of the patient.

Powered brushes have been available for more than 50 years and feature various mechanical movements of the brush head, such as side-to-side, counter or rotational oscillation, ultrasonic, circular, and so on (see Figure 2). Recent improvements, such as 2-minute timers, pressure control, visual

CHAPTER 5 Gingival Diseases

Table 4. Clinical Practice Guidelines for Recall and Maintenance of Patients with Implant-Borne Dental Restorations

Number	Topic	Guideline	Strength of Evidence*
1.	Patient recall	Patients with implant-borne restorations (fixed or removable) should be advised to obtain a dental professional examination visit at least every 6 months as a lifelong regimen.	D
		Patients categorized by the dentist as higher risk based on age, ability to perform oral self care, biological or mechanical complications of remaining natural teeth, tooth-borne restorations or implant-borne restorations should be advised to obtain a dental professional examination more often than every 6 months, depending upon the clinical situation.	D
2A.	Professional maintenance: (biological): Implant-borne removable restorations (implant-supported partial removable dental prostheses and implant-supported overdenture prostheses)	Professional biological maintenance for patients with implant-borne removable restorations should include an extra- and intraoral health and dental examination, oral hygiene instructions, hygiene instructions for the prostheses, and oral hygiene intervention (cleaning of any natural teeth, tooth-borne restorations, implant-borne restorations, or implant abutments).	A, C, D
		Professionals should use chlorhexidine gluconate as the oral topical agent of choice when antimicrobial effect is needed clinically.	A, C
		Professionals should use cleaning instruments compatible with the type and material of the implants, abutments, and restorations, and powered instruments such as the glycine powder air polishing system.	A, C, D
		Implant-supported partial removable dental prostheses and implant-supported overdenture prostheses should be professionally cleaned extraorally using professionally accepted mechanical and chemical cleaning methods.	D
		Professionals should recommend and/or prescribe appropriate oral topical agents and oral hygiene aids suitable for the patient's at-home maintenance needs.	A, C, D
2B.	Professional maintenance: (mechanical): Implant-borne removable restorations (implant-supported partial removable dental prostheses and implant-supported overdenture prostheses)	Professional mechanical maintenance for patients with implant-borne removable restorations should include a detailed examination of the prosthesis, intra- and extraoral prosthetic components, and patient education of foreseeable problems that could impair optimal function of the restoration.	C, D
		Professionals should recommend and perform adjustment, repair, replacement, or remake of any or all parts of the prosthesis and prosthetic components that compromise function.	C, D
2C.	Professional maintenance (biological): Implant-borne fixed restorations (implant-supported single crowns, partial fixed dental	Professional biological maintenance for patients with implant-borne fixed restorations should include an extra- and intraoral health and dental examination, oral hygiene instructions, and oral hygiene intervention (cleaning of any natural teeth, tooth-borne restorations, implant-borne restorations, or implant abutments).	A, C, D
		Professionals should use chlorhexidine gluconate as the oral topical agent of choice when antimicrobial effect is needed clinically.	A, C
		Professionals should use cleaning instruments compatible with the type and	A, C, D

(Continued on next page)

Table 4. Clinical Practice Guidelines for Recall and Maintenance of Patients with Implant-Borne Dental Restorations (cont'd)

Number	Topic	Guideline	Strength of Evidence*
	prostheses, and implant-supported complete arch fixed prostheses)	material of the implants, abutments, and restorations, and powered instruments such as the glycine powder air polishing system.	
		In patients with implant-supported fixed prostheses, the decision to remove the prosthesis for biological maintenance should be based on the patient's demonstrated inability to perform adequate oral hygiene. The prosthesis contours should be reassessed to facilitate at-home maintenance.	D
		Professionals should consider using new prosthetic screws when an implant-borne restoration is removed and replaced for professional biological maintenance.	D
2D.	Professional maintenance (mechanical):	Professional mechanical maintenance for patients with implant-borne fixed restorations should include a detailed examination of the prosthesis, prosthetic components, and patient education about any foreseeable problems that compromise function.	C, D
	Implant-borne fixed restorations (implant-supported single crowns, partial fixed dental prostheses, and implant-supported complete arch fixed prostheses)	Professionals should recommend and perform adjustment, repair, replacement, or remake of any or all parts of the prosthesis and prosthetic components that impair the patient's optimal function.	C, D
		Professionals should consider using new prosthetic screws when an implant-borne restoration is removed and replaced for professional mechanical maintenance.	D
		When clinical signs indicate the need for an occlusal device, professionals should educate the patient and fabricate an occlusal device to protect implant-borne fixed restorations.	D
		Professional maintenance of the occlusal device should include hygiene instructions, detailed examination of the occlusal device, and patient education about any foreseeable problems that impair optimal function with the occlusal device. The occlusal device should be professionally cleaned extraorally using professionally accepted mechanical and chemical methods.	D
		Patients with multiple and complex restorations on existing teeth should be advised to use oral topical agents such as toothpaste containing 5,000-ppm fluoride, toothpaste with 0.3% triclosan, and supplemental short-term use of chlorhexidine gluconate when indicated.	A, C, D
		Patients prescribed with occlusal devices should be educated to wear the occlusal device during sleep.	D
		Patients prescribed with occlusal devices should be educated about cleaning their occlusal device before and after use with a soft brush and the prescribed cleaning agent. Patients should also be educated about proper methods for storage of the occlusal device when not in use.	D
3A.	At-home maintenance:	Patients with implant-supported partial removable dental prostheses should be educated about brushing existing natural teeth and restorations twice daily, and the use of oral hygiene aids such as dental floss, water flossers, air flossers, interdental cleaners, and electric toothbrushes.	C, D
	Implant-borne removable restorations (implant-supported partial removable	Patients with implant-borne removable restorations should be advised to clean their intraoral implant components at least twice daily, using a soft brush and the professionally recommended oral topical agent.	D

(Continued on next page)

Table 4. Clinical Practice Guidelines for Recall and Maintenance of Patients with Implant-Borne Dental Restorations (cont'd)

Number	Topic	Guideline	Strength of Evidence*
	dental prostheses and implant-supported overdenture prostheses)	Patients with implant-borne removable restorations should be advised to clean their prosthesis at least twice daily using a soft brush with a professional recommended denture-cleaning agent.	D
		Patients with implant-borne partial or complete removable restorations should be advised to remove the restoration while sleeping. The removed prosthesis should be stored in a prescribed cleaning solution.	D
3B.	At-home maintenance:	Patients with implant-borne fixed restorations should be educated about brushing twice daily, and the use of oral hygiene aids such as dental floss, water flossers, air flossers, interdental cleaners and electric toothbrushes.	C, D
	Implant-borne fixed restorations (implant-supported single crowns, partial fixed dental prostheses, and implant-supported complete arch fixed prostheses)	In patients with multiple and complex implant-borne fixed restorations, professionals should recommend use of oral topical agents like toothpaste containing 0.3% triclosan and supplemental short-term use of chlorhexidine gluconate when indicated.	A, C, D
		Patients prescribed with occlusal devices should be advised to wear the occlusal device during sleep.	D
		Patients prescribed with occlusal devices should be educated about cleaning their occlusal device before and after use with a soft brush and the prescribed cleaning agent. Patients should also be educated about proper methods for storage of the occlusal device when not in use.	D

ppm, parts per million.
*Strength of evidence to support the guideline.
Source: J Prosthodont. 2016;25(suppl 1):S32–S40.[77]

display enhancements, traveling cases, and Bluetooth technology, make these brushes popular with consumers. Compliance rates are also good with powered brush use, with reports that 62% of people continue to use them daily over time.[82]

When compared with manual brushes, powered toothbrushes produce statistically significantly greater short-term and long-term reduction in plaque indices and gingival inflammation.[81] Although a 2003 systematic review reported that powered toothbrushes with a rotation oscillation action achieved a modest reduction in plaque and gingivitis compared with manual toothbrushing, a 2005 review concluded that there was no significant difference between the two.[82,83] A 2010 review compared powered toothbrushing modes for plaque reduction and gingival health.[84] The conclusion was that while there was some evidence that rotation oscillation brushes reduce plaque and gingivitis more than side-to-side, the studies were of short duration and the difference, and

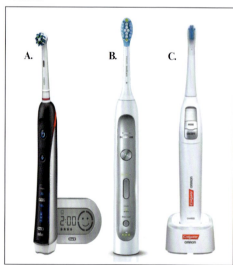

Figure 2. Powered Toothbrushes with Advanced Features

Source: **A.** Courtesy of Procter & Gamble. Cincinnati, OH, USA.
B. Courtesy of Philips Oral Healthcare, Bothell, WA, USA.
C. Courtesy of Colgate-Palmolive Company, New York, NY, USA.

thus clinical significance, was not clear. Safety of toothbrushes has also been reported, with no indication that manual or powered tooth brushing causes gingival recession.[81]

Interdental Biofilm Removal

Interdental mechanical removal of biofilm is essential to maintain interproximal gingival health. Different devices may be used by patients, including dental floss, interdental brushes, oral irrigators, and wood sticks.

Dental floss is available in many forms, including waxed, unwaxed, polytetrafluoroethylene, spongy, woven, and so on. Any form is safe for use as long as it is used appropriately. The disadvantage to floss is that it is technique sensitive, making it difficult to achieve high patient compliance.[75] A systematic review comparing toothbrushing and flossing with toothbrushing alone concluded that there is *some* evidence that flossing and toothbrushing reduces gingivitis in comparison with brushing alone. Regarding plaque reduction, weak evidence was reported at 1 and 3 months in favor of adjunctive flossing.[85] However, the majority of studies do not support effective plaque removal or a reduction of gingival inflammation with use of dental floss.[81]

Interdental brushes contain soft nylon filaments that are twisted into a conical or cylindrical shape on a fine stainless steel wire (see Figure 3). The width varies to match the interdental space. Slot and colleagues conducted a systematic review to determine the plaque and inflammation outcomes of using interdental brushes and toothbrushing versus toothbrushing alone or other interdental cleaning devices.[86] Interdental brushes removed more plaque than toothbrushing alone in outcomes of bleeding index, gingival index, and PPD. They also showed superior results when compared to dental floss in plaque index scores but not gingival index. Patient acceptance of interdental brushes for biofilm removal is generally good; therefore they should be recommended for daily patient use if indicated. However, Chapple and associates emphasize caution in recommending interdental brushes at healthy sites where attachment loss is not evident, as trauma may result from improper selection or use of the brush.[81]

Powered Interdental Cleaning Devices

Powered interdental cleaning devices have been introduced in recent years (see Figures 4 and 5). The dental water jet or irrigator was first introduced in the 1960s and has been studied in

Figure 3. Use of an Interdental Brush for Biofilm Removal

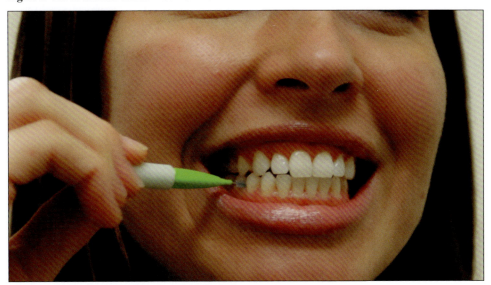

Source: Courtesy of Sunstar Americas, Inc., Chicago, IL, USA.

Figure 4. A Dental Water Flosser

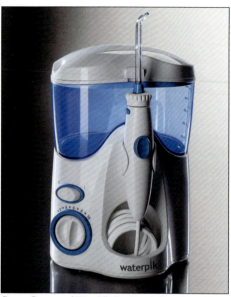

Source: Courtesy of WaterPik, Inc. Fort Collins, CO, USA.

Figure 5. An Interdental Cleaning Device that Delivers a Burst of Air and Microdroplets

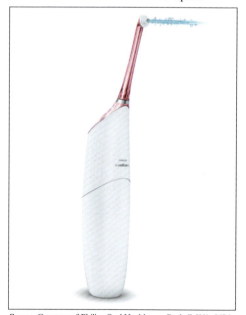

Source: Courtesy of Philips Oral Healthcare, Bothell, WA, USA.

numerous clinical trials for the reduction of bleeding and gingivitis. Patients shown to benefit from use of the water jet are people in periodontal maintenance; those with orthodontic appliances, implants, or prosthodontic work; people with diabetes; and those who are noncompliant with flossing.[87] The physical action of the dental water jet or irrigator is pulsation and pressure. This combination provides for phases of compression and interpulse decompression of the tissue to help expel contaminants. Although an early study showed that attached gingiva can withstand high amounts of pressure without damage, supragingival irrigation forces are much lower, at 80 to 90 pounds per square inch (psi).[88]

The water jet can be used for supragingival or subgingival therapy. The depth of delivery for the supragingival irrigation tip was reported by Eakle and coworkers in 1986 and found to be about 3 mm or half the pocket depth.[89] Using a 90-degree angle of application, they found that pocket penetration was 71% for shallow sites, 44% for moderately deep sites, and 67% for deep sites. Maximum pocket penetration of 4 to 5 mm was achieved. Braun and Ciancio studied the pocket penetration with use of a tip designed for subgingival irrigation and reported penetration of 90% of the depth of a 6-mm pocket and 64% of a 7-mm pocket[90] (see Figure 6).

Greenstein published a review on supra- and subgingival irrigation for the AAP in 2005.[64] Conclusions were that supragingival and marginal irrigation will continue to have a role in the treatment of gingivitis and the maintenance of periodontal patients.

Figure 6. Subgingival Irrigation Tip in Use

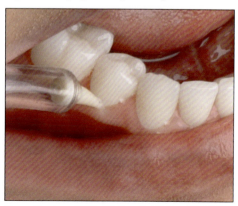

Source: Courtesy of WaterPik, Inc., Fort Collins, CO, USA.

The author noted that one of the advantages of self-administered subgingival irrigation is that it allows patients to participate in maintaining the bacterial reduction achieved by mechanical therapy.

A systematic review that was published in 2008 reported on the adjunctive effect of oral irrigation in addition to toothbrushing on plaque and clinical parameters of periodontal inflammation. The authors reported that as an adjunct to brushing, oral irrigation does not visibly reduce plaque but tends to improve gingival health, as evidenced by improved gingival index, bleeding scores, and pocket depth compared with toothbrushing alone. In addition, the periodontal index of the toothbrush only group worsened over time, but that of the oral irrigation group did not.[91]

Clinicians should always instruct patients in the proper use of the water jet for at-home use, reinforcing proper force and placement of the tip. The supragingival tip should be directed at a 90-degree angle to the long axis of the tooth and about 3 mm away from the gingival margin. Patient adherence is vital to efficacy of treatment. (See Chapter 2, Behavioral Science.)

Antimicrobial Dentifrice
Systematic reviews have shown evidence for significant improvements in plaque and gingivitis scores when chemical antiplaque agents are used in addition to toothbrushing.[81] Since most individuals claim to brush their teeth at least once or twice a day, an antimicrobial dentifrice is an easy and efficient way to provide additional plaque and gingivitis benefit to patients.

Dentifrice formulations available include stannous fluoride/sodium hexametaphosphate, amine fluoride/stannous fluoride, triclosan (2´-hydroxy-2,4,4´-tricholordiphenyl ether), essential oils, sodium bicarbonate, quaternary ammonium compounds, zinc citrate, or zinc chloride.[29] Few systematic reviews have been reported to provide evidence for use of the different formulations. However, systematic reviews have been published and reported evidence for the use of triclosan for reducing supragingival plaque and gingivitis.[92-94] Gunsolley also reported on positive plaque and gingivitis reduction with dentifrices containing stannous fluoride.[94] (See Chapter 16, Chemotherapeutic Agents.)

Antimicrobial Mouthrinses
Mechanical biofilm removal is difficult for some patients making the use of antimicrobial rinses appealing. They are easy and quick to use and are relatively inexpensive. Therapeutic mouthrinses have been widely investigated for plaque and gingivitis reduction and control. The most studied mouthrinses are those containing chlorhexidine gluconate (CHX), essential oils, and cetylpyridinium chloride (CPC). Systematic reviews have reported substantial plaque and gingivitis reduction.[94,95] Gunsolley concluded that there is strong evidence supporting the efficacy of CHX and essential oils as antiplaque, antigingivitis mouthrinses.[94] (See Chapter 16, Chemotherapeutics in Prevention.)

Use of antimicrobial rinses has been studied as an adjunct to mechanical plaque control. When compared with adjunctive flossing or flossing alone, essential oils had a significant effect as an antigingivitis and antiplaque treatment and, in some cases, performed better than floss alone.[96] Currently, a combination of daily toothbrushing, interdental cleaning, and antimicrobial rinsing is recommended by clinicians throughout the world.

Other factors that may influence patient acceptance of daily use of a mouthrinse include the potential for taste alteration, staining, burning, increase in calculus formation, and cost.[97] However, the advantages are many; among them, mouthrinses are quick and easy to use and inexpensive in most cases. CHX 0.12% mouthrinse requires a prescription in the United States, but other formulations are available elsewhere over the counter. The 0.12% formulation available in the United States is recommended as a 15-mL rinse. In Europe, the formulation is 0.2% and recommended as a 10-mL rinse. The two concentrations have equal efficacy and should be used for 20 seconds twice a day.[98] Essential oil rinses should be used undiluted (20 mL) for 30 seconds twice daily.

Another consideration with potential to impact

efficacy and compliance with the use of antimicrobial mouthrinses is the adverse interaction reported between dentifrice ingredients and CHX or CPC. Sheen and colleagues reported that a dentifrice may adversely affect the activity of CHX and CPC if used immediately after the rinse.[99] Kolahi and Soolari reported on a systematic review that found CHX and dentifrice ingredients such as sodium laurel sulfate and sodium fluoride were not compatible, "although the evidence does not allow for a definitive conclusion."[100] Recommendations for use from the review are that the interval between brushing and rinsing with CHX should be at least 30 minutes and perhaps close to 2 hours after brushing.[100] No interaction effect between essential oils and dentifrice has been reported.

Patient adherence to oral health instruction is vital to efficacy of treatment, and an evidence-based recommendation by clinicians is important to preventing disease. Considerations for daily use of an antimicrobial rinse include patient acceptance of taste and potential for staining.

New Therapies
Probiotics, an herbal patch, and antioxidants are all in various phases of investigation as adjunctive products for the treatment of gingivitis, periodontitis, and peri-implant diseases. A recent systematic review by Yanine and colleagues concluded that the effectiveness of probiotics on the prevention and treatment of periodontal diseases is questionable.[101]

An herbal patch is available to relieve the signs and symptoms of inflammation caused by gingivitis and periodontitis. It has two layers, with the outer layer composed of a nonabsorptive matrix that allows for slow dissolution of an inner layer. The patch provides a protective seal over inflamed gingival and oral mucosa while promoting wound healing by absorbing the local inflammatory exudate from the inflamed tissue.[102] Recently, the herbal patch has been investigated for the adjunctive management of chronic periodontitis and shown to have efficacy (R. Wilder, personal communication).

Antioxidants are also of interest to clinicians. San Miguel and coworkers studied the in vitro effects of antioxidants in human oral fibroblasts and concluded that they may have beneficial effects on gingival healing and periodontal repair.[103] However, a 2015 systematic review concluded that while the use of some antioxidants has the potential to improve periodontal clinical parameters, more investigation is needed.[104]

PATIENT LIFESTYLE AND EFFECT ON PREVENTION OF GINGIVAL DISEASES

The most important risk factor for gingivitis and periodontitis is the accumulation and maturation of plaque biofilm at and below the gingival margin. However, patient lifestyle factors may also contribute to the incidence and severity of gingivitis and periodontitis.[81]

Tobacco Use
Tobacco use is an undeniable risk factor for periodontal disease. Numerous studies have been published on the effect of smoking on the periodontal tissues and on the outcomes of treatment. As a preventive measure, clinicians may consider providing counseling for tobacco cessation in the dental setting. Rosa and colleagues reported on the effect of smoking cessation on nonsurgical periodontal therapy after 24 months.[105] Subjects received nonsurgical periodontal therapy and a concurrent smoking cessation intervention. Periodontal maintenance was performed every 3 months. The subjects who quit smoking showed significantly better improvement in CAL than subjects who did not quit.[105] Ramseier and Suvan published a systematic review supporting the use of brief interventions in the dental setting to increase the smoking cessation rate. Six of the eight studies in the review were conducted in dental offices.[106]

Patients appreciate and expect involvement from clinicians regarding smoking cessation.[9] Even though dental clinicians may not feel comfortable with conducting a full tobacco cessation program with a patient, most professionals can learn to provide a "brief intervention," which is a short conversation with the patient of up to 5 minutes to provide advice and limited counseling.[9]

In their consensus report on prevention of

periodontal diseases, Tonetti and coworkers emphasize that brief interventions in the dental setting increase the smoking cessation rate and recommend that clinicians minimally adopt a brief intervention using the Ask, Advise, and Refer approach.[9]

Nutrition and Obesity

Obesity rates have escalated in recent years, resulting in 500 million obese adults worldwide, including 30% of American adults.[107,108] Investigators have suggested that proinflammatory molecules may be altered by obesity and that obese individuals have an increased prevalence of periodontitis.[109] Suvan and colleagues studied 286 individuals to determine the odds of an association between overweight/obesity and diagnosis of periodontitis. Subjects with a body mass index (BMI) of 24.32 or greater were 1.6 times more likely to have a diagnosis of periodontitis than a subject with a lower BMI.[109] Another systematic review has reported a positive association between weight gain and new cases of periodontitis.[110] A third review suggested that overweight, obesity, weight gain, and increased waist circumference may be risk factors for the development of periodontitis or worsening of periodontal measures.[111]

Dental clinicians can educate patients about the potential risk of overweight and obesity, and their link to periodontal conditions. They can deliver nutrition and carbohydrate education to patients and, if trained, can participate in programs focused on weight reduction.[108] In addition, they can refer patients to other providers within the healthcare system for assistance with their condition. Not only will this potentially improve periodontal health, but it may improve overall systemic risk of disease.

Stress and Psychological Factors

Only one systematic review was located that investigated the scientific evidence for stress and psychological factors as risk factors for periodontal disease. Peruzzo and coworkers identified 58 articles of which 14 met the selection criteria. Fifty-seven percent found a positive outcome between psychosocial factors/stress and periodontal disease.[112]

Dental clinicians should consider stress as a risk factor for periodontal disease and discuss options for stress reduction with patients. Referrals to healthcare or psychological professionals should be considered, as indicated.

CASE 1: Adolescent Female Patient

PATIENT OVERVIEW

The patient is a 16-year-old girl.
Chief Complaint: "My gum tissues are too big."
Health History: American Society of Anesthesiologists category 1 (ASA 1). Unremarkable findings.
Dental History: Orthodontic treatment with no history of dental caries. Patient with poor oral hygiene.
Main Periodontal Diagnosis: Plaque-induced gingivitis associated with gingival overgrowth with likely hormonal influence (see Figure 7).

OUTCOME

Figure 8 shows the patient 8 months later, after removal of orthodontic appliance, gingivectomy, and improved oral hygiene.

Figure 7. Case 1–Initial Presentation

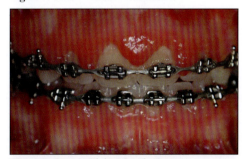

Figure 8. Case 1–Eight Months Later

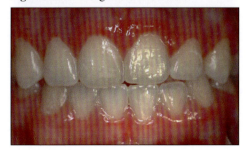

CHAPTER 5   Gingival Diseases

CASE 2: Adult Male Patient

PATIENT OVERVIEW
The patient is a 57-year-old man.
Chief Complaint: "I have bleeding gums and some pus also."
Health History: ASA 1. No known medical problems.
Dental History: Sporadic dental treatment.
Periodontal Diagnosis: Localized severe chronic periodontitis (see Figure 9).

OUTCOME
Figure 10 shows the patient 6 months later, after completion of nonsurgical and surgical therapy. The mandibular right second molar was lost due to severe periodontitis. Overall, there was significant improvement in probing depths and gain in clinical attachment.
Periodontal Maintenance Protocol: Every 3 months.

Figure 9. Case 2–Initial Presentation

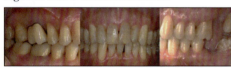

Figure 10. Case 2–Six Months Later

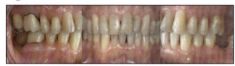

CASE 3: Elderly Male Patient

PATIENT OVERVIEW
The patient is a 75-year-old man.
Chief Complaint: "I have bleeding and pus on my lower left implant."
Health History: ASA 2. Moderate health issues, such as controlled hypertension.
Dental History: Frequent dental treatment and care. Implant-supported mandibular anterior fixed bridge was placed 3 years ago.
Periodontal Diagnosis: Peri-implantitis of the implant region, mandibular left canine. Excess implant crown cement was noted, leading to bacterial accumulation, swelling of oral mucosa, and alveolar bone loss (see Figure 11).

OUTCOME
Figure 12 shows the same area as Figure 11, immediately after debridement. Six weeks later, healing is visible (see Figure 13). Use of an interproximal brush was recommended to improve plaque control (see Figure 14).

Figure 11. Case 3–Initial Presentation

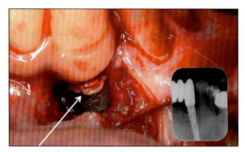

Figure 12. Case 3–Immediately After Debridement

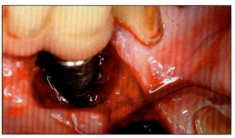

Figure 13. Case 3–Six Weeks Later

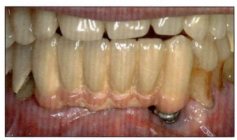

Figure 14. Case 3–Oral Health Instruction Preventive Technique

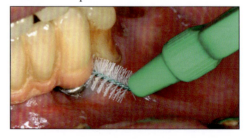

REFERENCES

1. American Academy of Periodontology. Glossary of periodontal terms 2001. 4th ed. Available at: https://www.perio.org/sites/default/files/files/PDFs/Publications/GlossaryOfPeriodontalTerms2001Edition.pdf. Accessed December 27, 2015.
2. Armitage GC. Development of a classification system for periodontal diseases and conditions. *Ann Periodontol.* 1999;4:1–6.
3. American Academy of Periodontology Task Force Report on the update to the 1999 classification of periodontal diseases and conditions. *J Periodontol.* 2015;7:835–838.
4. Eke PI, Dye BA, Wei L, et al. Update on the prevalence of periodontitis in adults in the United States: NHANES 2009 to 2012. *J Periodontol.* 2015;86:611–622.
5. Albandar JM, Kingman A. Gingival recession, gingival bleeding, and dental calculus in adults 30 years of age and older in the United States, 1988–1994. *J Periodontol.* 1999;70:30–43.
6. Li Y, Lee S, Hujoel P, et al. Prevalence and severity of gingivitis in American adults. *Am J Dent.* 2010;23:9–13.
7. Stamm JW. Epidemiology of gingivitis. *J Clin Periodontol.* 1986;13:360–370.
8. Kassebaum NJ, Bernabé E, Dahiya M, et al. Global burden of severe periodontitis 1990–2010: a systematic review and meta-regression. *J Dent Res.* 2014;93:1045–1053.
9. Tonetti MS, Eickholz P, Loos BG, et al. Principles of prevention of periodontal diseases. Consensus report of group 1 of the 11th European Workshop on Periodontology on effective prevention of periodontal and peri-implant diseases. *J Clin Periodontol.* 2015;42(suppl 16):S5–S11.
10. Löe H, Theilade E, Jensen SB. Experimental gingivitis in man. *J Periodontol.* 1965;36:177–187.
11. Buduneli N, Kinane DF. Host-derived diagnostic markers related to soft tissue destruction and bone degradation in periodontitis. *J Clin Periodontol.* 2011;38(suppl 11):85–105.
12. Listgarten MA, Loomer PM. Microbial identification in the management of periodontal diseases. A systematic review. *Ann Periodontol.* 2003;8:182–192.
13. Chatzopoulos GS, Doufexi AE, Kalogirou F. Association of susceptible genotypes to periodontal disease with the clinical outcome and tooth survival after non-surgical periodontal therapy: a systematic review and meta-analysis. *Med Oral Patol Oral Cir Bucal.* 2016;21:e14–e29.
14. Aljehani YA. Diagnostic applications of cone-beam CT for periodontal diseases. *In J Dent.* 2014;2014:865079.
15. Lang NP, Suvan JE, Tonetti MS. Risk factor assessment tools for the prevention of periodontitis progression: a systematic review. *J Clin Periodontol.* 2015;42(suppl 16):S59–S70.
16. Kwok V, Caton JG. Commentary. Prognosis revisited: a system for assigning periodontal prognosis. *J Periodontol.* 2007;78:2063–2071.
17. Lang NP, Tonetti MS. Periodontal Risk Assessment (PRA) for patients in supportive periodontal therapy (SPT). *Oral Health Prev Dent.* 2003;1:7–16.
18. Peri-implant mucositis and peri-implantitis: a current understanding of their diagnoses and clinical implications. *J Periodontol.* 2013;84:436–443.
19. Sanz M, Chapple IL. Clinical research on peri-implant diseases: consensus report of working group 4. *J Clin Periodontol.* 2012;39(suppl 12):202–206.
20. Mombelli A, Müller N, Cionca N. The epidemiology of peri-implantitis. *Clin Oral Implants Res.* 2012;23(suppl 6):67–76.
21. Atieh MA, Alsabeeha NHM, Faggion CM Jr, et al. The frequency of peri-implant diseases: a systematic review and meta-analysis. *J Periodontol.* 2013;84:1586–1598.
22. Belibasakis GN. Microbiological and immune-pathological aspects of peri-implant diseases. *Arch Oral Biol.* 2014;59:66–72.
23. de Waal, YC, Winkel EG, Meijer HJ, et al. Differences in peri-implant microflora between fully and partially edentulous patients: a systematic review. *J Periodontol.* 2014;85:68–82.
24. Clementini M, Rossetti PHO, Penarrocha D, et al. Systemic risk factors for peri-implant bone loss: a systematic review and meta-analysis. *Int J Oral Maxillofac Surg.* 2014;43:323–334.
25. Saffii SH, Palmer RM, Wilson RF. Risk of implant failure and marginal bone loss in subjects with a history of periodontitis: a systematic review and meta-analysis. *Clin Implant Dent Rel Res.* 2009;12:165–173.
26. Chrcanovic BR, Albrektsson T, Wennerberg A. Periodontally compromised vs. periodontally healthy patients and dental implants: a systematic review and meta-analysis. *J Dentistry.* 2014;42:1509–1527.
27. Naert I, Duyck J, Vandamme K. Occlusal overload and bone/implant loss. *Clin Oral Implants Res.* 2012;23(suppl. 6):95–107.
28. Van der Weijden F, Slot DE. Oral hygiene in the prevention of periodontal diseases: the evidence. *Periodontol 2000.* 2011;55:104–123.
29. Drisko CL. Periodontal self-care: evidence-based support. *Periodontol 2000.* 2013;62:243–255.
30. Beirne P, Worthington HV, Clarkson JE. Routine scale and polish for periodontal health in adults. *Cochrane Database Syst Rev.* 2007;(4):CD004625.
31. Patel S, Bay RC, Glick M. A systematic review of dental recall intervals and incidence of dental caries. *J Amer Dent Assoc.* 2010;141:527–539.
32. Flemmig TF, Beikler T. Control of oral biofilms. *Periodontol 2000.* 2011;55:9–15.
33. Cobb CM. Non-surgical pocket therapy: mechanical. *Ann Periodontol.* 1996;1:443–490.
34. Sanz I, Alonso B, Carasol M, et al. Nonsurgical treatment

of periodontitis. *J Evid Based Dent Pract.* 2012;12:76–86.
35. Van der Weijden GA, Timmerman MF. A systematic review on the clinical efficacy of subgingival debridement in the treatment of chronic periodontitis. *J Clin Periodontol.* 2002;29(suppl 3):55–71.
36. Hallmon WW, Rees TD. Local anti-infective therapy: mechanical and physical approaches. A systematic review. *Ann Periodontol.* 2003;8:99–114.
37. Rabbani GM, Ash MM Jr, Caffesse RG. The effectiveness of subgingival scaling and root planing in calculus removal. *J Periodontol.* 1981;52:119–123.
38. Stambaugh RV, Dragoo M, Smith DM, et al. The limits of subgingival scaling. *Int J Periodontics Restorative Dent.* 1981;1:30–41.
39. Waerhaug J. Healing of the dento-epithelial junction following subgingival plaque control. II: as observed on extracted teeth. *J Periodontol.* 1978;49:119–134.
40. Sherman PR, Hutchens LH, Jewson LG. The effectiveness of subgingival scaling and root planing II. Clinical responses related to residual calculus. *J Periodontal.* 1990;61:16–20.
41. Baderstein A, Nilveus R. Egelberg J. Effect of nonsurgical periodontal therapy. Moderately advanced periodontitis. *J Clin Periodontol.* 1981;8:57–72.
42. Drisko, CH. Nonsurgical periodontal therapy. *Periodontol 2000.* 2001;25:77–88.
43. Tunkel J, Heinecke A, Flemmig TF. A systematic review of efficacy of machine-driven and manual subgingival debridement in the treatment of chronic periodontitis. *J Clin Periodontol.* 2002;29:72–81.
44. Walmsley AD, Lea SC, Landini G, Moses AJ. Advances in power driven pocket/root instrumentation. *J Clin Periodontol.* 2008;35:22–28.
45. Aykol G, Baser U, Maden I, et al. The effect of low-level laser therapy as an adjunct to non-surgical periodontal treatment. *J Periodontol.* 2011;82:481–488.
46. Smiley CJ, Tracy SL, Abt E, et al. Systematic review and meta-analysis on the nonsurgical treatment of chronic periodontitis by means of scaling and root planing with or without adjuncts. *J Am Dent Assoc.* 2015;146:508–524.
47. Smiley CJ, Tracy SL, Michalowicz BS, et al. Evidence-based clinical practice guideline on the nonsurgical treatment of chronic periodontitis by means of scaling and root planing with or without adjuncts. *J Am Dent Assoc.* 2015;146:525–535.
48. ADA Center for Evidence Based Dentistry. Clinical practice guidelines. Available at: http://ebd.ada.org/en/evidence/guidelines/nonsurgical-treatment-of-chronic-periodontitis. Accessed January 9, 2016.
49. Eberhard J, Jervoe-Storm PM, Needleman I, et al. Full-mouth treatment concepts for chronic periodontitis: a systematic review. *J Clin Periodontol.* 2008;35:591–604.
50. Zijnge V, Meijer HF, Lie M-A, et al. The recolonization hypothesis in a full-mouth or multiple-session treatment protocol: a blinded, randomized clinical trial. *J Clin Periodontol.* 2010;37:518–525.

51. Knöfler GU, Purschwitz RE, Eick S, et al. Microbiologic findings 1 year after partial- and full-mouth scaling in the treatment of moderate chronic periodontitis. *Quintessence Int.* 2011;42:e107–e117.
52. Fang H, Han M, Li QL, et al. Comparison of full-mouth disinfection and quadrant-wise scaling in the treatment of adult chronic periodontitis: a systematic review and meta-analysis *J Periodontal Res.* 2015 Oct 19. doi: 10.1111/jre.12326. [Epub ahead of print.]
53. Stambaugh RV, Myers G, Ebling W, et al. Endoscopic visualization of the submarginal gingiva dental sulcus and tooth root surfaces. *J Periodontol.* 2002;73:374–382.
54. Geisinger ML, Mealey BL, Schoolfield J, et al. The effectiveness of subgingival scaling and root planing: an evaluation of therapy with and without the use of the periodontal endoscope. *J Periodontol.* 2007;78:22–28.
55. Michaud RM, Schoolfield J, Mellonig JT, et al. The efficacy of subgingival calculus removal with endoscopy-aided scaling and root planing: a study on multirooted teeth. *J Periodontol.* 2007;78:2238–2245.
56. Osborn JB, Lenton PA, Lunos SA, et al. Endoscopic vs. tactile evaluation of subgingival calculus. *J Dent Hyg.* 2014;88:229–236.
57. Petersilka GJ. Subgingival air-polishing in the treatment of periodontal biofilm infections. *Periodontol 2000.* 2011;55;124–142.
58. Petersilka GJ, Bell M, Haberlein I, et al. In vitro evaluation of novel low abrasive air polishing powders. *J Clin Periodontal.* 2003; 30;9–13.
59. Flemmig TF, Arushanov D, Daubert D, et al. Randomized controlled trial assessing efficacy and safety of glycine powder air polishing in moderate to deep periodontal pockets. *J Periodontol .* 2012;83:444–452.
60. Wennström JL, Dahlén G, Ramberg P. Subgingival debridement of periodontal pockets by air polishing in comparison with ultrasonic instrumentation during maintenance therapy. *J Clin Periodontol.* 2011;38:820–827.
61. Moëne R, Décaillet F, Andersen E, et al. Subgingival plaque removal using a new air-polishing device. *J Periodontol.* 2010;81:79–88.
62. Sculean A, Bastendorf ,KD, Becker C, et al. A paradigm shift in mechanical biofilm management? Subgingival air polishing: a new way to improve mechanical biofilm management in the dental practice. *Quintessence Int.* 2013;44:475–477.
63. Schmage P, Thielemann J, Nergiz I, et al. Effects of 10 cleaning instruments on four different implant surfaces. *Int J Oral Maxillofac Implants.* 2012;27:308–317.
64. Greenstein G. Research, Science and Therapy Committee of the American Academy of Periodontology. Position paper: the role of supra- and subgingival irrigation in the treatment of periodontal diseases. *J Periodontol* 2005:76:2015–2027.
65. Sbordone L, Ramaglia L, Guletta W, et al. Recolonization of the subgingival microflora after scaling and root planing in human periodontitis. *J Periodontol.*

66. Elworthy A, Greenman J, Doherty FM, et al. The substantivity of a number of oral hygiene products determined by the duration of effects on salivary bacteria. *J Periodontol.* 1996;76:572–576.
67. Jeffcoat MK, Bray KS, Ciancio SG, et al. Adjunctive use of a subgingival controlled-release chlorhexidine chip reduces probing depth and improves attachment level compared with scaling and root planing along. *J Periodontol.* 1998;69:989–997.
68. Stoller NH, Johnson LR, Trapnell S, et al. The pharmacokinetic profile of a biodegradable controlled release delivery system containing doxycycline compared to systemically delivered doxycycline in gingival crevicular fluid, saliva, and serum. *J Periodontol.* 1998;69:1085–1091.
69. Christersson LA. *Tissue Response and Release of Minocycline After Subgingival Deposition by Use of a Resorbable Polymer.* Warminster, PA: OraPharma Inc; 1988.
70. Finkelman RD, Polson AM. Evidence-based considerations for the clinical use of locally delivered, controlled-release antimicrobials in periodontal therapy. *J Dent Hyg.* 2013;87:249–264.
71. Sgolastra F, Gatto R, Petrucci A, et al. Effectiveness of systemic amoxicillin/metronidazole as adjunctive therapy to scaling and root planing in the treatment of chronic periodontitis: a systematic review and meta-analysis. *J Periodontol.* 2012;83:1257–1269.
72. Farooqi OA, Wehler CJ, Gibson G, et al. Appropriate recall interval for periodontal maintenance: a systematic review. *J Evid Based Dent Pract.* 2015;15:171–181.
73. Worthington HV, Clarkson JE, Bryan G, et al. Routine scale and polish for periodontal health in adults. *Cochrane Database Syst Rev.* 2013;(11):CD004625.
74. Needleman I, Nibali L, Di Iorio A. Professional mechanical plaque removal for prevention of periodontal diseases in adults—systematic review update. *J Clin Periodontol.* 2015;42(suppl 16):S12–S35.
75. Wilder RS, Bray KS. Improving periodontal outcomes: merging clinical and behavioral science. *Periodontol 2000.* 2016;71:65–81.
76. Giannobile WV, Braun TM, Caplis AK, et al. Patient stratification for preventive care in dentistry. *J Dent Res* 2013;92:694–701.
77. Bidra AS, Daubert DM, Garcia LT, et al. Clinical practice guidelines for recall and maintenance of patients with tooth-borne and implant-borne dental restorations. *J Prosthodont.* 2016;25(suppl 1):S32–S40.
78. Van der Weijden GA, Hioe KP. A systematic review of the effectiveness of self-performed mechanical plaque removal in adults with gingivitis using a manual toothbrush. *J Clin Periodontol.* 2005;32:214–228.
79. Needleman I, Nibali L, Di Iorio A. Professional mechanical plaque removal for prevention of periodontal diseases in adults—systematic review update. *J Clin Periodontol.* 2015;42(suppl 16):S12–S35.
80. Beals D, Ngo T, Feng Y, et al. Development and laboratory evaluation of a new toothbrush with a novel brush head design. *Am J Dent.* 2000;13:5A–14A.
81. Chapple IL, Van der Weijden F, Doerfer C, et al. Primary prevention of periodontitis: managing gingivitis. *J Clin Periodontol.* 2015;42(suppl 16):S71–S76.
82. Heanue M, Deacon SA, Deery C, et al. Manual versus powered toothbrushing for oral health. *Cochrane Database Syst Rev.* 2003;(1):CD002281.
83. Robinson PG, Deacon SA, Deery C, et al. Manual versus powered toothbrushing for oral health. *Cochrane Database Syst Rev.* 2005;(2):CD002281.
84. Deacon SA, Glenny AM, Deery C, et al. Different powered toothbrushes for plaque control and gingival health. *Cochrane Database Syst Rev.* 2010;(12):CD004971.
85. Sambunjak D, Nickerson JW, Poklepovic T, et al. Flossing for the management of periodontal diseases and dental caries in adults. *Cochrane Database Syst Rev.* 2011;(12):CD008829.
86. Slot DE, Dörfer CE, Van der Weijden GA. The efficacy of interdental brushes on plaque and parameters of periodontal inflammation: a systematic review. *Int J Dent Hyg.* 2008;6:253–264.
87. Jahn CA. The dental water jet: a historical review of the literature. *J Dent Hyg.* 2010;84:114–120.
88. Bhaskar SN, Cutright DE, Frisch J. Effect of high pressure water jet on oral mucosa of varied density. *J Periodontol.* 1969; 40:593-598.
89. Eakle WS, Ford C, Boyd RL. Depth of penetration in periodontal pockets with oral irrigation. *J Clin Periodontol.* 1986;13:39–44.
90. Braun RE, Ciancio SG. Subgingival delivery by an oral irrigation device. *J Periodontol.* 1992;63:469–472.
91. Husseini A, Slot DE, Van der Weijden GA. The efficacy of oral irrigation in addition to a toothbrush on plaque and the clinical parameters of periodontal inflammation: a systematic review. *Int J Dent Hyg.* 2008;6:304–314.
92. Hioe KP, van der Weijden GA. The effectiveness of self-performed mechanical plaque control with triclosan containing dentifrices. *Int J Dent Hyg.* 2005;3:192–204.
93. Davies RM, Ellwood RP, Davies GM. The effectiveness of a toothpaste containing triclosan and polyvinyl-methyl ether maleic acid copolymer in improving plaque control and gingival health: a systematic review. *J Clin Periodontol.* 2004;31:1029–1033.
94. Gunsolley JC. A meta-analysis of six-month studies of antiplaque and antigingivitis agents. *J Am Dent Assoc.* 2006;137:1649–1657.
95. Van Strydonck DA, Slot DE, Van der Velden U, et al. Effect of a chlorhexidine mouthrinse on plaque, gingival inflammation and staining in gingivitis patients: a systematic review. *J Clin Periodontol.* 2012;39:1042–1055.
96. Sharma N, Charles CH, Lynch MC, et al. Adjunctive benefit of an essential oil-containing mouthrinse in reducing plaque and gingivitis in patients who brush and floss regularly: a six-month study. *J Am Dent Assoc.* 2004;135:496–504.

97. Addy M. Oral hygiene products: potential for harm to oral and systemic health? *Periodontol 2000*. 2008;48:54–65.
98. Rath SK, Singh M. Comparative clinical and microbiological efficacy of mouthwashes containing 0.2% and 0.12% chlorhexidine. *Dent Res J*. 2013;10:364–369.
99. Sheen S, Owens J, Addy M. The effect of toothpaste on the propensity of chlorhexidine and cetylpyridinium chloride to produce staining in vitro: a possible predictor of inactivation. *J Clin Periodontol*. 2001;28:46–51.
100. Kolahi J, Soolari A. Rinsing with chlorhexidine gluconate solution after brushing and flossing teeth: a systematic review of effectiveness. *Quintessence Int*. 2006;37:605–612.
101. Yanine N, Ayaya I, Brignardello-Petersen R, et al. Effects of probiotics in periodontal diseases: a systematic review. *Clin Oral Investig*. 2013;17:1627–1634.
102. Chaushu L, Weinreb M, Beitlitum I, et al. Evaluation of a topical herbal patch for soft tissue wound healing: an animal study. *J Clin Periodontol*. 2015;42:288–293.
103. San Miguel SM, Opperman LA, Allen EP, et al. Bioactive antioxidant mixtures promote proliferation and migration on human oral fibroblasts. *Arch Oral Biol*. 2011;56:812–822.
104. Muniz FW, Nogueira SB, Mendes FL. The impact of antioxidant agents complimentary to periodontal therapy on oxidative stress and periodontal outcomes: a systematic review. *Arch Oral Biol*. 2015;60:1203–1214.
105. Rosa EF, Corraini P, Inoue G, et al. Effect of smoking cessation on non-surgical periodontal therapy: results after 24 months. *J Clin Periodontol*. 2014;41:1145–1153.
106. Ramseier CA, Suvan JE. Behaviour change counselling for tobacco use cessation and promotion of healthy lifestyles: a systematic review. *J Clin Periodontol*. 2015;42(suppl 16):S47–S58.
107. Wang YC, McPherson K, Marsh T, et al. Health and economic burden of the projected obesity trends in the USA and the UK. *Lancet*. 2011;378:815–825.
108. Lamster IB, Eaves K. A model for dental practice in the 21st century. *Am J Pub Health*. 2011;101:1825–1830.
109. Suvan J, D'Aiuto F, Moles DR, et al. Association between overweight/obesity and periodontitis in adults. A systematic review. *Obesity Reviews*. 2011;12:3381–3404.
110. Nascimento GG, Leite FR, Do LG, et al. Is weight gain associated with the incidence of periodontitis? A systematic review and meta-analysis. *J Clin Periodontol*. 2015;42:495–505.
111. Keller A, Rohde JF, Raymond K, et al. Association between periodontal disease and overweight and obesity: a systematic review. *J Periodontol*. 2015;86:766–776.
112. Peruzzo DC, Benatti BB, Ambrosano GM, et al. A systematic review of stress and psychological factors as possible risk factors for periodontal disease. *J Periodontol*. 2007;78:1491–1504.

Chapter 6
Preventing Damage to Oral Hard and Soft Tissues
Marc Shlossman and Mark Montana

PART 1: DAMAGE TO ORAL SOFT TISSUES

EPIDEMIOLOGY

Wear and tear is damage that naturally, inevitably occurs with normal wear or aging but can be accelerated by various etiologic factors. Trauma of the marginal gingiva may result from different etiologies and clinical manifestations, causing apical migration of the gingiva that exposes root surfaces. Loss of soft tissue can be rapid and acute or slow and chronic. Both preventative measures to reduce damage and corrective procedures are available to improve esthetics or function.

The American Academy of Periodontology (AAP) 1999 Classification of Periodontal Disease includes a section on nonplaque-induced gingival disease, listing traumatic gingival lesions as a subcategory.[1] These lesions may result from self-inflicted (factitious), accidental, or iatrogenic injuries. They may present as localized gingival recession, abrasions, ulcerations, or burns. Traumatic lesions also may be induced by gingival exposure to chemicals or medication. Physical injury may result from an accident, ill-fitting appliance, or inappropriate oral hygiene procedures or agents. Self-inflicted lesions are also termed *gingivitis artefacta*. Self-inflicted gingival injuries in children and adolescents can result from accidental trauma, premeditated infliction, or chronic habits such as fingernail biting, digit sucking, or sucking on objects such as pens, pencils, or pacifiers.[2]

Very few studies discuss the epidemiology of trauma to gingiva, and they are primarily case reports. One recent case series presents a sampling of traumatic gingival lesions resulting from chemical, physical, and thermal insult.[3] Another paper describes 13 cases with chemical, physical, and thermal injuries to the oral tissues.[4] Several other case reports document trauma resulting from oral piercings. Another report presents unusual gingival recession caused by lip piercing.[5,6]

In one study, 52 adults with tongue piercings were examined for gingival recession on the lingual aspect of the 12 anterior teeth and for tooth chipping anywhere in the mouth. The authors reported that long-term use of a tongue barbell increased the prevalence of these complications. Tongue piercing was also associated with lingual recession of mandibular anterior teeth and chipping of posterior teeth. This paper also included a report of an 18-year-old man who developed gingival recession on the facial aspect of the mandibular right central incisor associated with lip piercing. A concurrent recession along the lingual aspects of the mandibular left lateral and central incisors plus the mandibular right lateral incisor were attributed to an unusually large-diameter tongue barbell the patient wore.[7]

Intraoral and perioral jewelry may be associated with the development of significant mucogingival deformities. Most periodontal lesions reported with oral piercings involved tongue jewelry (64.3%) and lip jewelry (35.7%). The site of gingival recession most frequently recorded with tongue piercing was the lingual aspect of the lower central incisors. Injuries caused by lip jewelry, when specified, were localized to the facial aspect of the mandibular right central incisor in 58.3% of the reported cases and to the mandibular central incisors in 41.7% of the reported cases[8] (see Figure 1).

The AAP Classification also recognizes developmental or acquired conditions that can lead to a localized tooth-related position that may predispose to plaque accumulation and inflammatory changes or mucogingival abnormalities. Prevalence and severity of gingival recession defects are associated with periodontitis. Unfortunately, there are few epidemiological studies dealing with gingival recession. A review of cross-sectional epidemiological studies of gingival recession correlates recession to trauma, gender, malpositioned teeth, tobacco consumption, and inflammation (see Figure 2). Gingival recession was found in patients with both good and poor oral hygiene. Recession is multifactorial, with one type being associated with anatomical factors and another type with physiological or pathological factors. Recession

Figure 1.

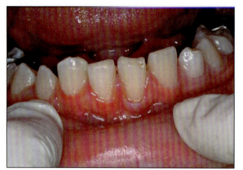

A 25-year-old woman recently removed a tongue piercing after 6 years and presented to her dentist with the complaint that "gum in front is sore and I think I chipped a tooth." Thin gingival tissue and shallow vestibule with gingival inflammation contributed to progression of recession. Treatment included gingival graft, repair of the chipped tooth, and counseling about oral jewelry.

Source: Photo courtesy of Marc Shlossman.

has been found more frequently on buccal surfaces than on other aspects of the teeth.[9]

Cross-sectional epidemiological studies indicate a high prevalence of gingival recession that increases with age and number of sites affected. According to data from the third National Health and Nutrition Examination Survey (NHANES III), 22.5% of US adults have one or more tooth surfaces with gingival recession of 3 mm or greater. Severity of gingival recession also increased with age. Men had significantly more gingival recession than women. Gingival recession was also greater and more severe on buccal surfaces of teeth.[10]

Two studies report a high level of gingival recession in Brazilian urban populations. This may correlate with destructive periodontal disease associated with calculus and cigarette smoking. Among 1,460 representative urban Brazilians, prevalence, extent, and severity of recession correlated with age. Men aged 30 years and older had significantly higher prevalence and extent of gingival recession than women. Slight recession (≥ 1 mm) was prevalent, with 83% affected, but recession defects of 3 and 5 mm or greater affected only a small percentage of teeth in subjects younger

Figure 2.

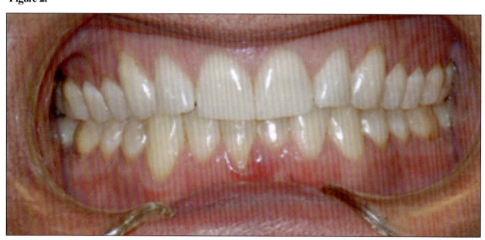

This 32-year-old man noted "the area in front is sore and bleeds, the gums on my right side are receding even though I brush several times a day." Tooth position and aggressive brushing have contributed to his current condition which was treated with localized scaling, modification of brushing technique, and regular monitoring of recession defects for intervention with grafting as needed.

Source: Photo courtesy of Marc Shlossman.

than age 40. On the other hand, moderate recession was pervasive in the older age groups. Among subjects aged 40 years or older, 79% or more of the subjects and 32% or more of teeth per subject had recession of 3 mm or greater. Periodontal disease, irregular dental care, cigarette smoking, and supragingival calculus were the factors most significantly associated with localized and generalized recession.[11] In a second study of 1,023 urban Brazilian adults aged 35 and older, recession of 1 mm or greater was found in 99.7% of subjects. The percentage of subjects with one or more teeth having recession of 3 mm or greater and 5 mm or greater was 75.4% and 40.7%, respectively. Study findings also indicated a more generalized pattern, with increasing age, male gender, smoking exposure, and the presence of calculus as significant risk indicators for recession.[12]

In a recent study of more than 800 Turkish patients, overall prevalence of gingival recession was 78.2%. Gingival recession for buccal surfaces measuring between 1 to 2 mm was found in 17.4% of the study population. Statistical analysis showed that age, smoking duration, traumatic toothbrushing, and high frenum are significant contributors to gingival recession.[13]

A cross-sectional survey was conducted in France with 2,074 subjects, aged 35 to 65 years, reflecting a nationally representative sample. All subjects had a full-mouth periodontal examination, and the buccal gingival recession status of each subject was assessed based on the severity and extent of gingival recession. Approximately 85% of the sample had at least one tooth with gingival recession. Extent of gingival recession was associated with such etiologic agents as age, gender, plaque index, and tobacco consumption.[14]

The influence of independent variables on recession including smoking status, glycemic index, plaque index, educational level, presence of supragingival calculus, and oral hygiene practices was studied in a population of young Greek adults. The overall prevalence of recession was 60.3%, with no statistically significant difference between men and women. Gingival inflammation and smoking were the most important associated risk factors for gingival recession.[15] Among Tanzanian adults, aged 20 to 34 years, the lingual surfaces of the lower anterior teeth were most frequently affected by gingival recession, and presence and extent increased with age.[16]

ETIOLOGY

Gingival recession is characterized by the apical migration of the gingival margin below the cementoenamel junction. Receded gingiva can be inflamed, healthy, localized to one tooth or several adjacent teeth, or generalized throughout the mouth (see Figure 3). Gingival recession increases with age; the prevalence varies from less than 10% in children to almost 100% in adults over the age of 50 years.[17] This has led some investigators to assume that recession may be a physiological process related to aging; however, no convincing evidence has been presented for a physiological shift of the gingival attachment. The gradual apical shift is most likely the result of the cumulative effect of minor pathological involvement and repeated minor direct trauma to the gingiva. The primary etiology remains the accumulation of dental plaque biofilm resulting in plaque-induced inflammation and gingival recession.[18] Clinically, many areas of recession associated with toothbrush abrasion will appear plaque-free, which is frequently observed in individuals with good oral hygiene.[17]

Figure 3.

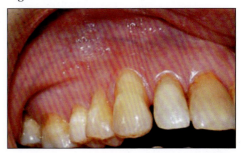

An aggressive toothbrushing habit in a healthy 42-year-old man who complained "my gums are receding and I don't like to smile." Treatment included gingival grafting for root coverage, modification of daily home care routine, and a 6-month recall schedule.

Source: Photo courtesy of Marc Shlossman.

Traumatic lesions may be self-inflicted and result from intentional or unintentional means. Toothbrush trauma may lead to gingival ulceration, recession, or both (see Figure 4). Iatrogenic trauma (i.e., induced by dentist or health professional) to gingiva can be caused by orthodontic appliances, dental materials, or instruments (see Figure 5). The health of gingival tissue also depends on properly designed and placed restorative materials. Pressure from a poorly designed partial denture, such as an ill-fitting denture clasp, can cause gingival trauma and recession[19] (see Figure 6A, B). Clinically, violation of the biological width typically manifests as gingival inflammation, deepened periodontal pockets, and gingival recession. Accidental damage to the gingiva may occur as a result of minor burns from hot foods and drinks.[18]

Local gingival tissue trauma or irritation can lead to inflammatory changes in the tissues, resulting in gingival recession. For example, when smokeless tobacco is used, the tobacco is kept in the vestibule adjacent to mandibular incisors or premolars for a prolonged time. Gingival tissues can experience mechanical or chemical injury, resulting in recession. Recession involving either mandibular or maxillary teeth is found in up to 80% of individuals with oral piercings.[18]

A mucogingival deformity describes an abnormality of the mucogingival junction and its relationship to the gingiva, the alveolar mucosa, and frenum attachments. A mucogingival deformity is a significant departure from the normal shape of the gingiva and the alveolar mucosa, and it may involve the underlying alveolar bone. Mucogingival defects affect the morphology, position, or amount of gingiva, which may result in aesthetic and functional concerns or difficulty with performing oral hygiene.[18]

A variety of factors can cause gingival recession. Predisposing and precipitating influences contribute to the initiation and progression of gingival recession. Tooth position, thin tissue biotype, bone dehiscence, minimal nonmobile keratinized tissue, shallow vestibular depth, or frenum pulls can all predispose to gingival recession (see Figures 7 and 8). Susceptibility to recession is also

Figure 4.

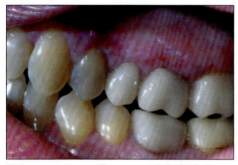

"My gums are really sore and I don't know why," commented this 57-year-old woman with medication-controlled hypertension and osteoporosis. She indicated that she had been away the previous week and had forgotten her regular toothbrush "so I picked one up at the hotel front desk—a harder toothbrush than I normally use." Discontinuing the hard toothbrush and palliative therapy during the acute phase resulted in resolution of gingival tenderness within 10 days, with no further sequelae.
Source: Photo courtesy of Marc Shlossman.

Figure 5.

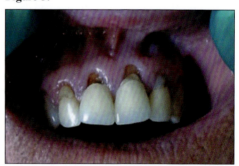

Gingival recession associated with older restorations and recurrent decay at gingival margins in a 73-year-old man. He complained "my teeth are getting longer and sensitive to temperature" and had dry mouth related to antihypertensive medication. His hygiene was adequate. Treatment included removing decay and replacing existing restorations with improved contours to cover areas of recession. Regular fluoride application and routine recall (every 3 to 4 months) were advised.
Source: Photo courtesy of Marc Shlossman.

influenced by the position of teeth in the arch, the root–bone angle, and the curvature of the clinical crown. Physical, thermal, and chemical trauma serve as precipitating factors along with excessive brushing, tobacco use, oral piercing, and iatrogenic dental treatment.[20]

Toothbrushing
Standard oral hygiene procedures, toothbrushing, or flossing may lead to frequent transient and minimal gingival injury.[21] Although toothbrushing is important for gingival health, faulty technique or brushing with hard bristles may cause significant injury. This injury may present as lacerations, abrasions, keratosis, and recession, with the facial marginal gingiva being the most affected.[22] The gingival changes attributable to toothbrush trauma may be acute or chronic. Signs of acute

Figure 6A and B.

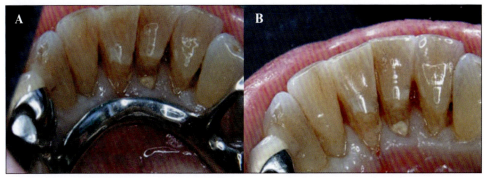

A 68-year-old woman noted "my gums are sore every time I put in my lower partial and it's only a few months old." Her lingual retainer was placing pressure at the gingival margin, which resulted in a tear and clefting of the minimal band of attached gingiva. A gingival graft was performed to increase tissue thickness and keratinized tissue prior to fabrication of a new appliance.
Source: Photo courtesy of Marc Shlossman.

Figure 7.

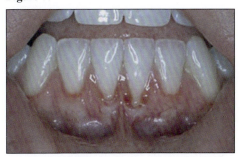

Recession in healthy 19-year-old woman taking oral contraceptives. Thin tissue, tooth position, frenal pull, and inflammation related to plaque accumulation have resulted in "gums that are sore to touch and bleed." Improved home care and gingival augmentation were completed, and more regular recalls (every 4 months) were recommended.
Source: Photo courtesy of Marc Shlossman.

Figure 8.

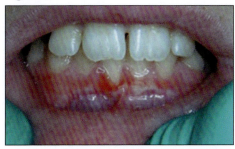

A strong frenal pull complicated by a thin tissue biotype and shallow vestibule has resulted in an inflammatory reaction with subsequent recession in this healthy 12-year-old girl. Her chief complaint was "my gums are sore and bleed when I brush." A frenectomy and gingival graft were completed to augment the tissue, increase the vestibular depth, and reduce tissue pull to assure long-term gingival health.
Source: Photo courtesy of Marc Shlossman.

gingival abrasion are frequently noted when the patient changes to a new brush. Chronic toothbrush trauma may result in gingival recession with exposure of the root surface. Interproximal attachment loss is generally a consequence of bacteria-induced periodontitis, whereas buccal and lingual attachment loss is frequently the result of toothbrush abrasion. The improper use of dental floss may cause lacerations of the interdental papilla, also known as "floss cuts."

Improper toothbrushing technique may be an important mechanical factor that contributes to the development of gingival recession (see Figure 9). Recession on buccal surfaces is commonly found in patients with a high standard of oral hygiene and among those with a history of hard toothbrush use.[23-25] Poor toothbrushing technique, including use of a horizontal scrubbing motion, brushing with a hard-bristled brush, or brushing too often or too long may all lead to mechanical destruction. One study examined the relationship between a history of use of hard-bristled toothbrushes and gingival recession. Recession was found to be more pronounced for subjects with a history of hard toothbrush use, with a mean of 9.4% receded surfaces versus 4.7% for those who had never used a hard brush. For users of hard toothbrushes, the percentage of surfaces with recession showed a significant and dramatic increase with increasing brushing frequency; this effect did not exist for those without a history of hard brush use. Furthermore, the relationship between amount of recession and age was highly significant.[26] Manual toothbrushes with hard bristles can remove plaque effectively but may also cause more soft tissue trauma compared to brushes with softer bristles.[27]

Several recent studies compare the clinical effects of manual and powered toothbrushes. A cross-sectional study of abrasion and recession in manual and oscillating–rotating power brush users focused on 181 participants. It was an uncontrolled observational study that reflected normal brushing behavior in young adults aged 18 to 35 years. In this population, gingival recession could not be explained by gingival abrasion associated with use of either the power brush or manual brush. The oral hygiene benefits of brushing with an advanced power brush are achieved at no more risk to gingival tissue than with a manual toothbrush.[28] Two studies have examined whether there are differences in the progression of existing gingival recession with use of either a manual or power brush. Neither type of brush led to an increase in recession defects during 12 months of daily use.[29,30]

Two recent systematic reviews reported on the influence of toothbrushing on gingival recession. The authors of the first paper stated that the presented evidence was "inconclusive" to support or refute an association between toothbrushing and gingival recession. Only one randomized clinical study concluded that power toothbrushes significantly reduced buccal surface recession. Other studies were observational and none satisfied all the specified criteria for quality appraisal. The authors concluded that a valid appraisal of the quality of the randomized controlled trials was not possible. However, they indicated other potential risk factors, including duration of toothbrushing, brushing force, frequency of

Figure 9.

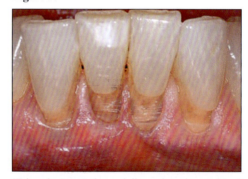

"I brush 4 to 5 times daily and can't get rid of the dark areas on my teeth," according to this healthy 52-year-old man. He presented with significant recession, generally healthy periodontal support, but evidence of aggressive brushing and thin tissues due to loss of keratinized gingiva. Gingival grafting was advised for root coverage and modification of brushing technique reviewed.

Source: Photo courtesy of Marc Shlossman.

changing the brush, bristle hardness, and toothbrushing technique.[31]

The second review reported that manual toothbrushing resulted in more recession than power brushing. Findings from two randomized, controlled clinical studies suggest that noninflammatory recession may be prevented through proper use of either a manual or power brush. Frequency and method of brushing are principal factors associated with progression of recession defects.[32]

Tooth Movement by Orthodontic Forces

Undergoing active orthodontic treatment or the post-treatment retention phase may also contribute to gingival recession. Orthodontic therapy can influence the development of gingival recession through several mechanisms. The movement of teeth to positions outside the labial or lingual alveolar plate could result in thinning of the alveolar plate or dehiscence formation, creating marginal gingiva without alveolar bone support (see Figure 10A, B). The unsupported tissue can migrate apically, leading to root exposure. Orthodontic patients are advised to maintain ideal oral hygiene to prevent plaque accumulation around orthodontic appliances. Active orthodontic treatment is typically followed by a retention phase with wire retainers in the anterior regions of the maxilla and mandible, around which plaque may accumulate, leading to an inflammatory response and recession.

A retrospective case-control study evaluated the development of labial gingival recession in orthodontic patients 6 years after therapy completion, compared to nontreated controls. The proportion of subjects with recession was consistently higher in those treated orthodontically compared with controls. The investigators concluded that orthodontic treatment or the retention phase may be risk factors for development of labial gingival recession. Mandibular incisors seemed to be most vulnerable to development of gingival recession.[33]

A study evaluating patients before, immediately after, and 2 and 5 years postorthodontic treatment found that prevalence of labial gingival recession correlates to age, treatment duration, and post-therapy time. Recession depends on age and increases from before orthodontic treatment to 5 years after therapy. The prevalence of gingival recession steadily increases after orthodontic treatment. Recession is more prevalent in older than younger patients. Canines, first premolars, first molars in the maxilla, central incisors, and first premolars in the mandible are at the highest risk for labial gingival recessions. No variable, except for age at the end of treatment, was associated with development of gingival recession.[34]

Figure 10A and B.

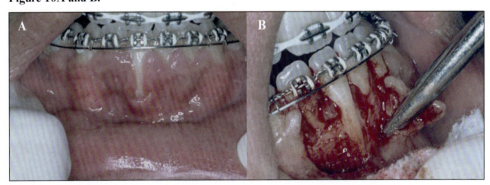

This 15-year-old girl undergoing orthodontic therapy noted "my gums disappeared and it is now very sore." Orthodontic movement compromised the thin buccal plate, resulting in alveolar dehiscence and subsequent recession. Treatment included modification of daily home care procedures, gingival graft with biological mediator, and 3-month recall during active orthodontic therapy.

Source: Photo courtesy of Marc Shlossman.

Studies about effects of orthodontic treatment on gingival recession typically suggest an incidence of 10% to 20% in patients evaluated for as long as 5 years after the completion of orthodontic therapy.[35] These rates of occurrence, considered relative to the overall high prevalence found in adults, suggest that orthodontic tooth movement may contribute minimally to the overall prevalence of gingival recession. Several recent studies even suggest that postorthodontic recession may affect only 10% of patients, with most cases being readily treatable as Miller class I lesions.[36]

Frenal Pull

Frenal pull is frequently cited as a predisposing factor to gingival recession. When the frenum attachment is proximate to the gingival margin, repetitious frenum stretch during oral function could exert forces that compromise mucosal tissue margins, leading to gingival recession. Plaque removal along affected marginal gingiva may also be impeded. However, cross-sectional studies failed to demonstrate an association of recession with high frenum attachment.[20] Previous studies examining the influence of frenal pull on recession are inconclusive. Only one study reported a correlation between high frenum and gingival recession, and this involved male participants in Turkey.[13]

Traumatic Lesions (Factitious, Iatrogenic, and Accidental)

Traumatic lesions may be accidental or result from inappropriate oral hygiene procedures, inadequate dental restorations, poorly designed dental appliances, or orthodontic bands and devices. Deficiencies in dental restorations or prostheses may also effect gingival inflammation and periodontal damage. Inadequate dental procedures that contribute to deterioration of periodontal tissues are referred to as iatrogenic factors. Laceration of the gingiva may result from the use of rubber dam clamps, matrix bands, and burs. Although such transient injuries generally heal, they are unnecessary patient discomforts. Orthodontic therapy may affect the periodontium by directly injuring the gingiva as a result of overextended bands or loose wires.[37] Maintenance of periodontal health focuses on specific characteristics of dental restorations and removable partial dentures. They include location of the gingival margin for the restoration, space between restorative margin and unprepared tooth, contour of restoration, occlusion, materials used in the restoration, type of restorative procedure, and design of the removable partial denture.

Chemical, physical, and thermal injuries in the oral, gingival, or palatal mucosa of iatrogenic origin can exhibit various clinical features. Management of traumatic injuries is dependent on the severity of involved periodontal tissues. Thirteen cases of chemical (ferric sulfate and formocresol), physical (due to orthodontic wires and appliances), and thermal (due to electrosurgery) injuries to the oral tissues have been reported. In most cases, elimination of the offending agent and symptomatic therapy are sufficient to allow for tissue repair; in severe cases, or when injury results in permanent defects, periodontal surgery and regenerative therapy may be necessary.[3,38]

Iatrogenic injuries are often acute and are generally self-limiting, whereas factitious injuries tend to be more chronic in nature. Patients may be unaware of self-inflicted injurious habits that may impact the initiation and progression of periodontal pathology. Mechanical forms of trauma can stem from the improper use of a toothbrush, toothpicks and other interdental aids between the teeth, dental floss, fingernail pressure, pizza burns, and other causes (see Figure 11). Sources of chemical irritation include the topical application of caustic agents, such as aspirin (see Figure 12) or cocaine; accidental contact with drugs, such as phenol or silver nitrate; allergic reactions to components in toothpaste and chewing gum; or the use of chewing tobacco, betel nut, bleaching agents, and concentrated mouthrinse.[37]

Use of smokeless tobacco is an important etiologic factor that can lead to gingival recession. Snuff and chewing tobacco constitute the two main forms of smokeless tobacco. Snuff is a fine-cut form of tobacco that is available loosely packed or in small sachets. Chewing tobacco is a more coarse-cut tobacco that is available in the form of loose leaves, a solid block, a plug, or as a twist of dried leaves. Increased incidences of gingival recession, cervical root abrasion, and root caries have been reported with smokeless tobacco. The incidence of gingival recession among adolescents who use smokeless tobacco has been reported at 42% as compared with 17% among nonusers. It can be concluded that use of smokeless tobacco is associated with at least localized gingival recession, clinical attachment loss, leukoplakia, and possibly enhanced susceptibility to severe periodontitis.[39,40]

Oral piercing jewelry in the lip or tongue is becoming increasingly common among teenagers and young adults. Both lip and tongue piercings are associated with high risk of gingival recession; tongue piercings are also correlated to tooth injuries. Increased wear time of tongue and lip piercings is also associated with greater prevalence of dental defects, gingival recession, and greater attachment loss and probing depth of teeth adjacent to pierced sites. Ornament morphology affects the prevalence of gingival recession.[7,8,41]

PATHOGENESIS

The normal gingiva covers the alveolar bone and tooth root to a level just coronal to the cementoenamel junction. The gingiva is divided into marginal, attached, and interdental areas. Each type of gingiva's unique structure allows it to function appropriately against mechanical and microbial insult, while exhibiting considerable variation in differentiation, histology, and thickness. The specific structure of different types of gingiva reflects each one's protective role as a barrier to the penetration of microbes and noxious agents into the deeper tissue.[42]

Getting "long in the tooth" is a phrase that links age to gingival recession. Gingival wear reflects the cumulative exposure to numerous potentially destructive processes. Wear and tear may result from chronic mechanical toothbrush trauma, habits, oral piercings, orthodontic treatment, and iatrogenic damage from dental procedures. Cumulative exposures result in an increased loss of attachment. Other factors are tissue morphology and anatomy, including thin soft tissues, frenum pulls, and a thin facial plate of bone with dehiscence or fenestrations. If a patient's oral hygiene is inadequate, secondary inflammation and eventually pocket formation

Figure 11.

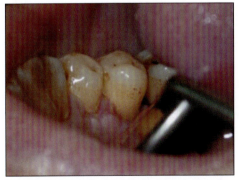

Improper use of an interproximal cleaning brush has resulted in tissue trauma in 58-year-old smoker. After a change to a smaller brush size and hygiene counseling, the irritation resolved.
Source: Photo courtesy of Marc Shlossman.

Figure 12.

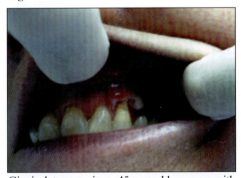

Gingival trauma in a 45-year-old woman with medication-controlled hypertension. "My tooth was sore so I put aspirin on it and now my gums really hurt" was her presenting complaint. Palliative treatment was provided during the acute phase, including mild saline rinses (1/2 tsp. salt in 8 oz. warm water) and an ultrasoft brush. The area was assessed for long-term damage and the need for gingival grafting, and she was counseled in the proper use of medication.
Source: Photo courtesy of Marc Shlossman.

may result. Five to ten percent of all periodontal attachment loss is termed "classical" recession.[18] Despite gingival margin recession, the interdental papillae usually fill the entire embrasure area in younger patients. The periodontal supporting structures in teeth exhibiting classical gingival recession generally have excellent health and minimal mobility.[43]

PREVENTION AND THERAPY

With scrupulous and proper oral hygiene, recession can be halted. Proper technique must be stressed for all patients who have preexisting defects or are more prone to recession. Manual and power brushes that carry the American Dental Association seal should be recommended. Chronic floss tearing requires educating patients in proper flossing technique to avoid further damage. Additional damage to soft and hard tissues from oral jewelry can only be prevented by educating patients who do not regard oral piercings as health hazards or who may be reluctant to remove them. Chewing tobacco has direct effects on the gingiva, so habit cessation and education efforts are critical. The potential for malignant change to the tissues must also be stressed (see Chapter 7).

Every effort by dental practitioners to avoid iatrogenic soft tissue damage during dental treatment is vital. Proper tissue isolation during endodontic and restorative procedures can minimize mechanical and chemical trauma. Use of appropriate retraction during surgical therapy can avoid tissue trauma and protect adjacent structures. Care must be taken not to violate the biological width during preparation of tooth surfaces. Despite efforts to prevent gingival recession, severe types of recession may require mucogingival surgery. Surgical correction of gingival recession is often considered when (1) a patient raises a concern about esthetics or tooth hypersensitivity (which cannot be managed using professional or consumer products that reduce dentin hypersensitivity), or when (2) evidence of ongoing active gingival recession persists despite other interventions. Successful treatment of recession-type defects is based on the use of predictable periodontal plastic surgery procedures.[20] Subepithelial connective tissue grafts, coronally advanced flaps, either alone or associated with other biomaterial, and guided tissue regeneration may be used as root coverage procedures for the treatment of localized recession-type defects.[44] Treatment options are discussed in detail in several recent workshop proceedings.

A comprehensive assessment of the relevant literature, performed as part of the 2014 American Academy of Periodontology Workshop on Periodontal Regeneration and Tissue Engineering, revealed a sizable volume of publications supporting most root coverage procedures. From this comprehensive assessment of the root coverage literature, a "decision tree" was generated. The ensuing consensus report should help clinicians in their daily practice to determine the best treatment modality to satisfy their patients' needs.[45] The scope of this consensus report was to assess the strength of the scientific evidence and make clinical and research recommendations for surgical interventions to cover exposed root surfaces and enhance soft tissues at implants. Emerging data indicate that it is possible to obtain complete root coverage at sites with some interdental attachment loss. The consensus of the report is that periodontal plastic procedures are complex, technique-sensitive interventions that require advanced skills and expertise.[46]

PART 2: DAMAGE TO ORAL HARD TISSUES

Damage to oral hard tissues may be categorized as biocorrosive (caries), impact trauma, and noncarious tooth surface loss, also known as tooth wear. Three processes result in tooth wear: attrition, abrasion, and erosion.[47] Tooth wear, which is the focus of this discussion, may be defined as physiological or pathological, and is typically dependent upon subjective interpretation as no clear set of criteria is currently available to assist the clinician. This section addresses several causes of damage to the hard tissues, with related discussions of etiology, pathogenesis, risk factors, and preventive strategies.

ATTRITION

Attrition is the act of wearing or grinding down by friction as a result of mastication, dysfunctional, or parafunctional activity, limited to the contacting surfaces of the teeth (see Figure 13). Attrition may be further categorized as physiological or pathological, depending on the rate of wear.[48] Unfortunately, an acceptable metric to diagnose a patient as having pathological attrition is not available; rather, it is up to the clinician to decide if the loss of structure is excessive relative to the age of the patient. Twenty percent loss of the incisal edge in an 80-year-old patient may be considered physiological, while the same measure of wear is cause for concern in a young adult. However, because pathological tooth-wearing behavior may begin at any time in life, age alone does not distinguish between health and disease. It is possible that a person of greater years may experience a physiological or psychological change that initiates a pathological wear potential. Accurate record keeping is a valuable tool for detecting early onset. Although it is impractical for most clinicians to store diagnostic casts indefinitely, scanning technology allows for permanent retention of both clinical and patient model images, enabling study of changing tooth morphology across time.

Etiology

When attrition is determined to be pathological, the cause is typically diagnosed as parafunctioning by the patient in the form of bruxism, an involuntary rhythmic or spasmodic nonfunctional grinding of the teeth, or increased bracing in athletic endeavors. Another etiology is dysfunctional occlusion, which includes excessive load or pressure on the remaining teeth in a shortened dental arch.

The causes of bruxism have been associated with tooth interferences, psychological components, lifestyle factors, and sleep apnea.[49] There are few data to support the historic occlusion argument.[50-52] Anxiety, stress, and adverse psychosocial factors are significantly related to nighttime grinding but are difficult to quantify, and therapeutic solutions rely on making positive changes to the patient's lifestyle, job, relationship, or other relevant stressors. Patients may adversely affect their condition through use of psychoactive substances, including alcohol, caffeine, tobacco, and antidepressive or antianxiety medications.

Patients who suffer obstructive sleep apnea (OSA) experience a closing of the airway, and bruxism is a compensatory mechanism of the upper airway to help overcome obstruction by activation of the clenching muscles, which brings the mandible, and therefore the tongue, forward. Often, attrition in the OSA patient is first noticeable on the anterior teeth, indicating a forward direction of movement of the mandible, the same as that required to open the airway. Studies have shown that treatment to reduce apneic episodes through continuous positive airway pressure (CPAP) or by mandibular

Figure 13.

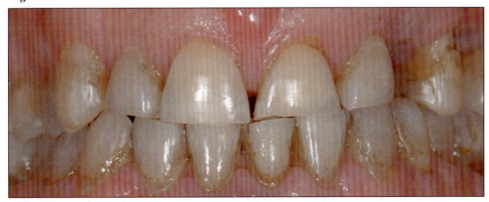

Attrition is tooth-to-tooth wear characterized by opposing surfaces fitting together tightly.
Source: Photo courtesy of Mark Montana.

advancement appliance therapy decreased or eliminated nocturnal bruxism. Once the patient is able to breathe, the body's need to protect the airway through posturing the jaw forward is reduced.[53]

Prevention

Prevention of pathological wear of the contacting surfaces of teeth resulting from nighttime bruxism is achieved through the reduction of apnea episodes by CPAP or a mandibular advancement appliance. By understanding that snoring is a sign of a body in distress, clinical intervention may occur before wear of teeth is exhibited. The consequences of OSA are serious and may affect young and old, slim and heavy alike.

Traditional nighttime appliance therapy for bruxism using a single arch occlusal splint may be effective for non-OSA patients but is not recommended for those with airway obstruction, as it may worsen the scenario by allowing the mandible to slide backward.[54] Diagnosis of the etiology of a patient's bruxism is crucial to determine if it is breathing related; consequently, an appropriate sleep study is required.

Wear from bruxism in the non-OSA patient is prevented through interference using a plastic occlusal splint or a soft mouthguard in the case of athletes who clench and grind during their activity. The goal is not to stop the grinding, but rather to avoid damage to the teeth.

For patients who have a reduced number of teeth and therefore wear away the remaining dentition at an accelerated rate, treatment consists of replacing proper masticatory function with harmonious bilateral contact to the first molar, if possible. Studies show that a reduction in the functional arch length increases pressure on the remaining dentition, often manifesting in wear to these teeth.[55] Prevention of this occurrence is of course best achieved by preserving the natural dentition, repairing it when damaged, and replacing it with dental implants when repair is unlikely.

ABRASION

Abrasion is the wearing away of tooth structure through some unusual or mechanical process other than mastication. In other words, something other than an opposing tooth is causing frictional wear.[56] Suspects include highly abrasive foods, contamination of food with abrasive particles, inhalation of abrasive particles, and iatrogenic abrading by the individual or by a dental professional.

Etiology

Historically, teeth were abraded by tough, fibrous diets and by eating food contaminated by gritty substances. Most wear occurred on the buccal cusps of the lower molars and the palatal cusps of the upper molars. These functional cusps often had scooped-out anatomy where the exposed dentin was worn away below the surface of the surrounding enamel by fibrous food or foreign particles. Interestingly, interstitial wear between teeth was a common finding as well, caused by teeth moving against each other with grit trapped between them. Modernization of food processing in industrialized society softened diets, dramatically reducing this cause of abrasion.[57,58]

People employed in historically dusty occupations, such as farmers, experienced accelerated wear of the chewing surfaces of their teeth due to the constant intake of ambient dust. The gritty feeling likely induced grinding, creating effective milling of the opposing surfaces. The result was characteristically flattened teeth. Abrasion may also be caused by habitual behavior, such as chewing on objects like pencils, nail biting, opening hair pins, or biting thread or fishing line, and by playing wind instruments. Abrasion may also occur as a result of dentally related actions, such as restoration of teeth with abrasive materials and purposeful sanding of dental structures.

The introduction of feldspathic porcelain crowns, starting in the mid-1960s, provided patients with an esthetically pleasing alternative to gold or silver-black restorations. Unfortunately, the surface of dental porcelain is extremely abrasive, resembling sandpaper when viewed under extreme magnification. The longer these crowns stay in the mouth, the more abrasive they become as the finer grains and glassy surface wear away, leaving behind the most abrasive particles. When placed on teeth with a longer range of sliding contact or articulation, such as a canine, the wear to their antagonist can be devastating (see Figure 14). Patients with a parafunctional activity such as bruxism are particularly at risk when restored with porcelain crowns as the incidence of contact is magnified greatly in these individuals. Significantly, it is not the hardness of the material that is important but rather the surface roughness; therefore, proper polishing of ceramic restorations is of utmost importance whether at completion in the dental laboratory or after adjustment in the patient's mouth.[59,60] Dental laboratories may substitute polishing by applying a glaze as the finishing step in making a crown because it is less time intensive than polishing, but studies suggest the net result is a more abrasive surface.[61-67] Dental procedures, including adjustment of opposing teeth to fit to a new crown or removing of residual brackets retaining resin following completion of orthodontic therapy, are also causes of abrasion, although they are limited to the event and are not ongoing phenomena.

Polishing of tooth surfaces in the dental office removes tooth stains; however, few commercial prophylaxis pastes have been shown to produce a smoother tooth surface when tested in vitro.[68] Selective polishing has been proposed as a safer approach to minimize potential damage to the hard tissues, given that early research documented that polishing procedures and products can abrade enamel, dentin, and cementum. However, the amount of reported tissue loss in these studies was inconsistent, making the clinical significance of this purported risk difficult to assess.[69-73] A more recent laboratory study simulated the effects of lifetime polishing on enamel thickness by polishing 24 extracted teeth 150 times using coarse grit prophylaxis paste. Matched unpolished teeth served as controls. When pre- and post-polishing micrometer measurements were compared using digital radiography, no differences in enamel thickness were noted between treated and untreated teeth, which suggests that polishing poses little clinically significant risk to enamel. However, root surface abrasion was noted on five of the treated molar teeth, which may be of greater concern, as cementum is softer and does not regenerate in areas exposed by recession. The authors suggest that alternative stain removal techniques be explored for affected root surfaces.[74]

In practice, many patients have come to expect a full polishing procedure at the end of their preventive care visits, believing that this procedure is of clinical benefit, causing reluctance among dental clinicians to adopt selective polishing.[75-77] Yet, routine polishing after scaling has not been shown to improve dental health beyond the effects of removing plaque and calculus.[78] While there is some evidence to show a slight reduction in

Figure 14.

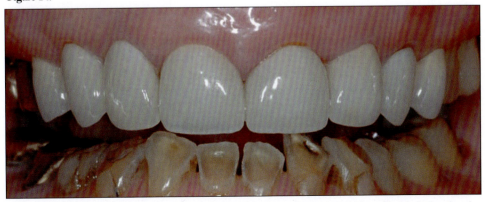

Abrasion is surface loss as a result of rubbing by a foreign substance. In this patient it is the abrasive porcelain crowns wearing away the lower natural teeth.
Source: Photo courtesy of Mark Montana.

gingivitis with regular (e.g., every 3 months) scaling and polishing, to date there is insufficient evidence to determine the benefits of routine scaling and polishing to improve periodontal health among adult patients.[79,80]

Air polishing is an alternative polishing technique that was first introduced in the 1970s. In general, air polishing can be used safely for both biofilm and stain removal, is more efficient than rubber cup polishing, and causes less operator fatigue.[81] Numerous devices and types of powders have been tested over the past three decades. As with traditional prophylaxis pastes, damage to enamel appears to be minimal, whereas abrasion is more likely to occur on dentin and cementum. The degree of damage to the tooth structure is affected by the type of powder, the powder to water ratio, length of contact time, and nozzle distance from the tooth surface.[82-86] A recent systematic review found that glycine powders cause significantly less damage to the oral hard and soft tissues as compared to sodium bicarbonate or calcium carbonate powders.[87]

Historically, both toothbrushing and dentifrice use have been associated with abrasion. Clinically, toothbrush abrasion is most often observed along the buccal/facial cervical third of the tooth, often with gingival recession, both of which are attributed to improper brushing technique (see Figure 15). Toothbrush abrasion is also site-dependent, with canine and premolar teeth most often affected.[88] Lesions are also more prominent on the contralateral side of the person's dominant hand used during toothbrushing.[17] Studies confirm that toothbrushing itself or toothbrushing with most dentifrice products cause clinically insignificant wear to enamel.[89-92] Variations in brush type, from soft to firm and manual to automated, have shown little to no difference in scratching of the enamel surface, but the use of hard brushes or of vigorous brushing may result in increased recession of the soft tissue and thus exposure of the at-risk, softer, underlying tooth structure. Thus, excessive force and improper technique with toothbrushing are risk factors for dentinal hypersensitivity.[17]

Dentifrices marketed for whitening, stain removal, and polishing properties have been shown to be effective in removing stain but produced some dentin abrasion when tested in vitro using standard nylon-bristle brushes. Degree of abrasion varied widely among tested products and was not directly related to stain-removal ability.[93] Findings from a recent workshop on dentifrice abrasiveness concluded that "the value of in vitro abrasivity data alone is not an appropriate measure to judge the safety and the risk of adverse effects of dentifrices on tooth hard substances under clinical conditions."[94] However, toothbrushing with dentifrice in combination with an acidic challenge causes additive effects to erosive enamel loss (see Erosion).[90]

Prevention
Preventing abrasion from daily home care involves teaching proper brushing technique using less

Figure 15.

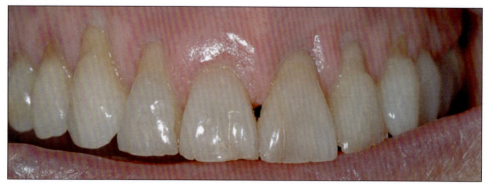

Figure 15. Loss of root surface attributed to abrasion from toothbrushing.
Source: Photo courtesy of Mark Montana.

force, a soft toothbrush, and a nonabrasive dentifrice.[17,95] Proper brushing technique should be assessed and reinforced at regular recare appointments. Clinicians should select the least abrasive prophylaxis paste or powder when polishing is deemed necessary for stain removal and use a technique that helps to prevent damage to the dentin and cementum.

EROSION

Dental erosion is the progressive loss of tooth substance by chemical processes that do not involve bacterial action. Erosion is divided into two causative categories: endogenic (intrinsic), from refluxed gastric juices; and exogenic (extrinsic), from dietary, medicinal, occupational, and recreational sources.[96] Teeth undergoing dissolution from acid may exhibit subtle external changes before diagnosis is finally made. Early signs include a dulling or matte appearance of the enamel followed by a noticeable smoothing of the contours.[97] The affected sites may begin to appear more yellow as the thinning enamel no longer masks the underlying dentin shade. If penetration through the enamel occurs, dimpling or deep cupping at these sights may follow as the exposed dentin will degrade at a faster rate than the surrounding enamel. The areas of the mouth most affected as well as the surfaces of the teeth involved are clinically helpful signs to aid in diagnosis. An endogenic etiology will manifest in changes to the lingual and possibly occlusal aspect of teeth while extrinsic erosion attacks the labial and buccal surfaces first. Sustained or repeated direct contact of the teeth by acidic substances (those with a pH below 5.5) is the common factor in all cases of dental erosion.

ENDOGENIC EROSION

Etiology

Endogenic erosion is due to bathing teeth in stomach acids through passive or active means. Passive introduction of digestive acid to the oral cavity can occur with gastroesophageal reflux disease (GERD), during which gastric and duodenal regurgitation may erode the teeth. Gastroesophageal reflux (GER) is considered normal and is characterized by physiological retrograde flow of gastric contents into the esophagus that occurs after meals for around 1 hour per day. In healthy individuals, esophageal reflux is cleared by esophageal peristalsis and saliva within 1 to 2 minutes.

When GER progresses to cause troublesome symptoms or complications, it is classified as GERD. This disease state can occur during both sleep and waking stages, but most patients who suffer from GERD report that it occurs during sleep. It is during this cycle that the body is ill prepared to offset the acid intrusion; the saliva in the mouth is reduced, diminishing the buffering effect, and swallowing is infrequent. The acid strips away the protective biofilm of the teeth, and the chemical action causes rapid dissolution of exposed tooth surfaces. As the person is in a supine position, it is typical and expected that the teeth most affected are those closest to the esophagus, the lower molars (see Figure 16).

GERD is a potentially dangerous condition that may manifest as Barrett's esophagus, a low-grade and high-grade dysplasia, and is the strongest risk factor for esophageal adenocarcinoma. Dentists may be the first professionals to diagnose the possibility of GERD, particularly when observing unexplained instances of tooth erosion, which might be accompanied by coexisting hyposalivation. The appearance is generally a smoothing of the tooth surface and potential exposure of underlying dentin, even where no antagonist articulates. Existing restorations, particularly amalgam fillings, are not affected by the acid washing and therefore may appear as islands protruding above the eroded surrounding tooth surface.[98–101]

The dental practitioner who is suspicious that a patient may be experiencing GERD should discuss his or her findings with the patient and refer to or consult with the patient's primary care physician for appropriate investigation. Evaluation of the patient for OSA is also advised.

Bulimia nervosa is an eating disorder characterized by frequent vomiting resulting in the dissolution of the tooth surface by gastric acid.[102,103] Because the action is violent, in contrast to GER,

Figure 16.

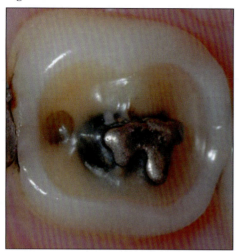

Erosion of a mandibular molar as a consequence of gastroesophageal reflux disease (GERD); note the "island" of amalgam filling unaffected by the acid.
Source: Photo courtesy of Mark Montana.

the acid is projected toward the anterior teeth, where loss of tooth structure is most commonly witnessed. Thin or missing enamel on the lingual aspect of the maxillary anterior teeth is almost pathognomonic for bulimia and is referred to as perimolysis (see Figure 17). When viewed from the facial aspect, teeth may appear more translucent than normal, with thinning edges. Viewed from the lingual aspect, the internal anatomy of the tooth may be visible through the smooth, thin surface layer. Compared with wear from attrition, faceting of the surface is absent as loss of structure from the erosive acid is faster than that from potential grinding, and therefore may mask a potential multifactorial etiology.

It is important to determine if the condition is ongoing or cessation has been achieved. Consultation with the patient's primary care physician is warranted. Extensive cosmetic restorative procedures are not practical for patients who have continuing, chronic problems with vomiting related to bulimia. Often temporary procedures are performed until therapy is conducted and the dysfunctional practices are managed. Clinicians should be aware that eating disorders do recur; therefore, restorative procedures that remove protective layering of teeth may be substituted by additive techniques such as composite bonding or veneering.[104,105]

Prevention

Clinicians should work closely with the patient and the patient's medical providers to identify and treat the underlying cause of the patient's systemic condition. Preventing continuing damage to the teeth is focused upon the act of diluting and preferably neutralizing the acidic incident. Therefore, rinsing with water immediately after vomiting is advised and, if available, adding a teaspoon of baking soda to a glass of water to neutralize the acid.[106] The patient should avoid toothbrushing

Figure 17.

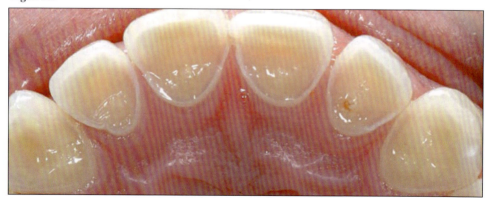

Acid erosion as a result of bulimia. This image is an example of perimolysis.
Source: Photo courtesy of Mark Montana.

for a minimum of 1 hour after vomiting. Individuals with bulimia should limit their intake of low pH drinks and use a straw whenever drinking such beverages. Application of daily neutral sodium fluoride by direct administration with a soft brush or a tray, a 0.05% fluoride rinse, or both, may aid areas that are sensitive or at risk for caries.

Effective communication is crucial to helping patients with bulimia as they may not be open to discussing their disorder. Dental health providers may be the first to discover the condition by detecting changes in the oral condition and therefore must take the first step in helping the individual. It is important to respect the confidentiality of the patient to develop trust, both of which may help to encourage the patient to disclose his or her behaviors and concerns. If the patient is a minor, the parents or guardians of the child should be informed of key dental findings and related concerns. Dental professionals can be instrumental in referring the patient to a psychologist, psychiatrist, licensed clinical social worker, or licensed professional counselor.[107]

EXOGENIC EROSION
Etiology
Exogenic erosion is a modern phenomenon correlating to changes in dietary habits.[108-112] As consumption of highly acidic beverages has dramatically increased, so has the occurrence of this form of structural loss; carbonated drinks and sports drinks are viewed as prime suspects. Although soft drinks (sodas) have been available for a century, it is the introduction of diet sodas that led to both increased, as well as slow and continuous "guiltless" consumption of these beverages, often directly from the container. Many sodas have a pH value (generally between 2 to 3.5) much closer to stomach acid (pH of 1) than to water (pH of 7) and diet sodas promote habitual change: consumers often drink them daily—sometimes throughout the day—as they do not add calories or become syrupy if not consumed immediately (see Figure 18). For many, sodas have become a substitute for other beverages, including water, tea, or coffee; sports drinks are often perceived as "healthy" because they are consumed by athletes.[113]

Exogenic erosion may also be attributed to fruit juices, wine, citrus fruits, chewable vitamin C tablets, yogurt, or any consumable product with a low pH, if ingestion is sustained or repeated. Many food choices that might have been historically regional or rare are now available in all places and times in most developed countries, enabling consistent consumption.

Saliva secretion will reflexively increase when acid enters the mouth to buffer the lower pH. However, this ability is not without limits and may be inadequate to buffer sustained acid attack. Also, many individuals suffer from a reduced saliva flow or a reduced quality of saliva and are therefore at greater risk for erosion of their teeth if acid is repeatedly introduced (see Figure 6A, earlier).

Prevention
Prevention of exogenous erosion is dependent upon educating patients about risk behaviors and providing appropriate suggestions for behavioral modification. Prognosis is entirely up to the willingness of individuals to modify their lifestyle. For all people, whether or not they are clinically diagnosed as having eroded teeth, the strategy for preventing erosion is as follows:

- Reduce intake of low pH foods and especially beverages, and limit the amount and prolonged or continuous intake of these beverages.

Figure 18.

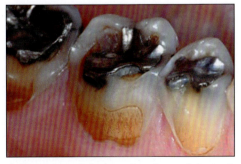

Acid erosion of the buccal surfaces of the teeth due to excessive soda consumption. The tooth surface is eroded away from the amalgam filling which is unaffected.

Source: Photo courtesy of Mark Montana.

- Whenever possible, consume acidic beverages using a straw.
- Dilute acidic intake at all times; this means sipping water with meals, and rinsing with water after meals or during or after consuming low pH beverages.
- Avoid brushing teeth for at least 30 minutes after meals to minimize the scrubbing away of temporarily softened tooth structure. [114-116]

ABFRACTION

Abfraction is defined as pathological loss of hard tooth substance caused by biomechanical loading forces resulting in flexure and chemical fatigue degradation of the enamel, dentin, or both, at a point remote from the loading force. [117,118] Whether abfraction is an actual process has been contested by those who believe that abrasion, specifically toothbrush abrasion with recession and dentin exposure, is the cause of the noncarious cervical lesion (NCCL) and not tooth flexure, and those who believe it occurs due to loading forces.

For clinicians, there are discoveries that are difficult to dismiss: one tooth is found with a notch-shaped lesion while the adjacent teeth have none, or a posterior tooth in cross-bite or edge-to-edge occlusion exhibits this defect, but not the surrounding teeth in norma-occlusion (see Figure 19). Another anomaly is the near absence of NCCL lesions on the lingual aspect of teeth, despite patients who brush this side as thoroughly.

In argument against the theory, some point to a lack of historical findings predating modern toothbrushing as proof that it is a scrubbing abrasion. Others state that there is a scarcity of such lesions in patients with bruxism; thus, occlusal stress cannot be the cause. In considering these viewpoints, we must recall that before modern diets, even our recent ancestors suffered significant wear of their occluding surfaces as well as interdental contacts, resulting in flattened anatomy and elimination of cusp inclines, reducing the chances of biomechanical loading forces. Also, the concept of abfraction requires the buildup of potential energy in the tooth (which then releases at the weakest point, the cementoenamel junction), where the enamel is

Figure 19.

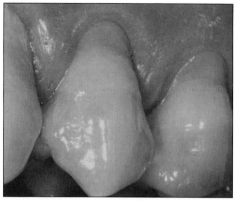

Abfraction lesions characterized by sharp edges and, in this patient, limited to few of the teeth.
Source: Photo courtesy of Mark Montana.

thinnest. Patients with bruxism are moving their jaws and so a necessary buildup of stress never occurs; thus, in theory, abfraction lesions would not be found in bruxing individuals.

There is currently no agreement on the existence of abfraction, and no viable means to test the veracity of these theories. The role of the clinician is to identify the lesion and distinguish it as either caries or an NCCL. In the absence of caries, the decision about whether to restore is typically based on the depth of the lesion and the dentist's interpretation of risk to the tooth. Because the majority of the defect occurs in the cementum and dentin, direct restorations are typically not placed unless the lesion is deep into the tooth. Clinicians should identify and document the presence of the lesion as well as the severity of the defect. Despite lack of consensus, toothbrush technique and materials, occlusal relationship, and possible parafunctional behavior must be considered as possible causes and patients advised accordingly.

MULTIFACTORIAL ETIOLOGY

It is possible that the aforementioned mechanisms of wear may act independently. However, the common finding is a combination of two or more of these causations at work, suggesting a multifactorial etiology of tooth wear (see Figure 20). For example, people who brush their teeth immediately after drinking an erosive beverage will suffer accelerated abrasion as the surface of the tooth is demineralized: an erosion-abrasion etiology. People with GERD may also exhibit nocturnal bruxism resulting in accelerated attrition of the softened occlusal surfaces: erosion-attrition etiology. Consider the example of a finding of attrition of the lower molars but not the opposing maxillary molars: a paradox unless the mandibular teeth are selectively softened during GERD and bruxism. Patients with bulimia may brush more vigorously in an attempt to rid their teeth of the yellowing appearance and, instead, hasten the color change they are seeking to reverse: erosion-abrasion etiology.

The dental team must therefore look beyond such simple diagnoses as wear, bruxism, or occlusal disease. Instead, a careful analysis of the mechanism of wear is required. Understanding these causes, their interactions, and manifestations will help the dental team institute proper prevention and treatment methods.

SUMMARY

Wear and tear to the periodontium primarily occurs as a result of trauma, the cause of which should be identified early, before significant tissue loss occurs. Trauma may be self-inflicted, such as that observed with overly aggressive toothbrushing technique; accidental, such as inadvertently allowing tooth-bleaching gels to come into contact with the gingiva; or iatrogenic, as observed with a poorly fitting oral appliance. Soft tissue trauma may present as localized recession, abrasion, ulcerations, or burns. Clinicians must perform a thorough history and clinical assessment to identify the etiology of the trauma. Trauma and irritation of the gingival tissue may lead to inflammatory changes, resulting in recession and exposure of the underlying tooth structure. A major contributing factor to chronic gingival inflammation is smoking, which provides clinicians with the opportunity to include smoking cessation education as a critical preventive message during oral health education.

Appropriate corrective measures should be implemented to prevent additional tissue loss. These measures include oral hygiene education using demonstration of proper techniques with toothbrushing, flossing, and other oral hygiene aids. Patients must be taught to use a soft bristled toothbrush, avoid use of a scrubbing motion, adapt the brush along the gingival margin, and apply only light pressure while brushing. Patients should also be encouraged to demonstrate their self-care techniques while cleaning between the teeth so that the clinician may evaluate dexterity and ability to remove biofilm effectively while preventing trauma to the interdental tissues.

Mucogingival deformities create challenges when performing effective biofilm removal along

Figure 20.

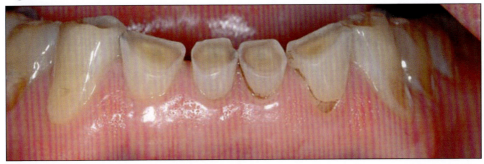

Most commonly, the clinical manifestations of wear represent more than one etiology. In this example, evidence of attrition and abrasion are evident; however, it is likely that acid erosion is a cofactor as well.

Source: Photo courtesy of Mark Montana.

the gingival margin. For these patients, corrective surgery may be warranted to help prevent additional tissue loss. Poorly constructed dental restorations, crowns, or both, need to be replaced to help restore tissue health and cleansibility. Correction of habits, such as fingernail biting or sucking on pens, should also be addressed with the patient, and the wearing of intraoral jewelry discouraged.

The loss of hard tooth structure may be attributed to one or more mechanisms, including attrition, abrasion, erosion, and abfraction. Most commonly, it is a combination of two or more of these factors. An accurate differential diagnosis is therefore essential to provide effective prevention and treatment. Because abrasion and exogenic erosion are largely preventable conditions requiring changes in habit and lifestyle, the emphasis from the dental community should be education and instruction of clinicians, patients, and the population at large.

Extrinsic erosion, in particular, plays a major synergistic role when combined with abrasion and attrition and is, without doubt, the most easily prevented. Simply making healthier beverage choices is a profound step, and when an acidic beverage is desired, patients should be taught to limit the number consumed and to drink quickly or use a straw to reduce the duration of acid attack. Drinking water with meals and alternating sips with an adjoining acidic beverage will dilute the acid and raise the pH in the oral cavity. Remembering to rinse with water after meals instead of brushing will remove acid and lingering sugars and allow time for dental structures to remineralize.

Abrasion may be reduced if as noted, erosion is prevented. Further, changing the schedule of brushing, choosing soft brushes, and using appropriate toothbrush technique are all simple and inexpensive steps to reducing this form of wear.

For patients suffering damage from abrasion and erosion, cessation of causation is of greater importance than restoration; it is more important to preserve what remains. Restoration without cessation caries a poorer prognosis as even the best fitting crown or filling margins are potential sites for breakdown, particularly from acids. Those patients who present with a history of oral damage resulting from GERD, bulimia, bruxism, alcoholism, and other nondental conditions require coordination of care with medical, physical, or psychosocial therapists to provide effective treatment.

The loss of tooth structure has been shown to be consistent with human history; however, the nature of wear today differs greatly from that in the past. Wearing away of enamel, dentin, and cementum are no longer consequences of the act of survival but commonly result from a marriage of poor choices, bad habits, and misinformation. Fortunately, prevention of most wear is simple, inexpensive, and available to everyone, requiring no painful sacrifices. By encouraging only limited consumption of acidic beverages, neutralization of the effects of acids by rinsing the mouth with water, and proper, nondestructive oral self-care, the dental team can negate the risk of most causes of tooth structure loss. Identifying the characteristics of the different causes of wear and the likelihood that more than one is at work in an individual enhances early diagnosis, and therefore management through prevention.

REFERENCES

1. Armitage GC. Development of a classification system for periodontal diseases and conditions. *Ann Periodontol.* 1999;4:1–6.
2. Holmstrup P. Non-plaque-induced gingival lesions. *Ann Periodontol.* 1999;4:20–29.
3. Rawal SY, Claman LJ, Kalmar JR, Tatakis DN. Traumatic lesions of the gingiva: a case series. *J Periodontol.* 2004;75:762–769.
4. Onur OM, Haytac C, Akkaya M. Iatrogenic trauma to oral tissues. *J Periodontol.* 2005;76:1793–1797.
5. Chambrone LI, Chambrone LA. Gingival recessions caused by lip piercing: case report. *J Can Dent Assoc.* 2003;69:505–508.
6. Dibart SI, De Feo P, Surabian G, Hart A, Capri D, Su MF. Oral piercing and gingival recession: review of the literature and a case report. *Quintessence Int.* 2002;33:110–112.
7. Campbell AI, Moore A, Williams E, Stephens J, Tatakis DN. Tongue piercing: impact of time and barbell stem length on lingual gingival recession and tooth chipping. *J Periodontol.* 2002;73:289–297.
8. Brooks JK, Hooper KA, Reynolds MA. Formation of mucogingival defects associated with intraoral and peri-

oral piercing. *J Am Dent Assoc.* 2003;134:837–843.
9. Kassab MM, Cohen RE. The etiology and prevalence of gingival recession. *J Am Dent Assoc.* 2003;134: 220–225.
10. Albandar JM, Kingman A. Gingival recession, gingival bleeding, and dental calculus in adults 30 years of age and older in the United States. *J Periodontol.* 1999;70:1988–1994.
11. Susin C, Haas AN, Oppermann RV, Haugejorden O, Albandar JM. Gingival recession: epidemiology and risk indicators in a representative urban Brazilian population. *J Periodontol.* 2004;75:1377–1386.
12. Rios FS, Costa RSA, Moura MS, Jardim JJ, Maltz M, Haas AN. Estimates and multivariable risk assessment of gingival recession in the population of adults from Porto Alegre, Brazil. *J Clin Periodontol.* 2014;41:1098–1107. doi: 10.1111/jcpe.12303.
13. Toker H, Ozdemir H. Gingival recession: epidemiology and risk indicators in a university dental hospital in Turkey. *Int J Dent Hyg.* 2009;7:115–120.
14. Alexandre S, Bourgeois D, Katsahian S, et al. Risk assessment for buccal gingival recession defects in an adult population. *J Periodontol.* 2010;81:1419–1425.
15. Chrysanthakopoulos NA. Prevalence and associated factors of gingival recession in Greek adults. *J Invest Clin Dent.* 2013;4:178–185.
16. Pradeep K, Rajababu P, Satyanarayana D, Sagar, V. Gingival recession: review and strategies in treatment of recession. *Case Rep Dent.* 2012;2012:563421. doi: 10.1155/2012/563421.
17. Dababneh RH, Khouri AT, Addy M. Dentine hypersensitivity—an enigma? A review of terminology, epidemiology, mechanisms, aetiology and management. *Br Dent J.* 1999;187:606–611.
18. Hinrichs, JE, Kotsakis G. Classification of diseases and conditions affecting the periodontium. In: Newman MG, Takei H, Klokkevold PR, Carranza FA, eds. *Carranza's Clinical Periodontology.* 12th ed. St Louis, MO: Elsevier/Saunders; 2015:45–67.
19. Zlataric DK, Celebic A, Valentic-Peruzovic M. The effect of removable partial dentures on periodontal health of abutment and non-abutment teeth. *J Periodontol.* 2002;73:137.
20. Chan HL, Chun YP, MacEachern M, Oates TW. Does gingival recession require surgical treatment? *Dent Clin North Am.* 2015;59:981–996.
21. Danser MM, Timmerman MF, IJzerman Y, et al: Evaluation of the incidence of gingival abrasion as a result of toothbrushing. *J Clin Periodontol.* 1998;25:701.
22. Offenbacher S, Barros SP, Singer RE, et al: Periodontal disease at the biofilm-gingival interface. *J Periodontol.* 2007;78:1911.
23. Serino G, Wennstrom JL, Lindhe J, Eneroth L. The prevalence and distribution of gingival recession in subjects with a high standard of oral hygiene. *J Clin Periodontol.* 1994;21:57–63.
24. Carlos MC, Muyco MM, Caliwag ML, Fajardo JA, Uy HG. The prevalence and distribution of gingival recession among U.E. dental students with a high standard of oral hygiene. *J Philipp Dent Assoc.* 1995;47:27–48.
25. Goutoudi P, Koidis PT, Konstantinidis A. Gingival recession: a cross-sectional clinical investigation. *Eur J Prosthodont Rest Dent.* 1997;5:57–61.
26. Khocht A, Simon G, Person P, Denepitiya JL. Gingival recession in relation to history of hard toothbrush use. *J Periodontol.*1993;64:900–905.
27. Zimmer S, Öztürk M, Barthel CR, Bizhang M, Jordan RA. Cleaning efficacy and soft tissue trauma after use of manual toothbrushes with different bristle stiffness. *J Periodontol.* 2011;82:267–271.
28. Rosema NA, Adam R, Grender JM, Van der Sluijs E, Supranoto SC, Van der Weijden GA. Gingival abrasion and recession in manual and oscillating–rotating power brush users. *Int J Dent Hyg.* 2014;12:257–266.
29. McCracken GI, Heasman L, Stacey F, et al. The impact of powered and manual toothbrushing on incipient gingival recession. *J Clin Periodontol.* 2009;36:950–957.
30. Sälzer S, Graetz C, Plaumann A, et al. Effect of a multidirectional power and a manual toothbrush in subjects susceptible to gingival recession: a 12-month randomized controlled clinical study. *J Periodontol.* 2016;16:1–15.
31. Rajapakse PS, McCracken GI, Gwynnett E, Steen ND, Guentsch A, Heasman PA. Does tooth brushing influence the development and progression of non-inflammatory gingival recession? A systematic review. *J Clin Periodontol.* 2007;34:1046–1061.
32. Heasman PA, Holliday R, Bryant A, Preshaw PM. Evidence for the occurrence of gingival recession and non-carious cervical lesions as a consequence of traumatic toothbrushing. *J Clin Periodontol.* 2015;42(suppl 16):S237–S255. doi: 10.1111/jcpe.12330.
33. Renkema AM, Fudalej PS, Renkema AAP, Abbas F, Bronkhorst E, Katsaros C. Gingival labial recessions in orthodontically treated and untreated individuals—a pilot case–control study. *J Clin Periodontol.* 2013;40:631–637. doi: 10.1111/jcpe.12105.
34. Renkema AM, Fudalej PS, Renkema A, Kiekens R, Katsaros C. Development of labial gingival recessions in orthodontically treated patients. *Am J Ortho Dentofac Orthop.* 2013;143:206–212.
35. Aziz T, Flores-Mir C. A systematic review of the association between appliance-induced labial movement of mandibular incisors and gingival recession. *Aust Orthod J.* 2011;27:33–39.
36. Joss-Vassalli I, Grebenstein C, Topouzelis N, et al: Orthodontic therapy and gingival recession: a systematic review. *Orthod Craniofac Res.* 2010;13:127–141.
37. Hinrichs JE, Math VT. The role of dental calculus and other local predisposing factors. In: Newman MG, Takei H, Klokkevold PR, Carranza FA, eds. *Carranza's Clinical Periodontology.* 12th ed. St. Louis, MO: Elsevier/Saunders; 2015:116–131.

38. Ozcelik, O, Haytac MC, Akkaya M. Iatrogenic trauma to oral tissue. *J Periodontol.* 2005;76:1793-1797.
39. Monten U, Wennstrom JL, Ramberg P. Periodontal conditions in male adolescents using smokeless tobacco (moist snuff). *J Clin Periodontol.* 2006;33:863–868.
40. Tomar SL, Winn DM. Chewing tobacco use and dental caries among U.S. men. *J Am Dent Assoc.* 1999;130:1601–1610.
41. Plessas, A, Pepelassi E. Dental and periodontal complications of lip and tongue piercing: prevalence and influencing factors. *Aust Dent J.* 2012;57:71–78. doi: 10.1111/j.1834-7819.2011.01647.x.
42. Fiorellini JP, Stathopoulou PG. Anatomy of the periodontium. In: Newman MG, Takei H, Klokkevold PR, Carranza FA, eds. *Carranza's Clinical Periodontology.* 12th ed. St. Louis, MO: Elsevier/Saunders; 2015:9–39.
43. Wolf HF, Hassell TM. *Color Atlas of Dental Hygiene.* Stuttgart, Germany: Thieme; 2006:155–164.
44. Chambrone L, Sukekava F, Araújo MG, Pustiglioni FE, Chambrone LA, Lima LA. Root coverage procedures for the treatment of localised recession-type defects. *Cochrane Database Syst Rev.* 2009(2):CD007161. doi: 10.1002/14651858.CD007161.pub2.
45. Richardson CR, Allen EP, Chambrone L, et al., Periodontal soft tissue root coverage procedures: practical applications from the AAP regeneration workshop. *Clin Adv Perio.* 2015;5:1,2–10.
46. Tonetti MS, Jepsen S. Clinical efficacy of periodontal plastic surgery procedures: consensus report of group 2 of the 10th European Workshop on Periodontology. *J Clin Periodontol.* 2014;41(suppl 15):S36–S43. doi:10.1111/jcpe.12219.
47. Addy M, Shellis RP. Interaction between attrition, abrasion and erosion in tooth wear. *Monogr Oral Sci.* 2006;20:17–31.
48. Kaidonis, JA. Tooth wear: the view of the anthropologist. *Clin Oral Investig.* 2008;12(suppl 1):21–26.
49. Bader G, Lavigne G. Sleep bruxism; an overview of an oromandibular sleep movement disorder. *Sleep Med Rev.* 2000;4:27–43.
50. Butler JH. Occlusal adjustment. *Dent Dig.* 1970;76 422–426.
51. Frumker SC. Occlusion and muscle tension. *Basal Facts.* 1981;4:85–87.
52. Holmgren K, Sheikholeslam A. Occlusal adjustment and myoelectric activity of the jaw elevator muscles in patients with nocturnal bruxism and craniomandibular disorders. *Scand J Dent Res.* 1994;102:238–243.
53. Landry ML, Rompré PH, Manzini C, Guitard F, de Grandmont P, Lavigne GJ. Reduction of sleep bruxism using a mandibular advancement device: an experimental controlled study. *Int J Prosthodont.* 2006;19:549–556.
54. Clark GT, Beemsterboer PL, Solberg WK, Rugh JD. Nocturnal electromyographic evaluation of myofascial pain dysfunction in patients undergoing occlusal splint therapy. *J Am Dent Assoc.* 1979;99:607–611.
55. Sarita PTN, Kreulen CM, Witter DJ, van't Hof M, Creugers NHC. A study on occlusal stability in shortened dental arches. *Int J Prosthodont.* 2003;16:375–380.
56. Smith BGN, Knight JK. Toothwear: aetiology and diagnosis. *Dent Update.* 1989;16:204–212.
57. Benazzi S, Nguyen HN, Schulz D, et al. The evolutionary paradox of tooth wear: simply destruction or inevitable adaptation? *PLoS ONE.* 2013;8:e62263.
58. Eliasson S, Richter S. Tooth wear in medieval Icelanders. The XXth Nordic Medical Congress, Program Abstracts, pp. 49, Abstract 32, 2005.
59. Seghi RR, Rosenstiel SF, Bauer P. Abrasion of human enamel by different dental ceramics *in vitro. J Dent Res.*1991;70:221–225.
60. Dahl BL, Oilo G. *In vivo* wear ranking of some restorative materials. *Quintessence Int.* 1994;25:561–565.
61. Janyavula S, Lawson N, Cakir D, Beck P, Ramp LC, Burgess JO. The wear of polished and glazed zirconia against enamel. *J Prosthet Dent.* 2013;109:22–29.
62. Park JH, Park S, Lee K, Yun KD, Lim HP. Antagonist wear of three CAD/CAM anatomic contour zirconia ceramics. *J Prosthet Dent.* 2014;111:20–29.
63. Luangruangrong P, Cook NB, Sabrah AH, Hara AT, Bottino MC. Influence of full-contour zirconia surface roughness on wear of glass-ceramics. *J Prosthodont.* 2014;23:198–205.
64. Hmaidouch R, Weigl P. Tooth wear against ceramic crowns in posterior region: a systematic literature review. *Int J Oral Sci.* 2013;5:183–190.
65. Miyazaki T, Nakamura T, Matsumura H, Ban S, Kobayashi T. Current status of zirconia restoration. *J Prosth Res.* 2013;57:236–261.
66. Olivera AB, Matson E, Marques MM. The effect of glazed and polished ceramics on human enamel wear. *Int J Prosthodont.* 2006;19:547–548.
67. Jagger DC, Harrison A. An in vitro investigation into the wear effects of unglazed, glazed, and polished porcelain on human enamel. *J Prosthetic Dent.*1994;72: 320–323.
68. Avey KD, DeBiase CB, Gladwin MA, Kao EC, Bagby MD. Development of a standardized abrasive scale: an analysis of commercial prophylaxis pastes. *J Dent Hyg.* 2006;80:21.
69. Biller IR, Hunter EL, Featherstone MJ, Silverstone LM. Enamel loss during a prophylaxis polish in vitro. *J Int Assoc Dent Child.* 1980;11:7–12.
70. Rühling A, Wulf J, Schwahn C, Kocher T. Surface wear on cervical restorations and adjacent enamel and root cementum caused by simulated long-term maintenance therapy. *J Clin Periodontol.* 2004;31:293–298.
71. Stookey GK. In vitro estimates of enamel and dentin abrasion associated with a prophylaxis. *J Dent Res.* 1978;57:36.
72. Christensen RP, Bangerter VW. Immediate and long-term in vivo effects of polishing on enamel and dentin. *J Prosthet Dent.* 1987;57:150–160.

73. Thompson RE, Way DC. Enamel loss due to prophylaxis and multiple bonding/debonding of orthodontic attachments. *Am J Orthod.* 1981;79:282–295.
74. Pence SD, Chambers DA, van Tets IG, Wolf RC, Pfeiffer DC. Repetitive coronal polishing yields minimal enamel loss. *J Dent Hyg.* 2011;85:348–357.
75. Barnes CM. The science of polishing. *Dimensions of Dental Hygiene.* 2009;7(11):18–20.
76. Nagel Beebe S. To polish or not to polish: understanding the principle and the pros and cons of selective polishing. *Dimensions of Dental Hygiene.* 2009;7(3):32–35.
77. Frame PS, Sawai R, Bowen WH, Meyerowitz C. Preventive dentistry: practitioner's recommendations for low-risk patients compared with scientific evidence and practice guidelines. *Am J Prev Med.* 2000;18:159–162.
78. Zanatta FB, Pinto TMP, Kantorski KZ, Rösing CK. Plaque, gingival bleeding and calculus formation after supragingival scaling with and without polishing: a randomised clinical trial. *Oral Health Prev Dent.* 2011;9:275–280.
79. Worthington HV, Clarkson JE, Bryan G, Beirne PV. Routine scale and polish for periodontal health in adults. *Cochrane Database Syst Rev.* 2013;(11):CD004625. doi:10.1002/14651858.CD004625.pub4.
80. Slot DE. Insufficient evidence to determine the effects of routine scale and polish treatments. *Evid Based Dent.* 2014;15:74–75.
81. Graumann SJ, Sensat ML, Stoltenberg JL. Air polishing: a review of current literature. *J Dent Hyg.* 2013;87:173–180.
82. Petersilka GJ, Bell M, Mehl A, Hickel R, Flemming TF. Root defects following air polishing. An in vitro study on the effects of working parameters. *J Clin Periodontol.* 2003;30:165–170.
83. Agger MS, Hörsted-Bindslev P, Hovgaard O. Abrasiveness of an air-powder polishing system on root surfaces in vitro. *Quintessence Int.* 2001;32:407–411.
84. Pikdoken ML, Ozcelik C. Severe enamel abrasion due to misuse of an air polishing device. *Int J Dent Hyg.* 2006;4:209–212.
85. Tada K, Kakuta K, Ogura H, Sato S. Effect of particle diameter on air polishing of dentin surfaces. *Odontology.* 2010;98:31–36.
86. Tada K, Wiroj S, Inatomi M, Sato S. The characterization of dentin defects produced by air polishing, *Odontology.* 2012;100:41–46.
87. Bühler J, Amato M, Weiger R, Walter C. A systematic review on the effects of air polishing devices on oral tissues. *Int J Dent Hyg.* 2015;14:15–28.
88. Addy M, Griffiths G, Dummer P, Kingdon A, Shaw WC. The distribution of plaque and gingivitis and the influence of brushing hand in a group of 11-12 year old school children. *J Clin Periodontol.* 1987;14:564–572.
89. Addy M. Tooth brushing, tooth wear and dentine hypersensitivity—are they associated? *Int Dent J.* 2005;55(suppl 1):261–267.
90. Addy M, West NX. The role of toothpaste in the aetiology and treatment of dentine hypersensitivity. *Monogr Oral Sci.* 2013;23:75–87.
91. Abrahamsen TC. The worn dentition pathognomonic patterns of abrasion and erosion. *Int Dent J.* 2005;55:268–276.
92. Grippo JO, Simring M, Schreiner S. Attrition, abrasion, corrosion and abfraction revisited: a new perspective on tooth surface lesions. *J Am Dent Assoc.* 2004;135:1109–1118.
93. Schemelhorn BR, Moore MH, Putt MS. Abrasion, polishing, and stain removal characteristics of various commercial dentifrices in vitro. *J Clin Dent.* 2011;22:11–18.
94. Dörfer CE, Hefferren J, Gonz lez-Cabezas C, Imfeld T, Addy M. Methods to determine dentifrice abrasiveness. Summary proceedings of a workshop in Frankfurt, Germany. *J Clin Dent.* 2010;21(suppl):S1–S16. Available at: http://www.gaba-dent.de/data/docs/en/6848/JCD-21-Suppl-RDA-Suppl.pdf.
95. Wiegand A, Egert S, Attin T. Toothbrushing before or after an acidic challenge to minimize tooth wear? An in situ/ex vivo study. *Am J Dent.* 2008;21:13–16.
96. ten Cate JM, Imfeld T. Dental erosion, summary. *Eur J Oral Sci.* 1996;104(part 2):241–244.
97. Johansson AK, Omar R, Carlsson GE, Johansson A. Dental erosion and its growing importance in clinical practice: from past to present. *Int J Dent.* 2012;2012.632907.
98. Wang GR, Zhang H, Wang ZG, Jiang GS, Guo CH. Relationship between dental erosion and respiratory symptoms in patients with gastro-oesophageal reflux disease. *J Dent.* 2010;38:892–898.
99. Schlueter N, Hardt M, Klimek J, Ganss C. Influence of the digestive enzymes trypsin and pepsin in vitro on the progression of erosion in dentine. *Arch Oral Biol.* 2010;55:294–299.
100. Bartlett DW, Evans DF, Anggiansah A, Smith BG. A study of the association between gastro-oesophageal reflux and palatal dental erosion. *Br Dent J.* 1996;181:125–131.
101. Ranjitkar S, Kaidonis JA, Smales RJ. Gastroesophageal reflux disease and tooth erosion. *Int J Dent.* 2012;2012:479850.
102. Öhrn R, Enzell K, Angmar-Månsson B. Oral status of 81 subjects with eating disorders. *Eur J Oral Sci.* 1999;107:157–163.
103. Johansson AK, Norring C, Unell L, Johansson A. Eating disorders and oral health: a matched case-control study. *Eur J Oral Sci.* 2012;120:61–9.
104. Briggs P, Bishop K, Kelleher M. Case report: the use of indirect composite for the management of extensive erosion. *Eur J Prosthodont Rest Dent.* 1994;3:51–54.
105. Burke FJ, Kelleher MG, Wilson N, Bishop K. Introducing the concept of pragmatic esthetics, with special reference to the treatment of tooth wear. *J Esthetic Rest Dent.* 2011;23:277–293.
106. Messias DC, Turssi CP, Hara AT, Serra MC. Sodium

bicarbonate solution as an anti-erosive agent against simulated endogenous erosion. *Eur J Oral Sci.* 2010;118:385–388.
107. Burkhart NW. Bulimia: decreasing the damage to enamel. Available at: http://www.rdhmag.com/articles/print/volume-31/issue-1/columns/bulimia-decreasing-the-damage-to-enamel.html. Accessed August 10, 2016.
108. Khan F, Young WG, Law V, Priest J, Daley TJ. Cupped lesions of early onset dental erosion in young southeast Queensland adults. *Aust Dent J.* 2001;46:100–107.
109. Hemingway CA, Parker DM, Addy M, Barbour ME. Erosion of enamel by non-carbonated soft drinks with and without toothbrushing abrasion. *Br Dent J.* 2006;201:447–450.
110. Jacobson MF. Liquid candy: how soft drinks are harming Americans' health. 2005. Available at: http://www.cspinet.org/new/pdf/liquid_candy_final_w_new_supplement.pdf. Accessed August 10, 2016.
111. Harnack L, Stang J, Story M. Soft drink consumption among US children and adolescents: nutritional consequences. *J Am Dietetic Assoc.* 1999;99:436–441.
112. Messer LB, Young WG. Childhood diet and dental erosion. In: Khan F, Young WG, eds. *Tooth Wear. The ABC of the Worn Dentition.* Chichester, UK: Wiley-Blackwell; 2011:34–49.
113. Milosevic A. Sports drinks hazard to teeth. *Br J Sports Med.* 1997;31:28–30.
114. Jaeggi T, Lussi A. Toothbrush abrasion of erosively altered enamel after intraoral exposure to saliva: an in situ study. *Caries Res.* 1999;33:455–461.
115. Rios D, Honorio HM, Magalhães AC, et al. Influence of toothbrushing on enamel softening and abrasive wear of eroded bovine enamel: an in situ study. *Braz Oral Res.* 2006;20:148–154.
116. Johansson AK, Lingstrom P, Imfeld T, Birkhed D. Influence of drinking method on tooth-surface pH in relation to dental erosion. *Eur J Oral Sci.* 2004;112:484–489.
117. Grippo JO. Abfraction: a new classification of hard tissue lesions of teeth. *J Esth Dent.* 1991;3:14–18.
118. Aubry M, Maffart B, Donat B, Brau JJ. Brief communication: study of noncarious cervical tooth lesions in samples of prehistoric, historic and modern populations from the South of France. *Am J Phys Anthropol.* 2003;121:10–14.

Chapter 7
Head and Neck Cancers

Jacquelyn Fried

Oral health professionals have a responsibility to help reduce the morbidity and mortality associated with head and neck cancers (HNCs). Globally, head and neck carcinomas are the sixth most common cancer in developed countries.[1,2] In the United States, HNCs rank eighth among men, with men experiencing twice as many cases as women.[3] Survival rates for oral cancers have been relatively unchanged for three decades. Early detection remains elusive. In the United States, between 2005 and 2011, only 62.5% of all patients with HNCs survived for 5 years.[4] Oropharyngeal cancers (OPCs) associated with the human papillomavirus (HPV) have shown more promising survival rates than HPV-negative oral cancers, but early detection is difficult because a premalignant state is as yet unidentifiable and lesion sites are less accessible visually.

Oral health professionals must understand the threats posed by HNCs, take positive actions to combat them, and strive to educate other healthcare providers about the importance of screening for HNCs and referring, when appropriate. HNC is a condition that affects many aspects of a patient's life. Ensuring a patient's ability to eat, speak, realize psychosocial well-being, and maintain strength falls within the purview of many healthcare providers. Speech pathologists, oncologists, nurses, dentists, dietitians, and dental hygienists are healthcare providers who can work together to make basic patient needs attainable. Through awareness, education, and action, the collaborative healthcare team can help address and prevent HNCs. This chapter provides a comprehensive framework to guide oral and nonoral health professionals as they strive to reduce the incidence and prevalence of HNCs and their associated morbidity and mortality.

EPIDEMIOLOGY

HNCs are a broad grouping of malignancies that include cancers of the oral cavity and cancers of the oropharynx (OPCs). The latter are commonly associated with HPV. Since the etiologic pathways for "traditional" carcinogen-induced oral cancers and HPV-driven OPCs are different, some researchers have designated them as two different disease entities.[5] While the incidence of oral cavity cancers in the United States has decreased over the past 15 years, the number of new OPCs has risen at an alarming rate.[6] An incidence of approximately 15,500 new cases of HPV-associated oropharynx cancer is anticipated in the United States per year.[4] Between 1988 and 2004, in the United States, oral cancers declined by 50% while OPCs increased by 225%.[7] These statistical findings have been attributed to changes in lifestyle, decreased tobacco use, and increased practices of high-risk sexual behaviors (see Figure 1).

In 2012, an estimated 291,108 people were living with oral cavity and pharyngeal cancer in the United States.[4] Oral and oropharyngeal cancer rates are higher for men than for women. Hispanic and black men suffer more oral cancers than do whites. Oral cancers have long been associated with African-American elderly men of low socioeconomic status who use tobacco and alcohol, whereas the typical HPV-OPC patient is a white man, in his early 50s, of the middle-income bracket, with little to no history of alcohol and tobacco use.[5] Although HNC rates increase with age, the median age for HPV-OPCs is lower than that for "traditional" carcinogen-induced oral cancers. Additionally, comorbidities such as tobacco use do lessen survival rates for HPV-induced HNCs.[8] Figure 2 and Table 1 show the number of new cases between 2008 and 2012 by age and ethnicity, while Figure 3 displays mortality rates by age for the same time period.

OPC rates have risen dramatically in economically developed countries, including Canada, England, Sweden, and Australia.[7] OPC is the 11th most common cancer worldwide.[9] In light of the rampant increase in OPCs with no plateau in sight, the late stage of HNC detection,

CHAPTER 7   Head and Neck Cancers

low survival rates, an aging population more vulnerable to cancer, and the prevalence of HNCs globally, addressing measures to prevent, detect, and reduce HNCs and associated morbidity and mortality are critical.

ETIOLOGY AND RISK FACTORS

The specific etiologic factors that give rise to HNCs and the degree to which they contribute vary from person to person. A combination of lifestyle habits, genetics, epigenetics, and many unknowns may be

Figure 1. New Cases, Deaths, and 5-Year Relative Survival for Oral Cavity and Pharynx Cases*

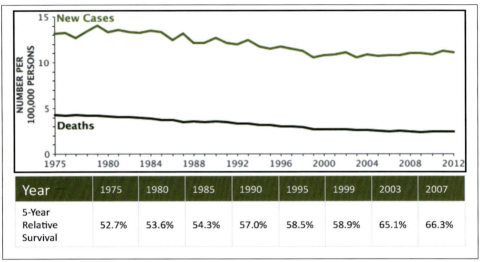

Year	1975	1980	1985	1990	1995	1999	2003	2007
5-Year Relative Survival	52.7%	53.6%	54.3%	57.0%	58.5%	58.9%	65.1%	66.3%

*Using statistical models for analysis, rates for new oral cavity and pharynx cancer cases have been stable over the last 10 years. Death rates have been stable over 2003–2012. 5-year survival trends are shown below the graph.
Source: National Cancer Institute. SEER stat fact sheets: oral cavity and pharynx cancer. Available at: http://seer.cancer.gov/statfacts/html/oralcav.html. Accessed March 24, 2016.

Figure 2. Percent of New Cases by Age Group: Oral Cavity and Pharynx Cancer, 2008–2012, All Races, Both Sexes

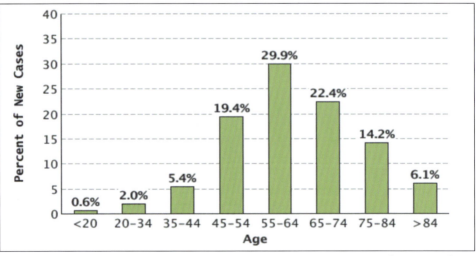

Source: National Cancer Institute. SEER stat fact sheets: oral cavity and pharynx cancer. Available at: http://seer.cancer.gov/statfacts/html/oralcav.html. Accessed March 24, 2016.

Table 1. Number of New Cases per 100,000 Persons by Race/Ethnicity and Sex: Oral Cavity and Pharynx Cancer, 2008–2012

Male	Race	Female
16.5	All races	6.3
17.1	White	6.4
14.6	Black	5.2
11.0	Asian/Pacific Islander	4.9
13.2	American Indian/Alaska Native	5.2
10.1	Hispanic	4.0
17.6	Non-Hispanic	6.6

Source: National Cancer Institute. SEER stat fact sheets: oral cavity and pharynx cancer. Available at: http://seer.cancer.gov/statfacts/html/oralcav.html. Accessed March 24, 2016.

Table 2. Etiology and Risk Factors for Head and Neck Cancers

- Tobacco use (smoked or smokeless)*
- Alcohol use*
- Combined tobacco and alcohol use*
- Use of any nicotine acquisition product*
- Practice of high-risk sexual behaviors*
- Exposure to ultraviolet light*
- Exposure to environmental or consumption of toxins*
- Family history of cancer
- Personal history of cancer
- Age
- Gender
- Race
- Immunosuppression
- Oral mucosal conditions

*Modifiable risk factors.

part of the equation. Some oral cavity and oropharyngeal cancers have no clear cause. They may be linked to other as yet unknown risk factors. Others may have no external cause and result from DNA mutations within a cell. Regardless of a viral or carcinogenic etiology, HNCs are associated with biological and behavioral risk factors that cause or contribute to cancer prevalence. Some of these factors are modifiable; others are not (see Tables 2 and 3).

Carcinogen-induced oral cancers and OPCs have different associated risk factors. HPV-associated OPCs are transmitted during skin-to-skin contact and are highly correlated with sexual behavior. Specific characteristics of sexual practices that may increase an individual's vulnerability to HPV-positive HNC include anal sex, oral sex, early sexual debut, autoinoculation, number of lifetime vaginal and oral sex partners, and sex with someone who has a history of HPV.[5,10,11] Oral cancers, the majority of which are not HPV related, are associated with tobacco and alcohol use or a combination thereof.[1]

Figure 3. Percent of Deaths by Age Group: Oral Cavity and Pharynx Cancer, 2008–2012, All Races, Both Sexes*

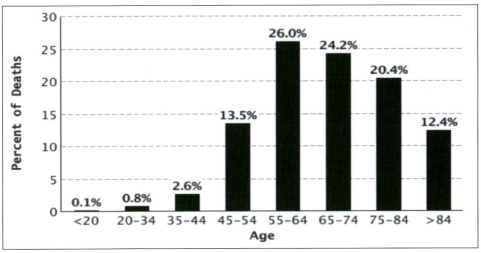

*Median age at death = 67. The percentage of oral cavity and pharynx cancer deaths is highest among people aged 55–64.
Source: National Cancer Institute. SEER stat fact sheets: oral cavity and pharynx cancer. Available at: http://seer.cancer.gov/statfacts/html/oralcav.html. Accessed March 24, 2016.

Table 3. Levels of Evidence for Increased Risk

Adequate for all HNCs	Adequate for OPCs
• Tobacco use • Alcohol use • Combined tobacco and alcohol use • Betel quid chewing	• Human papillomavirus infection

HNC, head and neck cancer; OPC, oropharyngeal cancer.
Source: National Cancer Institute: Oral cavity and oropharyngeal cancer prevention—health professional version (PDQ®). http://www.cancer.gov/types/head-and-neck/hp/oral-prevention-pdq#link/_206_toc. Accessed November 13, 2015.

High-risk sexual practices and the use of tobacco or electronic nicotine delivery systems (ENDS) and alcohol are modifiable behavioral risk factors. Sexual practices that can help prevent the transmission of HPV-positive HNCs include routine use of condoms and abstinence from higher risk sex acts. Abstinence from tobacco and alcohol use will reduce the risk of carcinogen-induced HNCs. Other behaviors such as healthful eating, sufficient exercise, and adopting a generally healthy lifestyle appear to help prevent cancers. Choosing to alter lifestyle patterns may help an individual become less vulnerable to HNCs. Exposure to sunlight and ultraviolet rays is another risk factor for HNCs. The use of hats, sunscreen, avoiding tanning beds, and limiting time in the sun can reduce the effect of this risk factor.

Nonmodifiable risk factors include age, race, and gender. Certain physical conditions that weaken the immune system are not modifiable and may increase a person's risk for cancer development. A weakened immune system can be present at birth or result from conditions such as the acquired immunodeficiency syndrome (AIDS) and certain medicines (e.g., those given after organ transplantation). Among the genetic conditions that predispose to HNC is Fanconi's anemia, a condition that exhibits inherited defects in several genes contributing to repair of DNA. Dyskeratosis congenita is a genetic syndrome that puts individuals at very high risk of developing cancer of the mouth and throat at an early age. Graft-versus-host disease (GVHD) is a condition that sometimes occurs after stem cell transplantation. GVHD can affect many tissues of the body, including those in the mouth. A severe case of lichen planus may increase the risk of HNC. Lichen planus occurs mainly in middle-aged people and manifests as white lines, dots, or striations on the oral mucosal or gingival tissue.[11]

Hypothetical etiologies for HNCs that are not evidence based have been mentioned in the literature. These include denture irritation and the effects of alcohol-containing mouthrinses. Any potential risk posed by mouthrinses would be due to misuse (i.e., overuse). Ill-fitting dentures could possibly cause carcinogenic agents to linger in the oral cavity, potentially increasing risk. Neither of these hypotheses is grounded in science.[12-14]

PATHOGENESIS[13-15]

Multiple genetic events culminate in carcinogenesis. Although carcinogen-induced HNCs and HPV-positive oropharyngeal cancers have unique pathogenic processes, some genetic events are similar for both conditions. Alteration or damage to host DNA cells within the oropharyngeal and oral cavity areas occurs. Genetic alterations that cause tumor development are of two major types: tumor suppressor genes, which promote tumor development when inactivated; and oncogenes, which promote tumor development when activated. Microenvironmental changes result in alterations in tumor suppressor behavior and oncogenes in tumor cells. Tumor suppressor genes can be inactivated through genetic events such as mutation, loss of heterozygosity, or deletion, or by epigenetic modifications such as DNA methylation or chromatin remodeling. Oncogenes can be activated through overexpression due to gene amplification, increased transcription, or changes in structure due to mutations that lead to increased transforming activity. Compensatory actions manifest through changes in molecular markers such as epidermal growth factor, transcription factors, and vascular endothelial growth factors. Questions remain concerning the exact timing of genetic events that transpire to cause head and neck neoplasia. Not all genetic events occur in all squamous oral

Table 4. Molecular Biological and Histopathologic Comparisons by Etiology

	HPV-Positive	Carcinogen-Induced
Biology and mutation, p53 and Rb	p53: increased catabolism of E6 pRb: increased catabolism of E7	p53: inactivation by mutation; evidence for loss of pRB
Biology and mutation, p16	Compensatory increase in p16 expression	p16 lost; p16-mediated pathways inactive
Histopathology	Poorly differentiated or basaloid squamous cell carcinoma	Usually moderately to well-differentiated squamous cell carcinoma; keratinizing histology

HPV, human papillomavirus; Rb, retinoblastoma protein.
Source: Modified from Dok R, Nuyts S. HPV positive head and neck cancers: molecular pathogenesis and evolving treatment strategies. Cancers (Basel). 2016 Apr; 8(4): 41. Published online 2016 Mar 29. doi: http://dx.doi.org/10.3390%2Fcancers8040041"10.3390/cancers8040041. Accessed 6/15/2016.

Table 5. Common Locations of Head and Neck Cancers

Oral Cavity	Oropharyngeal
•Lateral border of tongue •Floor of mouth •Lips •Gingivae	•Uvula •Tonsil •Base of tongue •Posterior pharyngeal wall •Soft palate

carcinomas, and similar genetic alterations may occur at different times in the process of carcinogenesis.[3]

Carcinogens and viruses are both instrumental in the etiology of HNCs, but their pathogenic pathways differ (see Table 4). Carcinogens cause direct damage to DNA while viruses such as HPV tend to disrupt the normal functioning of tumor suppressor cells. Specifically, *p53*, a host tumor suppressor, is mutated in carcinogen-induced HNCs while it is suppressed in HPV-positive HNCs. In HPV-positive oropharyngeal cancers, a compensatory action is increased transcription of *p16*. Thus, *p16* is considered a key biomarker for the presence of HPV-positive cancer. Although little is known about the biological mechanism and life cycle of HPV, the behavior of its oncoproteins and their transcription have been well documented.

Histologically, HPV has an affinity for basaloid tissue. Lesions originate in the oropharyngeal areas in the protected sites of the Waldeyer ring. These sites include the tonsils, base of tongue, soft palate, uvula, and posterior pharyngeal walls. Oral cancers are found most commonly on the lateral borders of the tongue and the floor of the mouth. Other sites include the dorsal and ventral surfaces of the tongue, buccal mucosa, gingiva, lips, hard palate, and retromolar areas (see Table 5). Since OPCs have no premalignant state, no precursor lesions can be identified. Given their location in protected epithelial tissue, keratinization is atypical. Nodular metastasis is not uncommon (see Figures 4 through 7).

Since HPV-positive oropharyngeal lesions do not have a bona fide premalignant state, staging of lesions cannot occur. Malignant transformation occurs through expression of two viral oncogenes, E6 and E7. HPV oncoproteins E6 and E7 are early arrivers to the tissue site, and they institute tumor suppression activity that then allows for increased transcription of oncogenic proteins that overtake the host DNA (see Figure 8).

Figure 4. Tonsillar Cancer

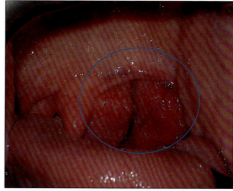

Source: Courtesy of Dr. Martin Tyler, McGill University, and Dr. Nancy Burkhart, PennWell Corporation.

Figure 5. Squamous Cell Carcinoma of Posterior Oropharyngeal Wall

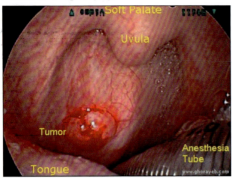

Source: Reproduced with permission from Otolaryngology Houston, http://www.ghorayeb.com.

Figure 6. Cervical Metastasis from Squamous Cell Carcinoma of Left Tonsil and Tongue Base

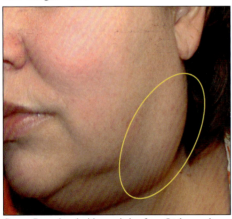

Source: Reproduced with permission from Otolaryngology Houston, http://www.ghorayeb.com.

Oral cancers that are not HPV-positive typically arise through a breach in the basement membrane separating the epithelial and mesenchymal compartments. Molecular alterations result in visible tissue change and potential metastasis. Stages of tissue change range from initial dysplasia, to leukoplakia (see Figures 9 and 10) or erythroplakia and mixed lesions (see Figures 11 and 12), to cancer in situ (see Figure 13) or invasive cancer. Unlike HPV-positive oropharyngeal lesions, premalignant oral cancer lesions can be identified and staged. Table 5 lists common locations of lesions.[11]

Figure 7. Tonsillar Cancer

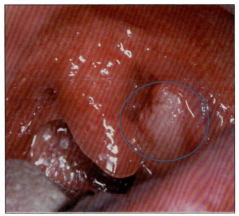

Source: Courtesy of Dr. Martin Tyler, McGill University, and Dr. Nancy Burkhart, PennWell Corporation.

Figure 8. Oncoproteins E6 and E7

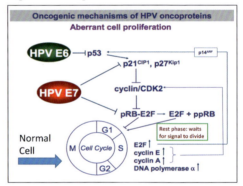

Hypotheses explaining how oral cancer arises include the role of combustion byproducts and their interaction with saliva, a possible diminution of anticancer protective agents in saliva, and genetic polymorphisms. The role of heat and its effect of mucosal tissue also is a consideration. Squamous cell carcinomas of the oral cavity are characterized by their ability to spread locally and regionally.[12-14]

SIGNS AND SYMPTOMS

Common signs of HNC include a sore in the mouth that does not heal; persistent mouth, tooth, or jaw pain; a lump or thickening in the cheek or neck; a white or red lesion on the gums, tongue, tonsil, or buccal mucosa; a sore throat or feeling that something is caught in the throat that

Figure 9. Flat, White Leukoplakia of Tongue in a Smoker

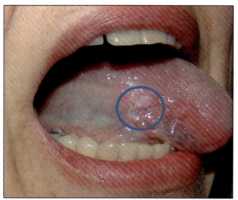

Source: Reproduced with permission from Otolaryngology Houston, http://www.ghorayeb.com.

Figure 10. Leukoplakia on Lateral Border and Ventral Surface of Tongue

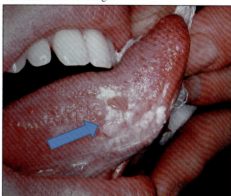

Source: Courtesy of Dr. Karen Garber.

Figure 11. (1) Speckled (Red and White) Lesion on Floor of Mouth and Alveolar Ridge, (2) Fissured Erythroplakic Lesion on Lateral Border of Tongue

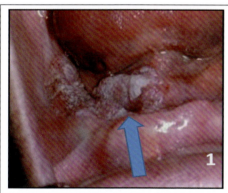
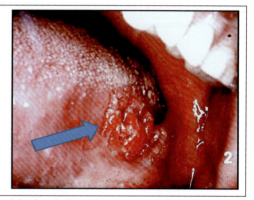

Source: (1) Courtesy of Dr. John Basile. (2) Reproduced with permission from Otolaryngology Houston, http://www.ghorayeb.com.

Figure 12. Subtle Mixed, Crusty Ulcerated Lesion of Upper Lip Diagnosed as Squamous Cell Carcinoma

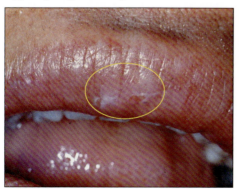

Source: American Cancer Society; National Cancer Institute.

Figure 13. Keratinized Carcinoma of Floor of Mouth

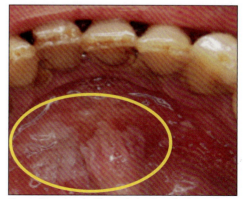

Source: Reproduced with permission from Otolaryngology Houston, http://www.ghorayeb.com.

does not go away; difficulty swallowing, chewing, or moving the jaw or tongue; numbness of the tongue or elsewhere in the mouth; jaw swelling; loosening of the teeth; hoarseness or voice changes; weight loss; and persistent bad breath (see Table 6). Although many of the signs and symptoms of HNCs are shared, OPCs are specifically characterized by odynophagia (painful swallowing), dysphagia (difficulty swallowing), and otalgia (ear pain). Bleeding, decreased tongue mobility, and trismus may be accompanying signs. Base of tongue cancers are associated with submucosal spread. Table 7 shows clinical differences by etiology.

Carcinogen-induced precancerous or cancerous lesions may be described as leukoplakic, erythroplakic, or speckled. Leukoplakic lesions have the lowest conversion rates and clinically may appear flat and white. As the lesions increase in size, terms such as *exophytic, pedunculated, verrucous,* and *sessile* are used to describe them. Neoplasms may appear keratinized, nodular, warty, fissured, or ulcerated (see Figures 11 through 14).

DIAGNOSTIC TESTS

Survival rates for OPC vary depending on the tumor's stage when it is detected.[4] A thorough and accurate diagnosis is the first step in developing a targeted and effective patient care plan. Many diagnostic tests and techniques are available to assess the presence of HNCs. Some are conducted clinically but most require laboratory analysis. Only a handful of diagnostic tests are evidence based, but several are used in dental practices and clinics.

A comprehensive head and neck examination and screening must be a component part of routine risk assessment. It is considered a standard of care for detecting early HNCs and premalignant lesions, yet no evidence supports its role in reducing mortality in the general population.[16] All intraoral and extraoral head and neck structures, including all lymph nodes and lymph node chains, must be palpated manually and visually

Table 6. Symptoms of Oral and Oropharyngeal Cancer

•Ear or jaw pain, or both	•Fatigue
•Chronic bad breath	•Difficulty chewing, swallowing, or moving jaws or tongue
•Changes in speech	•Loss of appetite
•Loose teeth or toothache	•Unexplained weight loss
•Dentures that no longer fit	•Trismus
•Sore that does not heal	•Red or white patch
•Hoarseness	•Lump or thickening in cheek
•Numbness of mouth or tongue	•Headaches
•Pain or bleeding in mouth	

HPV, human papillomavirus; Rb, retinoblastoma protein.
Source: Modified from: Cantrell et al. (2013); Dufour et al. (2012). National Cancer Institute; Centers for Disease Control.

Table 7. Comparison of Head and Neck Cancers by Etiology

	HPV-Positive	Carcinogen-Induced
Incidence	Increasing	Decreasing
Age	Younger (~ 50s)	Older (~ 60+)
Sex	Male	Male (smoking)
Risk factors	Sexual: number of partners, early first sexual encounters, smoking, and immunosuppression may play role	Alcohol and smoking, other host factors
Prognosis	Good	Poor
Vaccine	Yes (for some types)	No

Source: Courtesy of Dr. John Basile.

Figure 14. Clinical Images and CT Scan of Patient with Tonsillar Cancer

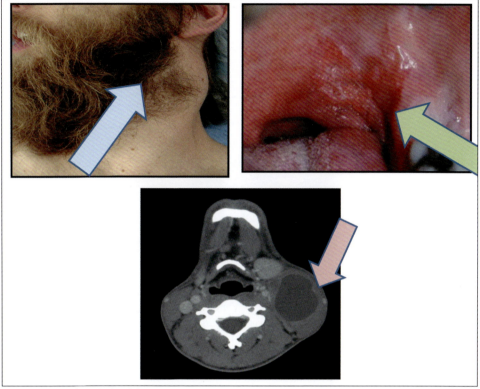

Source: Courtesy of Dr. Andrew Salame.

examined. Specific techniques for conducting these examinations have been published.[17] With the increasing incidence of HPV-associated HNCs, oral healthcare providers have been advised to scrutinize the soft palate and oropharyngeal areas thoroughly. Seating a patient supinely enables better viewing of the oropharyngeal area, whereas palpation of the cervical lymph nodes is best accomplished when the patient is sitting upright. The use of light, a tongue blade or dental mirror for tongue retraction, and proper patient positioning enhance the accuracy of the exam.[17] Because of their defined premalignant state, oral cancers are more easily seen than OPCs. OPCs also present in less accessible areas. Although screenings can be discriminatory, most oral cancers are detected in late stages, reducing the possibility of positive prognoses or high survival rates.[18] Evidence indicates that visual examination as part of a population-based screening program in India may reduce the mortality rate of oral cancer in high-risk individuals.[18,19] A key benefit of manual, oral, and visual HNC screenings is raising patient awareness.

Dental radiographs, particularly panoramic images, have the potential to identify suspicious lesions. Further examination would be necessary for a differential diagnosis. Other imaging techniques include computed tomography (CT; see Figures 14 and 15), magnetic resonance imaging (MRI), and positron emission tomography (PET) scans (see Table 8). Chemiluminescence and autofluorescence are optical diagnostic tests that require the use of specialized equipment and reagents. Meta-analyses have found little evidence to support the diagnostic value of these two methods.[19,20] The use of exfoliative cytology was deemed to have "potential merit" as its sensitivity and specificity were found to be superior to chemiluminescence and autofluorescence. However, oral

Figure 15. Clinical Images and CT Scan of Patient with Cancer of Tongue Base

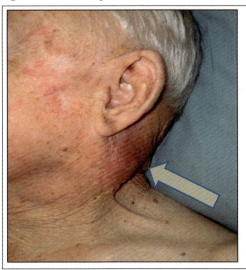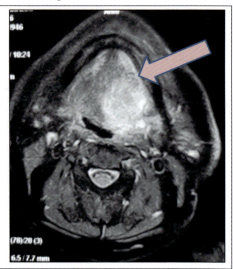

Source: Courtesy of Dr. Andrew Salame.

Table 8. Selected Methods for Detecting and Diagnosing Head and Neck Cancers

•Manual palpation and visualization	•Endoscopy
•Optical testing: autofluorescence and chemolumination	•Ultrasound
•Cytological testing	•Computed tomography (CT) scan
•X-ray or panoramic radiograph (PanorexTM)	•Magnetic resonance imaging (MRI)
•Chairside salivary testing	•Positron emission tomography (PET) scan
•Laboratory assays	•Barium swallow
	•Pharyngoscopy
	•Blood serum analysis

cancer detection using exfoliative cytology can be challenging, and some cancers may be missed or confused with abnormal but noncancerous cells. A biopsy would be needed to make a definitive diagnosis. This technique remains the gold standard for histological assessment and a definitive diagnosis.[19]

Blood tests are used to identify HPV antibodies, although their presence may not be detectable in everyone exposed to HPV. The L1 antibody has long been a marker for HPV. Since it indicates exposure, and not necessarily current disease, its value is limited. The presence of serum *p16* is another biomarker for HPV-positive OPCs. HPV-16 antibodies indicate a higher risk for OPC, but their identification may reflect cumulative exposure and does not reveal the cancer site. *P16* has been correlated with subsequent HPV-positive HNCs.[21]

Current salivary testing for HPV indicates the presence or absence of the oral virus. Positive findings provide little guidance for diagnosis. The stealthy nature of HPV could result in conflicting salivary test reports. The sophistication of current testing is limited. New salivary and blood tests that identify HPV tumor DNA are under study.[22] These tests could provide more specific information to aid in diagnosis and prognosis.

Several sophisticated laboratory testing methods (i.e., immunohistochemistry, polymerase chain reaction, and in situ hybridization) provide tumor information at the molecular biological level. These tests enable pathogen profiling, functional analysis of genes, and the identification of abnormal gene expression through the use of DNA and RNA. Each provides information relevant to tumor inception, growth, location, and type.

Other medical tests diagnose tumors. Barium swallows stain suspicious areas. Endoscopy, direct and indirect pharyngoscopy, and laryngoscopy permit visualization of the patient in real time. During indirect pharyngoscopy, small mirrors are placed at the most posterior portion of the throat to clearly examine the throat, the base of tongue, and part of the larynx. Direct scoping requires a fiber-optic source directed to the site of interest. Scalpel biopsy and subsequent histological assessment is still the gold standard for diagnosing oral cancers, but more advanced imaging and laboratory diagnostic tests may be necessary to identify less obvious lesions or those that manifest no premalignant state (see Table 8).

PATIENT MANAGEMENT AND INTERVENTIONS
Preventive Strategies

Oral health professionals are well-positioned to prevent HNCs. It is one of the most important services they can provide. Regardless of age and population served, certain preventive strategies and provider services that target HNCs are universal. Others may be more age specific. Communication techniques and the delivery of educational content will depend on the recipient of the messages. Regardless of the scenario, patients must be fully engaged in all discussions. By personalizing risk factors, patients may become more inquisitive about signs and symptoms of disease and preventive behaviors. All patients must become familiar with the appearance of their oral cavities through self-screening; if changes should occur, they then may have a better chance of noticing them. Patients must become their own advocates and make certain that they receive HNC screenings whenever they visit their oral health professionals.

For all patients and target populations, behavioral and biological risk factors for HNCs must be assessed and addressed. These include tobacco or nicotine dependence, excessive use of alcohol, and their combination, and engagement in high-risk sexual practices. Health education topics with almost universal applicability include prevention of HNCs, tobacco and nicotine use prevention and cessation (see Table 9), measured consumption of alcohol, the oral–systemic link, and the adoption of healthy lifestyle behaviors related to nutrition and weight control. Individuals of any age must know that tobacco use not only increases their risk for most cancers, but negatively affects their abilities to engage in physical activity, whether it be playing on a sports team, dancing, or climbing stairs. Individuals with family histories of cancers and those with conditions associated with cancer must understand the cumulative effect of additional risk factors. Those who are immunocompromised or may have genetic or clinical conditions associated with HNCs must receive tailored messages related to their status. Manual and visual screenings and radiographic imaging are routine assessment tools for all age groups. If a suspicious lesion is detected, follow-up or referral to a specialist for biopsy and further testing is warranted.

Primary and middle school curricula typically include sex education and content on misuse of drugs, alcohol, and tobacco. Echoing and reinforcing concepts learned in school is appropriate and needed. However, young students may not learn that high-risk sexual behaviors can promote the acquisition and transmission of HPV. They also may not be told that timely vaccination against HPV will prevent it. Oral health professionals may need to broach topics such as risk factors for HPV (which could include discussions of

Table 9. Levels of Evidence for Interventions to Reduce Risk

Adequate for all HNCs: Tobacco cessation
Inadequate for all HNCs: Cessation of alcohol consumption
Inadequate for OPCs: Vaccination against HPV-16 and other high risk subtypes

HNC, head and neck cancer; OPC, oropharyngeal cancer.
Source: National Cancer Institute: Oral cavity and oropharyngeal cancer prevention—health professional version (PDQ®). http://www.cancer.gov/types/head-and-neck/hp/oral-prevention-pdq#link/_206_toc. Accessed November 13, 2015.

safe sex) and the importance of HPV vaccination for prevention. Conversations related to sensitive topics can be seamlessly raised in the context of the risks they pose for HNCs. Since children as young as 9 years of age are encouraged to be vaccinated against HPV, these conversations should begin at an early age. Likewise, tobacco prevention and cessation counseling should begin when children are young, as most individuals begin smoking before the age of 18 years.

Parents or caretakers must be made aware of age-appropriate HNC prevention strategies. Significant others often make choices for their infants, toddlers, children, and adolescents. Caretakers must be shown how important their roles are in shaping an individual's growth and development. Providers should encourage caretakers to role model and promote healthy lifestyles that include nutritious food plans, exercise, and avoidance of cancer risk factors. Older children and teenagers with concerns about their appearances must be advised to limit their sun exposure, avoid tanning beds, use sunscreen, and wear hats and visors for protection if outdoors. Similar rules must be enforced with young children to ensure compliance.

Other issues may facilitate behavioral change in adults. In the context of aesthetics, providers may be able to help adults make lifestyle changes. Tobacco use has been associated with premature skin wrinkling, low sperm counts, spontaneous abortion, and difficulties conceiving. Oral effects include halitosis, staining, and calculus buildup. Cumulative years of sun exposure may cause premalignant or cancerous skin lesions, necessitating a dermatologist's care. The HPV vaccine is posited to be effective in individuals up to the age of 26 years. A discussion of the vaccine is thus relevant to young adults and adults. Pregnant women should be aware that HPV can be transmitted to an infant during delivery through the birth canal. They should also understand that good prenatal nutrition and abstinence from tobacco and alcohol use during pregnancy may favorably shape their child's development.

Adults may have a better understanding of the host–response relationship and its relevance to their risk of HNC. Individuals with long histories of tobacco and alcohol use, those who are immunocompromised, and others with genetic conditions associated with HNCs must understand that they are at increased risk for disease. Oral conditions such as lichen planus also have been associated with oral cancer. The most important preventive behavior a healthcare provider can assume is advocacy for prevention of HNCs, patient wellness, and public awareness. A very small percentage of the public is aware of HNC, and few recognize its relationship to sexual behaviors. Only a small percentage of younger aged children are being vaccinated against HPV. Many adults may not understand the value of vaccination, fear immunizations in general, or think that vaccination promotes sexual behaviors. Oral health professionals must endorse HPV vaccination and promulgate the message that HNCs can be prevented through adherence to healthy lifestyles and the adoption of judicious health behaviors.

Therapeutic Interventions Prior to Treatment
Therapeutic interventions may help prevent HNCs from developing. Aside from tailored and poignant preventive educational messages, therapeutic interventions for tobacco prevention and cessation and for assisting recovering alcoholics are available. Much research has considered interventions for cessation of tobacco use. Some are evidence based while others may work effectively for certain individuals. An evidence-based approach to tobacco cessation, referred to as the 5 A's, is endorsed by the Agency for Healthcare Research and Quality. In this approach, patients are *asked* about tobacco use, *advised* to stop, their readiness to abstain is *assessed*, they are *assisted* in their attempts to refrain, and follow-up is *arranged*.[23] Advising is a critical piece of the 5 A's. During this phase of the five-step process, patients are shown the effects of their tobacco habits in their mouths, enabling their ownership of the problem. The 5 A's also advocates the use of pharmacological adjuncts to assist the patient in

Figure 16. Behavioral Change Stages in Process of Tobacco Cessation

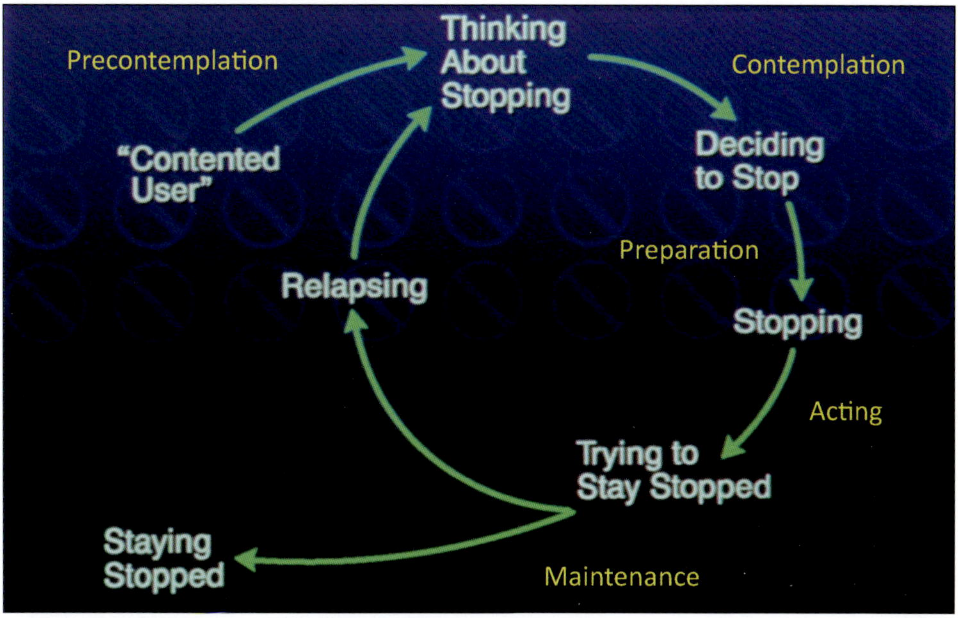

Source: National Cancer Institute: *How to Help Your Patients Be Tobacco-free.*

successful abstinence.

Nicotine replacement therapies and non-nicotine medications can be recommended and prescribed, depending on the patient's individual needs.[24] Many nicotine replacement therapies are available over the counter (e.g., gum, patches, lozenges), allowing patients to self-medicate. Providers should offer support and encourage patients to seek professional oversight as they make their cessation plans. In some instances, pharmacists, physicians, dentists, and dental hygienists may work together in helping patients abstain from tobacco use. For patients who have tried science-based approaches without success, alternative measures may be considered. For example, the use of hypnosis is not grounded in science but it has been helpful for some. The goal for healthcare providers is to work with patients to successfully help them stop using tobacco. In this effort, evidence-based approaches are preferred, but other strategies that pose no harm to the patient may need to be employed.

Motivational interviewing (MI) is an evidence-based counseling and communication technique that is used to addresses a patient's ambivalence to change.[25] The goal of MI is to heighten patients' self-awareness so that they independently identify the plusses and minuses of their habit, in this case tobacco use, and ultimately decide for themselves when it is time to stop.

Well-trained facilitators are crucial to successful MI. Oral healthcare providers may already use some aspects of this technique with other patient behavior change. Tobacco or nicotine users who seek behavioral change move through phases in the cessation process (see Figure 16). When patients first present they may be contented users. Then with a facilitator's guidance they begin to contemplate the wisdom of their habit, prepare for possible cessation, take action by setting a quit date, and continue working to maintain their abstinence. Oral healthcare providers may recommend referral to a psychologist or individual well-versed in the MI technique to help the patient.

Self-help groups, behavioral counseling, counseling combined with medications, and referrals to quit lines have all been useful for helping individuals abstain from tobacco use. Research indicates that the use of medication without counseling is less effective than with counseling. Referral to Alcoholics Anonymous might be appropriate for problem drinkers who need or request assistance. The 12-step programs have successfully aided individuals with addictions. Other in-patient programs or self-help groups are available through local hospitals and the American Cancer Society.

All of the detection tests previously mentioned in this chapter offer the therapeutic benefit of making patients more aware. If a patient has had genital HPV or has had sexual relationships with someone who is HPV positive, education will help that individual monitor himself or herself. Frequent Pap smears may be required, which could be beneficial in diminishing patient anxiety or discovering an early-stage malignancy. Other blood serum markers can indicate the presence of HPV antibodies. Although the time from their identification to the development of a carcinoma could take decades,[21] the patient and his or her providers will be vigilant and could detect a lesion at an early stage.

Members of the oral healthcare team should work together to endorse a practice or clinic philosophy that promotes cancer prevention. Health professionals who collaborate on interprofessional teams should reinforce positive messages for prevention of disease and promotion of wellness. When more providers work together, the chances for patient success are greater.

Therapeutic Interventions[26-28]

Oral health professionals are instrumental in therapeutic interventions prior to, during, and following surgery, radiation, or chemotherapy. Treatments for HNCs often have oral ramifications, reinforcing the need to educate patients and provide therapy during all phases of care. Some recommended therapies, such as practicing good oral hygiene, are universal, regardless of treatment rendered. Other protocols and therapeutic interventions must be based on the patient's level of tolerance, medical status, type of cancer, treatment rendered, and response to treatment.

Prior to treatment, all patients should receive thorough clinical examinations. The dentist and dental hygienist should examine the soft tissues to identify inflammation or infection, assess plaque levels and dental caries, review oral hygiene and oral care protocols, and prescribe antimicrobial therapy as indicated. Implementing periodontal debridement and the use of adjunctive therapies can help reduce the patient's oral bacterial load. Therapeutic interventions can help minimize the severity of a patient's pain and oral infection, thereby preventing a disruption or termination of treatment.

Treatment interventions for HNCs include surgery, chemotherapy, radiation therapy, combination therapies, and biological and targeted therapies. Oral healthcare providers should be aware of the side effects associated with each approach so that individualized patient therapeutic interventions can be designed and implemented. Most patients with HNC present with locally advanced stage III or IV disease. These stages typically require a combination of chemotherapy, radiation, or surgery. For patients who present with early stage I or II disease, radiation or surgery is the commonly recommended course of care. These patients have an excellent prognosis.

Side effects of surgical procedures may include swelling, loss of voice, speech impairment, difficulty chewing or swallowing, ear numbness, impaired movement in lower lip, limited ability to raise the arms over the head, and facial disfigurement. Reconstructive surgery may be needed if large masses of tissue are removed. Healthy tissue and bone may be taken from other parts of the body to compensate. Prosthodontists may design and fabricate artificial dental and facial parts and obturators to improve aesthetics. In these instances, oral health professionals may be working collaboratively with speech pathologists and registered dieticians who, respectively, will help patients relearn speech patterns and design acceptable and healthy food plans.

Radiation therapy may be the primary form of treatment or used following surgery to further ensure the complete destruction of the cancer cells. Radiation therapy remains a mainstay of curative therapy for oropharyngeal cancer. Side effects of radiation therapy can include skin redness, xerostomia, difficulty swallowing or speaking, mucositis and oral lesions, loss of appetite, bone pain or dental problems (e.g., osteoradionecrosis), nausea, fatigue, ear wax buildup, and hearing loss. Chemotherapy is an integral part of treating locally advanced HNC. Side effects of chemotherapy may include fatigue, nausea, loss of appetite, hair loss, xerostomia, difficulty eating, mucositis, infection, and diarrhea.

Patients and their caretakers must understand the importance of working to maintain good oral hygiene to minimize infection and reduce patient discomfort throughout any type of cancer treatment. Basic oral self-care should include brushing in a nontraumatic fashion with a soft brush and flossing or other interdental cleansing as tolerated. Oral health professionals must provide patients with recommendations for treating dry mouth, such as sipping water frequently, sucking on ice chips or sugar-free candy, using moisturizing agents, chewing sugar-free gum with xylitol, and using a saliva substitute spray or gel or a prescribed saliva stimulant. For caries prevention, the use of fluorides may be warranted. The strength and delivery agent should be adjusted to meet the patient's comfort level. Prescribing topical anesthetics or analgesics for oral pain may be necessary. The Cochrane Oral Health Group considered interventions for preventing and reducing the severity of oral mucositis in cancer patients. Agents and therapeutic interventions were evaluated in patients with different forms of cancer, undergoing different types of treatment, so benefits may pertain to only the disease and treatment combinations evaluated.[27] Cryotherapy (ice chips) and keratinocyte growth factor (palifermin) showed some benefit in preventing mucositis, and sucralfate was deemed effective in reducing the severity of mucositis. Seven additional interventions—aloe vera, amifostine, intravenous glutamine, granulocyte colony-stimulating factor (G-CSF), honey, laser, and antibiotic lozenges containing polymyxin/tobramycin/amphotericin (PTA)—showed weaker evidence of benefit.[27] The Multinational Association of Supportive Care in Cancer and International Society of Oral Oncology (MASCC/ISOO), in a more recent systematic review, established no guidelines regarding the use of these seven interventions due to insufficient or conflicting findings.[28] The use of sucralfate also was not recommended for the prevention or treatment of chemotherapeutic or radiation-induced mucositis, as opposed to the earlier Cochrane report. Based on the evidence supporting the MASCC/ISOO Guidelines, the following interventions were deemed most effective, given the specific circumstances indicated: oral cryotherapy, palifermin, and low-level laser therapy. (See Appendix 1.) To help reduce the risk of oral and potentially systemic infection, essential surgical or restorative dental care should be completed prior to treatment. Patients with lichen planus or other treatable risk factors may require prescription therapy.

The goal of any treatment is to prolong life, but quality of life, preservation of function, and appearance must be considered. Treatments are continually being researched and refined to minimize invasiveness. Surgical techniques have continued to evolve, with greater focus on minimally invasive procedures where appropriate. Current research suggests that therapies less intensive than those used for HPV-negative HNCs may be effective for HPV-positive tumors. HPV-positive cancers tend to be more sensitive to radiation, chemotherapy, and combined therapies, prompting some researchers to suggest a reexamination of prescribing similar treatments regardless of etiology.[29] Survival rates, in general, are higher and relapse rates lower for HPV-positive HNCs. Recurring cancers also may require modified approaches to treatment.

Patient Management Considerations
Throughout treatment, a team approach to patient care is essential. Dentists, oncologists, dental hygienists, speech pathologists, dieticians, and others must be aware of the potential oral side effects of surgery, radiation, and chemotherapy and work together to minimize them. Patients need to understand that side effects are treatable and that reconstructive surgery and rehabilitation

can help with facial disfigurements and speech or swallowing difficulties. When delivering preventive messages or communicating with patients diagnosed with HNCs, receiving treatment, recovering, or seeking palliative care, variations in approach are necessary. Patients diagnosed with HNCs of different etiologies should receive tailored educational messages regarding risk factors and management of the condition. Demographic factors such as ethnicity, health literacy level, and socioeconomic status will influence dialogues. Some cultural and religious groups hold health beliefs that may conflict with those of the provider, and they should be met with respect. The emotional impact of a cancer diagnosis can be profound. Oral health professionals can provide essential psychosocial support to patients with new diagnoses or to those experiencing side effects. Helping patients identify support systems may be another provider role.

Patients should be closely monitored post-treatment with periodic dental evaluations and prophylaxes as a mainstay of therapeutic interventions. Thorough examinations must be included at all recall appointments. Subsequent visits and follow-up should be based on patient need. Oral complications can continue or emerge long after radiation therapy has ended. High-dose radiation treatment carries a lifelong risk of xerostomia, dental caries, and osteonecrosis. Lifelong daily fluoride application, good nutrition, and conscientious oral hygiene are especially important for patients with salivary gland dysfunction. At any stage of diagnosis, patients remain at high risk for recurrence and second primary tumors. Oral health professionals should be mindful of these possibilities and remain proactive when treating patients who have had HNCs.[30]

Special Considerations
Children who have received radiation to craniofacial and dental structures should be monitored for abnormal growth and development. Developmental disturbances in children treated before age 12 years generally affect craniofacial development, including the size, shape, and eruption patterns of teeth. Common manifestations may include abnormal tooth formation, such as decreased crown size, shortened and conical shaped roots, and microdontia; delayed tooth eruption, including increased frequency of impacted maxillary canines; and diminished alveolar processes that lead to decreased occlusal vertical dimension. These changes tend to be symmetrical, so they may not be clinically evident. The child's age at the time of cancer therapy and the protocol followed influence the extent and location of dental and craniofacial anomalies. For children younger than 5 or 6 years of age at the time of treatment (particularly those who undergo treatment that involves concomitant chemotherapy and head and neck radiation), a higher incidence of dental and craniofacial anomalies tends to occur as compared to older children or those who undergo only chemotherapy. Managing oral complications in pediatric patients is challenging, as limited research addresses oral toxicities.[31,32]

FUTURE EPIDEMIOLOGICAL TRENDS
Future epidemiological trends will vary by global region. Based on current data, carcinogen-induced cancers will continue to decline or remain relatively stable in the United States and in select western European countries.[2,3] High tobacco use rates persist in areas of Eastern Europe, South Asia, and the Middle East.[2] Unless usage rates decline, the incidence, prevalence, and mortality rates for HNCs will not change substantially. The use of betel quid in India remains a significant risk factor for HNC, a disease that is the second leading cause of death in that country.[2,33]

Trends indicate that the rise in HPV-associated OPCs will remain unabated in the United States, Canada, Sweden, Great Britain, and other developed western European countries.[6] It is suggested that by 2020, the incidence of HPV-positive HNCs could reach epidemic proportions.[34] In Australia, where HPV vaccination is mandated, a reduction in HPV-positive HNCs is anticipated.[35] Despite lower compliance rates in the United States, a recent analysis of National Health and Nutrition Examination Survey (NHANES) data indicates a lower prevalence of certain HPV strains among girls who have been vaccinated.[36] To increase the vaccination rate in the United States, adolescents and adults must become more aware and better educated about the value of the vaccine and understand that already-contracted genital infections increase the risk of transmission when high-risk sexual behaviors are practiced. Greater dissemination of information related to HPV transmission could alter the practice of high-risk sexual behaviors, thereby decreasing transmission rates.

More public health campaigns and health professionals' advocacy is needed to enlighten society about the cancer threats that genital and oral HPV infections pose.[37] All health professionals should be educated about the genital–oral link associated with HPV, and they should promote early vaccination against HPV during patient care. Preventing and diminishing tobacco use and nicotine dependence must remain a high priority. Although tobacco rates have decreased in some countries, they remain high in others.[2] It behooves all professionals to stay engaged in the war on tobacco and nicotine addiction.

Epidemiological trends will also depend on the use of other, less traditional smoked products such as hookah, clove cigarettes (Bidi, Kretek), and marijuana. Unsmoked products such as spit tobacco also pose harm. ENDS may also affect the incidence and prevalence of HNCs. The long-term effect of these products on the development of HNCs is unknown.[38] It also is unknown if their use encourages or discourages smoking. The Food & Drug Administration recently developed regulations for e-cigarettes and other alternative nicotine products.[39] The legalization of recreational marijuana, an agricultural substance that could contain tobacco products and does produce combustion, may become more widespread in the United States.[40] Little research has examined the long-term effects of marijuana on the oral cavity or the oropharyngeal areas. The relationship between marijuana use and subsequent or concomitant adoption of a tobacco habit is also unclear. Another consideration that could affect future trends will be the oral health professional's philosophy on harm reduction versus total abstinence from tobacco and nicotine acquisition products.

FUTURE RESEARCH EFFORTS

New scientific discoveries and technological change will influence the screening, detection, and treatment of HNCs. Advances could improve screening methods and boost early detection, thereby increasing survival rates. More sophisticated salivary and serum blood tests under study may help identify HPV tumor DNA when the disease is in an incipient stage, also potentially improving survival rates.[22] The use of chairside salivary diagnostics is expected to grow, which could prove beneficial for screening, detection, and treatment.[41] With personalized genomic mapping, at-risk individuals could be identified before a malignancy develops.[42] Studies looking at the effectiveness of the current HPV vaccine against HPV oral infection have been undertaken, and the results appear promising. For some individuals, dosages lower than the three prescribed administrations proved effective.[43] Developing a vaccine that prevents oral HPV infection will occur.

In the area of treatment, research on minimally invasive surgical techniques continues.[44] Transoral endoscopic and robotic surgeries allow access to the tumor through the mouth, thereby avoiding incisions through the neck or face. Recent advances in radiotherapy have focused on fractionation schedules and the use of intensity-modulated radiation therapy, a form of high-precision radiotherapy that delivers radiation more precisely to the tumor while relatively sparing the surrounding normal tissues. Reconstruction and free-tissue-transfer techniques have also improved, resulting in better function and aesthetics. Biological (immunotherapy) and targeted therapies are relatively new and are still being researched. Biological therapies include drugs that boost the body's immune system.[42] Targeted therapies kill cancer cells and not healthy cells. An example would be antibodies against epidermal growth factor used with radiation therapy (EGFR). Another newer therapy is radiofrequency thermal ablation (RFA). RFA uses heat to destroy cancer cells. It is a minimally invasive treatment option that may be useful for localized tumors that cannot be removed with surgery.[45]

Advancements in science and research are difficult to predict. Given the global morbidity and mortality associated with HNCs, their late stage detection, and the rise in HPV-associated HNCs, one can assume that more answers will be found and more successful strategies will be developed.

CONCLUSIONS

Oral health professionals must continue to maintain a proactive, visible, and relevant role in the fight against HNC. Dentists and dental hygienists have many opportunities to engage with patients and reduce the morbidity and mortality associated with these cancers. As preventive health educators, oral health professionals have an ethical obligation to inform their patients about HNCs, the associated risk factors, and the measures to prevent them. They must be advocates for tobacco cessation and prevention and for the administration of the HPV vaccine. They must talk to their patient populations but also to the community at large about HNCs.

A critical role for oral health professionals is the screening for and detection of HNCs. All patients must receive routine head and neck oral and visual cancer screenings. Patients must be taught how to conduct self-examinations and be advised to request a screening when they present for routine care.

The oral health professional may be the first provider to come in contact with a patient who presents with a suspicious finding. Patient monitoring and triage with other specialists often follows. Oral health professionals must value their own contributions to the patient's well-being and maintain open communication with other involved healthcare providers. Therapeutic roles for oral health professionals are many and essential throughout the patient's treatment. Psychosocial support, palliative care, necessary interventions, and assistance with oral side effects help patients maintain their strength and continue their courses of treatment.

In summary, dentists and dental hygienists are leaders in preventing and combatting HNCs. Oral health professionals know best the head and neck regions and can help educate other healthcare providers about HNCs and the relationship between oral and systemic well-being. In interprofessional collaborations, oral healthcare providers should share their expertise and maintain key positions in discussions addressing patient care, the oral side effects of treatments, the need for possible oral health interventions, and the importance of maintaining good oral hygiene practices during treatment. Oral health professionals are needed in the preventive, therapeutic, and intervention phases of patient care. They must embrace and value their contributions.

In the next section, patient cases are included. They highlight information related to risk assessment, risk behaviors, and potential preventive and therapeutic interventions. Thoughts on how to interact with patients are presented.

CASE 1: Adolescent Patient Who Uses Spit Tobacco

PATIENT OVERVIEW

James S. is a 16-year-old Caucasian male. He has been a patient since he was 5 years old.

Chief Complaint: "A white area on my gum."

Medical History: Broken arm in 2014 while playing basketball on the high school varsity team. All else, within normal limits.

Risk Assessment/Risk Factors: Uses spit tobacco (ST) in sachet form; places sachet in the mandibular labial vestibule where lesion is located; uses during basketball season (October to March) but at no other time. Believes ST helps his concentration and improves his playing. Parents are unaware of his habit. Patient claims he does not engage in high-risk behaviors other than the occasional beer with his "buddies on the weekends."

If patient continues habit, he is at moderate risk for oral cancer and periodontal disease. If the current brand contains sugar or silicate particles, or both, the risk for caries, abrasion, and recession, respectively, is increased.

CLINICAL EXAMINATION

Extra-/Intraoral Examination: Leukoplakic lesion in labial vestibule adjacent to teeth #s 24–27; appears striated, diffuse, and measures 5 by 5 mm; classified as stage II lesion.

Caries Assessment: No lesions present; exposed roots adjacent to placement site are negative.

Periodontal Assessment: High plaque-free score (81%); 2 mm of recession found on teeth #s 26 and 27. No other findings.

Health Behaviors: Patient consumes fluoridated tap water (lives in community with fluoridated water supply); uses fluoridated toothpaste daily and flosses 4 times per week. Rinses 4 times per day with essential oils mouthrinse for breath freshening.

Risk Assessment: Potential for oral cancer could become high if habit is continued; low risk for caries and periodontal disease if ST habit is discontinued and if good oral hygiene and sound dietary practices are maintained. Risk rises to moderate in both categories with continuance of habit and decline in preventive home care measures.

Risk Reduction: Patient shown localized mandibular anterior recession areas; educational interventions focus on oral cancer, permanent tissue attachment loss and further recession, possible tooth mobility and tooth loss, physical appearance, and halitosis. Patient advised that overuse of mouth rinse could irritate soft tissues; recommendation of 2 times daily use for 30 seconds. Best method for eliminating halitosis would be discontinuation of habit.

OUTCOMES

The use of pharmacological adjuncts is recommended when *assisting* the patient using the 5 A's approach; however, in James's case, this option is unavailable due to his age. Regardless of age, because he limits his use to basketball season, his level of addiction may not warrant pharmacological assistance. If James becomes aware of the dangers associated with ST and learns what they are, he may want to quit "cold turkey" immediately. Age-appropriate emphases are needed, as indicated in the table. Another important factor to consider in behavioral interventions is patient–provider rapport, including communication comfort level, and

Interventions for Lesion

Preventive	Therapeutic	Alternatives
Lifestyle/behavioral change: to prevent cancer; tobacco abstinence, tapering	Employ the 5 A's	No use of pharmacological adjuncts due to patient age (under 18)
Content areas of 5 A's: Ask, Advise, Assess, Assist, Arrange	Ultimate goal: patient sets quit date	Refer for biopsy if no resolution
Education: risks of habit, nicotine addiction—oral cancer Age-relevant topics: • Effect of peer pressure on use • Aesthetics (appearance, halitosis) • Impact of use on athletic performance • Elevated high blood pressure	Show literature on head and neck cancer surgeries; disfigured survivors	
Patient ownership of habit and effects (employ "teachable moment")	Patient sees visual effects through use of mirror/self-examination; radiographs	
Patient goal-setting (some elements of motivational interviewing)	Patient moves from precontemplation to readiness for change	

Source: Treating Tobacco Use and Dependence: 2008 Update. June 2015. Agency for Healthcare Research and Quality, Rockville MD. http://www.ahrq.gov/professionals/clinicians-providers/guidelines-recommendations/tobacco/index.html. Accessed 6/16/2016.

the length and depth of the relationship.

Ethical considerations also must be weighed. Since James's parents are unaware of his habit, should the provider keep the findings confidential until the 2-week follow-up appointment? If no resolution is apparent, is that the time to engage the parents? Should informing the parents be used as an impetus for cessation?

James struggled with abstinence initially but at his follow-up appointment 2 weeks after the lesion identification, resolution had occurred. James was relieved to see the tissue change. He is aware that if he returns to his habit, a reversion to his former state will occur and dysplasia and malignancy could follow. Given his level of motivation, James's prognosis is good.

FUTURE CONSIDERATIONS

After his 2-week follow-up, James will be called to ensure he has maintained abstinence and not relapsed. Relapse is common when patients have a nicotine addiction. If he has adhered to the abstinence regimen, James will be rescheduled for a 3-month follow-up to reinforce his abstinence and reassess his tissue health. He will receive an interim call for support. If he remains tobacco-free and his lesion resolves, he will be placed on a 6-month maintenance schedule.

CASE 2: Young Adult Female Patient with History of E-Cigarette and Marijuana Use, Irregular Pap Smear, and Low Health Literacy

PATIENT OVERVIEW

Amanda B. is a 21-year-old Caucasian female who is new to the practice. She presents for her dental hygiene appointment.
Chief Complaint: "I want the stain removed from my teeth."
Health History: Takes birth control pills and multivitamins; has not seen her general physician for 2 years; saw OB/GYN 3 months ago.
Past Medical History: Irregular Pap smear last year—mild dysplasia noted; OB/GYN is monitoring condition; cryosurgery may be necessary. History of genital herpes.

Family History: Parents both alive, divorced; father has history of gout; mother uses tobacco but has no medical conditions.
Social History: Uses marijuana on weekends; occasional e-cigarette use; attends local community college; employed as legal secretary in large law firm.
Physical Assessment: Of average weight and size; pierced nose and obvious tattoo on right shoulder; hair color is purple.
Risk Assessment/Risk Factors: Marijuana use; sporadic use of e-cigarettes; irregular Pap smear; possibility of high-risk sexual behaviors; low health literacy regarding relationship between human papillomavirus (HPV) and head and neck squamous cell carcinomas (HNSCCs); no knowledge of HPV vaccine.

CLINICAL ASSESSMENT

Extra-/Intraoral Examination: Xerostomia; coated tongue.
Periodontal Assessment: Hyperplastic gingiva; minimal bleeding; localized moderate periodontal disease; generalized health.
Accretions: Generalized heavy stain; moderate calculus localized.
Plaque-Free Score: 52%.
Home Care Regimen: Patient brushes once daily with hard toothbrush; rinses 4 times per day with essential oils mouth rinse; uses water irrigator for interdental cleansing 2 times per week.
No diagnostic tests indicted.

RISK REDUCTION

See table on next page.

OUTCOMES

Amanda is at an age when many young people do not have well-shaped identities. These individuals sometimes exhibit edgy appearances and engage in risky behaviors. What is marked is Amanda's gynecological history and her marijuana and e-cigarette use. She also presents with low health literacy, so educating her is critical. Using motivational interviewing (MI) techniques may be helpful, but Amanda is defensive and it may take time for her to decide to abstain from her risky behaviors.

Risk Reduction

Preventive	Therapeutic	Alternatives
Improve health literacy: • Discussion of clinical findings—their relationship to e-cigarette and marijuana use • Are habits only random? • Education regarding risks of habit and nicotine addiction		
Patient ownership of habit and effects (employ "teachable moment")	Patient sees heavy stain—visual effects through use of mirror/self-examination; hyperplastic tissue; minimal blood flow; relate stain to appearance	
Lifestyle/behavioral change: abstinence from e-cigarette and marijuana use	Employ the 5 A's	Possible use of pharmacological adjuncts, depending on extent of habit and patient desire
Content areas of 5 A's: Ask, Advise, Assess, Assist, Arrange	Ultimate goal: patient sets quit date Return for follow-up 2 weeks after quit date	
Patient goal-setting (some elements of motivational interviewing)	Patient moves from precontemplation to readiness for change	Patient maintains habit; patient is monitored Refer for addictions counseling; refer to self-help groups
OB/GYN report related to cervical HPV?	Contact OB/GYN Educate OB/GYN about HNSCCs, if necessary	Refer back to OB/GYN
Discussion of relationship between high-risk sexual practices and HPV; HPV and HNSCC	Discuss HPV vaccine Recommend practice of low-risk sexual behaviors; condom use	Sexual abstinence

Source: Herbert H, Severson HH, Eakin EG, Stevens VJ, Lichtenstein E. Dental office practices for tobacco users: independent practice and HMO clinics. *Am J Public Health* 1990;80:1503–1505.

She is concerned about her irregular Pap smears, so the provider's effort to establish a relationship with her OB/GYN may enable a team approach for behavior change. Amanda's better understanding of genital HPV, the risk of oral infection, and the potential for HNSCCs may motivate her. Recommending the HPV vaccine for the prevention of oral infections or potential HNCs is not evidence based, but preliminary research shows promise for its effectiveness. Some researchers conclude that the vaccine may be effective in women up to 26 years of age. However, the vaccine is preventive; it does not treat. So, if Amanda has had previous exposure, no benefit will accrue. In-depth discussions regarding her sexual practices are best left to the OB/GYN.

The public is unclear about the risks of e-cigarettes as no federal guidelines exist to provide warnings, limit availability, standardize contents, and delineate appropriate usage. Since e-cigarettes are relatively new products, scientific reports remain controversial and provide little evidence for or against their use.

FUTURE CONSIDERATIONS

Amanda has been asked to return in 3 months. She agrees because she does not like the stain on her teeth. Whether that dislike and concern for her appearance will translate into behavior change is unknown. The fact that she is willing to return is a positive sign. Employing MI techniques during her visits and suggesting that she join a self-help group or see an addiction counselor if she needs help to refrain from marijuana and e-cigarette use will continue. Dialogue with the OB/GYN provider will be maintained as it may provide insight into future discussions with Amanda about her risk for HPV.

REFERENCES

1. National Institute of Dentistry and Craniofacial Research (NIDCR). Oral cancer. NIH Fact sheet. Available at: http://report.nih.gov/nihfactsheets/ViewFactSheet.aspx?csid=106. Accessed October 30, 2015.
2. Bray F, Ren J-S, Masuyer E, Ferlay J. Global estimates of cancer prevalence for 27 sites in the adult population in 2008. *Int J Cancer* 2013;132:1133–1145. doi: 10.1002/ijc.27711. (Cited in International Agency for Research on Cancer. *Globocan 2012: Estimated Cancer Incidence, Mortality and Prevalence Worldwide in 2012.* Lyon, France: IARC; 2012. World Health Organization; 2013.
3. American Cancer Society. *Cancer Facts & Figures 2015.* Atlanta, GA: American Cancer Society; 2015.
4. National Comprehensive Cancer Network. NCCN clinical practice guidelines in oncology: head and neck cancers. Vol 1. 2012. Available at: http://www.nccn.org/professionals/physician_gls/pdf/head-and-neck.pdf. Accessed October 2015.
5. Gillison ML, D'Souza G, Westra W, et al. Distinct risk factor profiles for human papillomavirus type 16-positive and human papillomavirus type 16-negative head and neck cancers. *J Natl Cancer Inst.* 2008;100:407–420.
6. Chaturvedi AK, Anderson WF, Lortet-Tieulent J, et al. Worldwide trends in incidence rates for oral cavity and oropharyngeal cancers. *J Clin Oncol.* 2013;31:1–10.
7. Chaturvedi AK, Engels EA, Anderson WF, Gillison ML. Incidence trends for human papillomavirus-related and unrelated oral squamous cell carcinomas in the United States. *J Clin Oncol.* 2008;26:612–619.
8. Gillison ML, Zhang Q, Jordan R, et al. Tobacco smoking and increased risk of death and progression for patients with p16-positive and p16-negative oropharyngeal cancer. *J Clin Oncol.* 2012;30:2202–2211.
9. Ferlay J, Soerjomataram I, Ervik M, Dikshit R, Eser S, et al. Globocan 2012 v1.0, Cancer Incidence and Mortality Worldwide: IARC CancerBase No. 11 (Internet). Lyon, France: International Agency for Research on Cancer; 2013. Available from: http://globocan.iarc.fr, accessed 15/6/2016. (Cited in International Agency for Research on Cancer. *Globocan 2012: Estimated Cancer Incidence, Mortality and Prevalence Worldwide in 2012.* Lyon, France: IARC; 2012. World Health Organization; 2013.)
10. D'Souza G, Kreimer AR, Viscidi R, et al. Case-control study of human papillomavirus and oropharyngeal cancer. *N Engl J Med.* 2007;356:1944–1956.
11. Vigneswaran N, Williams MD. Epidemiological trends in head and neck cancer and aids in diagnosis. *Oral Maxillofac Surg Clin North Am.* 2014;26:123–141.
12. Oral Cancer Foundation. Risk factors. Available from: http://www.oralcancerfoundation.org/cdc/cdc_chapter3.php. Accessed November 19, 2015.
13. Choi I, Myers JN. Molecular pathogenesis of oral squamous cell carcinoma: implications for therapy. *J Dent Res.* 2008;87:14–32.
14. Lassen P. The role of human papillomavirus in head and neck cancer and the impact on radiotherapy outcome. *Radiother Oncol.* 2010;95:371–380.
15. Ram H, Sarkar J, Kumar H, Konwar R, Bhatt MLB, Mohammed S. Oral cancer: risk factors and molecular pathogenesis. *J Maxillofac Oral Surg.* 2011;10:132–137.
16. Brocklehurst P, Kujan O, O'Malley LA, Ogden G, Shepherd S, Glenny AM. Screening programmes for the early detection and prevention of oral cancer. *Cochrane Database Syst Rev.* 2013;(11):CD004150.
17. National Institute of Dentistry and Craniofacial Research (NIDCR). Detecting oral cancer: a guide for health care professionals. [Poster.] Available at: http://www.nidcr.nih.gov/oralhealth/Topics/OralCancer/Documents/DetectingOralCancerPoster_100313_508C.pdf. Accessed February 27, 2016.
18. Ford PJ, Farah CS. Early detection and diagnosis of oral cancer: strategies for improvement. *J Canc Policy.* 2013;1:e2–e7.
19. Liu JLY, Walsh T, Kerr A, et al. Diagnostic tests for oral cancer and potentially malignant disorders in patients presenting with clinically evident lesions. *Cochrane Database Syst Rev.* 2012;(12):CD010276, 1–19.
20. Olson CM, Burda BU, Beil T, Whitlock EP. Screening for Oral Cancer: A Targeted Evidence Update for the U.S. Preventive Services Task Force. Evidence Synthesis No. 102. AHRQ Publication No. 13-05186-EF-1. Rockville, MD: Agency for Healthcare Research and Quality; April 2013.
21. Kreimer AR, Johansson M, Waterboer T, et al. Evaluation of human papillomavirus antibodies and risk of subsequent head and neck cancer. *J Clin Oncol.* 2013;31:2708–2715.
22. Agarawal N, VanHook A. Science Translational Medicine. Podcast. American Association for the Advancement of Science; June 24, 2015;7(293):293pc1. Available at: http://podcasts.aaas.org/science_transl_med/SciTranslMed_150624.mp3. Accessed November 30, 2015.
23. Fiore M, Bailey W, Cohen SJ, et al. Treating Tobacco Use and Dependence: Clinical Practice Guideline: *2008 Update.* Rockville, MD: U.S. Department of Health and Human Services, Agency for Healthcare Research and Quality; June 2015. Available at: http://www.ahrq.gov/profession-

als/clinicians-providers/guidelines-recommendations/tobacco/index.html. Accessed February 27, 2016.
24. Boyce JH, Stead, LF, Cahill K, Lancaster T. Efficacy of interventions to combat tobacco addiction: Cochrane update of 2013 reviews. *Addiction*. 2014;109:414–425.
25. Lindson-Hawley N, Thompson TP, Begh R. Motivational interviewing for smoking cessation. *Cochrane Database Syst Rev*. 2015;(3):CD006936.
26. National Institute of Dentistry and Craniofacial Research (NIDCR). Oral complications of cancer treatment: what the dental team can do. Available at: http://www.nidcr.nih.gov/oralhealth/Topics/CancerTreatment/OralComplicationsCancerOral.htm. Accessed November 15, 2015.
27. Worthington HV, Clarkson JE, Bryan G, et al. Interventions for preventing oral mucositis for patients with cancer receiving treatment. *Cochrane Database Syst Rev*. 2011;(4):CD000978.
28. Lalla RV, Bowen J, Barasch A, et al. MASCC/ISOO Clinical practice guidelines for the management of mucositis secondary to cancer therapy. *Cancer*. 2014;120:1453–1461.
29. Ramqvist T, Grün N, Dalianis T. Human papillomavirus and tonsillar and base of tongue cancer. *Viruses*. 2015;7(3);1332–1343.
30. Gregoire V, Lefebvre JL, Licitra L, Felip E; EHNS-ESMO-ESTRO Guidelines Working Group. Squamous cell carcinoma of the head and neck: EHNS–ESMO–ESTRO Clinical Practice Guidelines for diagnosis, treatment and follow-up. *Ann Oncol*. 2010;21(suppl 5):v184–v186.
31. Carrillo CM, Correa FN, Lopes NN, Fava M, Filho VO. Dental anomalies in children submitted to antineoplastic therapy. *Clinics*. 2014;69:433–437.
32. National Cancer Institute. Oral complication of chemotherapy and head/neck radiation–health professional version (PDQ®). Updated April 2014. Available at: http://www.cancer.gov/about-cancer/treatment/side-effects/mouth-throat/oral-complications-hp-pdq#section/_207. Accessed November 17, 2015.
33. Coelho KR. Review article: challenges of the oral cancer burden in India. *J Cancer Epidemiol*. 2012;(2012):701932.
34. Ramqvist T, Dalianis T. Oropharyngeal cancer epidemic and human papillomavirus. *Emerg Infect Dis*. 2010;16:1671–1677.
35. Cancer Council of Australia. HPV vaccine. Has the program been successful? Available at: http://www.hpvvaccine.org.au/the-hpv-vaccine/has-the-program-been-successful.aspx. Accessed February 27, 2016.
36. Markowitz LE, Liu G, Harairi S, Steinau M, Denne EF, Unger E. Prevalence of HPV after introduction of the vaccination program in the United States. *Pediatrics*. 2016;137(2):e20151968.
37. President's Cancer Panel. *Accelerating HPV Vaccine Uptake: Urgency for Action to Prevent Cancer*. Bethesda, MD: National Cancer Institute; 2014.
38. National Cancer Institute. Health risks of e-cigarettes, smokeless tobacco, and waterpipes. Available at: http://www.cancer.net/navigating-cancer-care/prevention-and-healthy-living/tobacco-use/health-risks-e-cigarettes-smokeless-tobacco-and-waterpipes. Accessed February 27, 2016.
39. http://www.fda.gov/TobaccoProducts/Labelling/RulesRegulationsGuidance/ucm394909.htm.
40. Lopes CFB, de Angelis BB, Prudente HM, et al. Concomitant consumption of marijuana, alcohol and tobacco in oral squamous cell carcinoma development and progression: recent advances and challenges. *Arch Oral Biol*. 2012;57:1026–1033.
41. Guerra ENS, Acevedo AC, Leite AF, et al. Diagnostic capability of salivary biomarkers in the assessment of head and neck cancer: a systematic review and meta-analysis. *Oral Oncol*. 2015;51:805–818.
42. Dorsey K, Agulnik M. Promising new molecular targeted therapies in head and neck cancer. *Drugs*. 2013;73:315–325.
43. Kreimer AR, Gonzalez P, Katki HA, Porras C, Schiffman M. Efficacy of a bivalent HPV 16/18 vaccine against anal HPV 16/18 infection among young women: a nested analysis within the Costa Rica Vaccine Trial. *Lancet Oncol*. 2011;12:862–870.
44. Lawson G, Matar N, Remacle M, Jamart J, Bachy V. Transoral robotic surgery for the management of head and neck tumors: learning curve. *Eur Arch Otorhinolaryngol*. 2011;268:1795–1801.
45. Chu KF, Dupuy DE. Thermal ablation of tumours: biological mechanisms and advances in therapy. *Nat Rev Cancer*. 2014;14:199–208.

Appendix 1: MASCC/ISOO Clinical Practice Guidelines for Oral Mucositis*

RECOMMENDATIONS IN FAVOR OF AN INTERVENTION (i.e., strong evidence supports effectiveness in the treatment setting listed):

1. The panel recommends that 30 minutes of oral cryotherapy be used to prevent oral mucositis in patients receiving bolus 5-fluorouracil chemotherapy (II).
2. The panel recommends that recombinant human keratinocyte growth factor-1 (KGF-1/palifermin) be used to prevent oral mucositis (at a dose of 60 mcg/kg per day for 3 days prior to conditioning treatment and for 3 days after transplant) in patients receiving high-dose chemotherapy and total body irradiation, followed by autologous stem cell transplantation, for a hematological malignancy (II).
3. The panel recommends that low-level laser therapy (wavelength at 650 nm, power of 40 mW, and each square centimeter treated with the required time to a tissue energy dose of 2 J/cm^2), be used to prevent oral mucositis in patients receiving HSCT conditioned with high-dose chemotherapy, with or without total body irradiation (II).
4. The panel recommends that patient-controlled analgesia with morphine be used to treat pain due to oral mucositis in patients undergoing HSCT (II).
5. The panel recommends that benzydamine mouthwash be used to prevent oral mucositis in patients with head and neck cancer receiving moderate dose radiation therapy (up to 50 Gy), without concomitant chemotherapy (I).

SUGGESTIONS IN FAVOR OF AN INTERVENTION (i.e., weaker evidence supports effectiveness in the treatment setting listed):

1. The panel suggests that oral care protocols be used to prevent oral mucositis in all age groups and across all cancer treatment modalities (III).
2. The panel suggests that oral cryotherapy be used to prevent oral mucositis in patients receiving high-dose melphalan, with or without total body irradiation, as conditioning for HSCT (III).
3. The panel suggests that low-level laser therapy (wavelength around 632.8 nm) be used to prevent oral mucositis in patients undergoing radiotherapy, without concomitant chemotherapy, for head and neck cancer (III).
4. The panel suggests that transdermal fentanyl may be effective to treat pain due to oral mucositis in patients receiving conventional or high-dose chemotherapy, with or without total body irradiation (III).
5. The panel suggests that 2% morphine mouthwash may be effective to treat pain due to oral mucositis in patients receiving chemoradiation for head and neck cancer (III).
6. The panel suggests that 0.5% doxepin mouthwash may be effective to treat pain due to oral mucositis (IV).
7. The panel suggests that systemic zinc supplements administered orally may be of benefit to prevent oral mucositis in oral cancer patients receiving radiation therapy or chemoradiation (III).

RECOMMENDATIONS AGAINST AN INTERVENTION (i.e., strong evidence indicates lack of effectiveness in the treatment setting listed):

1. The panel recommends that PTA (polymyxin, tobramycin, amphotericin B) and BCoG (bacitracin, clotrimazole, gentamicin) antimicrobial lozenges and PTA paste not be used to prevent oral mucositis in patients receiving radiation therapy for head and neck cancer (II).
2. The panel recommends that iseganan antimicrobial mouthwash not be used to prevent oral mucositis in patients receiving high-dose chemotherapy, with or without total body irradiation, for HSCT (II), or in patients receiving radiation therapy or concomitant chemoradiation for head and neck cancer (II).
3. The panel recommends that sucralfate mouthwash not be used to prevent oral

mucositis in patients receiving chemotherapy for cancer (I), or in patients receiving radiation therapy (I) or concomitant chemoradiation (II) for head and neck cancer.
4. The panel recommends that sucralfate mouthwash not be used to treat oral mucositis in patients receiving chemotherapy for cancer (I), or in patients receiving radiation therapy (II) for head and neck cancer.
5. The panel recommends that intravenous glutamine not be used to prevent oral mucositis in patients receiving high-dose chemotherapy, with or without total body irradiation, for HSCT (II).

SUGGESTIONS AGAINST AN INTERVENTION (i.e., weaker evidence indicates lack of effectiveness in the treatment setting listed):
1. The panel suggests that chlorhexidine mouthwash not be used to prevent oral mucositis in patients receiving radiation therapy for head and neck cancer (III).
2. The panel suggests that granulocyte-macrophage colony-stimulating factor mouthwash not be used to prevent oral mucositis in patients receiving high-dose chemotherapy, for autologous or allogeneic stem cell transplantation (II).
3. The panel suggests that misoprostol mouthwash not be used to prevent oral mucositis in patients receiving radiation therapy for head and neck cancer (III).
4. The panel suggests that systemic pentoxifylline, administered orally, not be used to prevent oral mucositis in patients undergoing bone marrow transplantation (III).
5. The panel suggests that systemic pilocarpine, administered orally, not be used to prevent oral mucositis in patients receiving radiation therapy for head and neck cancer (III), or in patients receiving high-dose chemotherapy, with or without total body irradiation, for HSCT (II).

Source: © Multinational Association of Supportive Care in Cancer (MASCC) and The International Society of Oral Oncology (ISOO). All rights reserved worldwide. Publication/adaptation of these guidelines in any form requires prior permission from the MASCC/ISOO Mucositis Study Group. http://www.mascc.org
Abbreviations: Gy, grays; HSCT, hematopoietic stem cell transplantation; MASCC/ISOO, Multinational Association of Supportive Care in Cancer and International Society of Oral Oncology; mW, milliwatt; nm, nanometers.
*Level of evidence for each guideline is in brackets after the guideline statement.

Chapter 8
Oral Malodor
P. Mark Bartold

Halitosis, *bad breath*, and *oral malodor* all are terms used interchangeably for breath malodor. Halitosis is defined as an unpleasant odor from the mouth and can be caused by the consumption of certain foods, poor oral hygiene, alcohol or tobacco use, dry mouth, or by some chronic medical conditions. Oral malodor originates from within the mouth, whereas bad breath may arise from sites other than the mouth. Indeed, *oral malodor* is a definitive term and should not be mistaken for transient breath malodor arising from various foods, alcohol, or smoking. It is also a separate condition from morning breath malodor, which is present upon waking as a result of diminished salivary flow during sleep and usually resolves following breakfast and morning oral hygiene regimens. Therefore, when discussing halitosis, it is necessary to distinguish between oral malodor and bad breath.

Oral malodor is considered to be the most common form of halitosis[1,2] and is generally attributed to the production of volatile sulfur compounds, which have a particularly unpleasant smell and are produced by oral bacteria.[3] Thus, oral malodor is considered a symptom of several oral conditions that need to be accurately diagnosed. Individuals who suffer from oral malodor consider the condition to be of considerable concern and importance, with significant impact on their daily activities. Indeed, this is not only an important oral condition but also an interesting sociological issue that has led to large-scale marketing, and consumption, of breath-freshening aids (lozenges, mouth rinses, toothpastes, etc.) that represent a billion-dollar industry.

EPIDEMIOLOGY OF HALITOSIS
Historically, halitosis has been recognized as an issue of considerable concern, with references to "pleasant breath" being found in ancient papyrus manuscripts as early as 1550 BC.[4] Throughout the ages and across cultures, halitosis has been featured as a social condition affecting individuals' quality of life.

The prevalence of chronic halitosis (including oral malodor) differs considerably across global populations due mainly to cultural differences in odor perception, lack of uniform guidelines and procedures for its measurement and evaluation, and poor correlation between self-reported and clinically evident halitosis.[5] In general, epidemiological studies have reported variable prevalence of halitosis ranging between 2% and 30% of the world's population.[6-9] The overall incidence in industrialized countries may be as high as 25% to 40% of the population.[8] Where halitosis has been identified, studies report that up to 90% of halitosis cases have oral origins that are usually associated with poor oral hygiene, periodontal disease (gingivitis and periodontitis), dental caries, and tongue coatings—all of which would be consistent with a diagnosis of oral malodor.[10] Approximately 10% of halitosis cases are of nonoral origin, with 5% of halitosis cases being associated with sinus or gastrointestinal problems, while other etiologies account for the remaining 5%.[10]

Several studies have investigated relationships among oral malodor, gender, and age.[10-13] In general, it has been concluded that oral malodor is three times higher in men than in women and three times higher in people over 20 years of age. The age distribution of individuals presenting for assessment of halitosis in a private periodontal practice is shown in Figure 1. These data confirm that halitosis appears to be a condition of concern to adults between 40

Figure 1. Age Distribution of Patients Attending a Private Halitosis Assessment Clinic

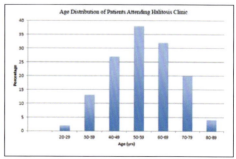

and 80 years of age rather than children (0%), adolescents (0%), and young adults between the ages of 20 and 40 years (15%). However, in this cohort of patients seeking treatment for halitosis, 54% were female and 47% were male (unpublished data).

CLASSIFICATION OF HALITOSIS

A useful classification system for halitosis focusing on the origin of the problem was first described and published in Japanese in 1999 by Miyazaki and colleagues[14] and was subsequently presented in English by Yaegaki and Coil.[15] This classification categorizes halitosis as temporary, intraoral, extraoral, pseudo, or halitophobia (see Table 1). In doing so, it encourages rational treatment decisions to be made depending on the overall diagnosis of the condition. Of the five categories in this classification, the two most important distinctions are between intraoral and extraoral halitosis because these are recognized to represent the presence of "real" halitosis. The term *intraoral halitosis* is used to describe cases in which the source of the problem can be found within the oral cavity and includes tongue coatings as well as pathological conditions such as gingivitis, periodontitis, ulcers, and dental caries. *Extraoral halitosis* can generally be subdivided into blood-borne and non–blood-borne halitosis. The terms *pseudohalitosis* and *halitophobia* are used to describe conditions in which patients believe they have halitosis but, following clinical assessment, no such condition can be confirmed. The condition of *temporary halitosis* is usually associated with various types of food, drink, or tobacco use.

PATHOGENESIS OF INTRAORAL HALITOSIS (ORAL MALODOR)

Historically, there have been numerous theories regarding the etiology and pathogenesis of halitosis. The most commonly accepted sources of halitosis have been considered to be nonoral (such as from the stomach) and poor oral hygiene.[16] Today, it is well-recognized that intraoral halitosis (oral malodor) is caused principally by the degradation of organic material by some of the anaerobic bacteria associated with periodontal disease.[16-18] These

Table 1. Categories of Oral Malodor

Temporary Halitosis
Smoking
Diet (garlic, spicy foods, dairy)
Intraoral Halitosis (Oral Malodor)
Oral bacteria
- Chronic gingivitis
- Periodontitis
- Tongue coating
Acute infections
- Abscess
- Necrotizing ulcerative periodontitis
- Pericoronitis
Dry mouth
- Sjögren's syndrome
- Medications
Extraoral Halitosis
Nasal, paranasal, or laryngeal origins
- Including acute viral or bacterial infection, tonsillitis, deep tonsillar crypts, tonsilloliths, chronic sinusitis, postnasal drip, foreign body in nasal cavity or sinus.
Pulmonary tract or upper gastrointestinal tract origins
- *Bronchi and lungs*, including chronic bronchitis, bronchial carcinoma, bronchiectasis
- *Gastrointestinal*, including regurgitation, hiatus hernia, *Helicobacter pylori* infection, achalasia, steatorrhea and other malabsorption conditions
Blood-borne and emitted via lungs
- Liver cirrhosis
- Kidney insufficiency
- Systemic metabolic disorders, including diabetes, trimethylaminuria, starvation
- Internal bleeding
- Menstrual cycle
Pseudohalitosis
Oral malodor does not exist, but patient believes he or she has halitosis
Halitophobia
After treatment for genuine halitosis or pseudohalitosis, patient continues to believe he or she suffers from halitosis

bacteria produce the bad smell that is attributed to the presence of volatile sulfur compounds, diamines, and phenyl compounds (see Table 2).[3,19] Of these, it is the volatile sulfur compounds that have been most extensively studied; in particular, methylmercaptan, hydrogen sulfide, and dimethyl sulphide have received the most attention. Specific bacteria demonstrated to produce volatile sulphur compounds include *Fusobacterium nucleatum, Treponema denticola, Prevotella intermedia, Porphyromonas gingivalis,* and *Bacteroides forsythus.*

Table 2. Volatile Malodorous Contributors to Oral Malodor

Volatile Sulfur Compounds
Methylmercaptan
Hydrogen sulfide
Dimethyl sulfide
Diamines
Putrescine
Cadaverine
Short-chain fatty acids
Butyric acid
Propionic acid
Phenols
Indole
Skatole
Pyridine

Examples of the ability of *P. gingivalis* and *F. nucleatum* to produce high levels of hydrogen sulphide and methylmercaptan (but not dimethyl sulphide) are shown in Figure 2. It is now generally accepted that oral malodor is particularly associated with elevated levels of methylmercaptan and hydrogen sulfide whereas halitosis from nonoral sources may be associated with another volatile sulfur compound, dimethyl sulfide.[20]

The bacteria mostly responsible for the production of methylmercaptan and hydrogen sulfide are associated with the subgingival plaque of gingivitis and periodontitis, although they are also commonly found on the dorsum of the tongue. Some studies have suggested that in addition to periodontal disease, oral malodor is directly related to the total bacterial load in both saliva and tongue coating.[21,22] Nonetheless, it is generally accepted that patients with oral malodor have significantly more pockets greater than 5 mm and heavier tongue coating than those without oral malodor.[7] Interestingly, it has been reported that oral malodor in adults is caused by both periodontal disease and heavy tongue coating whereas oral malodor in children may be more likely to be the result of tongue coating.[7]

PATHOGENESIS OF EXTRAORAL HALITOSIS

Extraoral halitosis can be further divided into non–blood-borne halitosis, which includes halitosis arising from the nasal passages and the respiratory tract, and blood-borne halitosis.[20] Most extraoral halitosis is of a blood-borne nature and occurs when volatile substances are absorbed into the bloodstream from many sites in the body—including the mouth, stomach, liver, and kidneys—and subsequently transported to the lungs, where they are secreted into the pulmonary alveoli, resulting in halitosis in exhaled air. The principal odorous volatile sulphur compound in blood-borne halitosis is dimethyl sulphide. It is estimated that extraoral halitosis accounts for between 5% and 10% of halitosis cases. Importantly, extraoral halitosis can be associated with serious diseases, including metabolic disorders, liver disease, and kidney disease.

Figure 2. Detection of Volatile Sulphur Compounds from Cultured Isolates of *Porphyromonas gingivalis* and *Fusobacterium nucleatum*

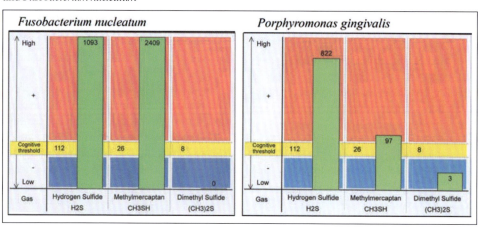

HOW CAN HALITOSIS BE ASSESSED?

A thorough history, both medical and dental, is an essential starting point when assessing for halitosis. The medical history should include questions relating to current medications, nasal and sinus conditions, snoring and sleep apnea, mouth breathing, throat infections, tonsilloliths, and an assessment of ingestion of foods that may contribute to bad odor.

The dental history should focus on general dental care through regular dental visits; oral hygiene practices, including frequency of toothbrushing; and use of other oral hygiene aids such as dental floss, interdental cleaning aids, mouthrinses, and tongue cleaning/scraping. Specific questions relating to the oral malodor must also be addressed, such as how long the problem has been present, whether it is worse at any particular time of day, and if anyone has commented on the problem. Following the initial interview, both an oral evaluation and breath analysis are required.[23]

The oral evaluation should include an assessment of the following: tonsils, oral debris, caries, exposed pulps, extraction wounds, interdental food impaction, gingivitis, periodontitis, necrotizing periodontal conditions, peri-implantitis, pericoronitis, and recurrent oral ulcerations.

An assessment of tongue coating is also an integral part of the oral assessment for halitosis. An index (Winkel Tongue Coating Index) for assessing tongue coatings has been used in which the dorsum of the tongue is divided into six sections (see Figure 3).[24] The presence of any tongue coating is then graded and recorded for each of the sextants. No coating is given a score of 0, a light–thin coating is given a score of 1 and a heavy–thick coating is given a score of 2 (see Figure 4). A score is then calculated by adding all six scores, thus obtaining a total score within a range of 0 to 12.

It is also important to assess the quantity and quality of saliva and any relationship this has to the presence of a dry mouth. An important consequence of reduced saliva and dry mouth is increased bacterial growth due to the absence or reduction in the antibacterial properties of saliva. With the increased bacterial load, there is an associated increase in release of volatile sulfur compounds and thus an increase in oral malodor.

Following the oral examination, breath odor should be evaluated. There are numerous ways in which this can be done, including organoleptic methods (smelling patients' exhaled breath) or use of purpose-built instruments (Halimeter®, Breathtron® or OralChroma™).

Organoleptic Measurement of Halitosis

Organoleptic measurement of halitosis requires a trained clinician to sniff and smell the patient's expired air and score the level of odor. This is considered the gold standard for assessing oral malodor. An intensity of odor range has been proposed based on the clinical rating of the odor and subsequently slightly modified (see Table 3).[25,26] However, there are a number of concerns with this very subjective approach to breath assessment. One concern is the potential for differences in scoring between different assessors. This can somewhat be overcome by using multiple assessors who have been calibrated in their scoring and assessment. Clearly the biggest problem with this form of assessment is that it is an unpleasant

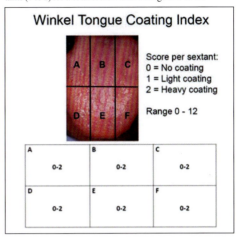

Figure 3. Winkel Tongue Coating Score

The dorsum of the tongue is divided into sextants, and the amount of tongue coating is subjectively graded for each sextant. The score is calculated by adding the scores for all sextants (0 to 2) for a total score within a range of 0 to 12.

Figure 4. Winkel Tongue Coating Score
Tongue coating is graded on a scale of 0 to 2.

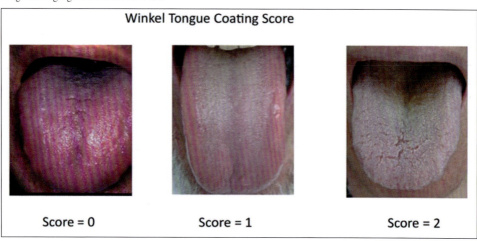

Table 3. Organoleptic Scoring of Halitosis

0 = No odor present
1 = Barely noticeable odor
2 = Slight but clearly noticeable odor
3 = Moderate odor
4 = Strong offensive odor
5 = Extremely offensive odor

Source: J Dent Res. 2004;83(1):81–85.[38]

experience for both the patient and the assessor. Therefore, more objective and sophisticated means of measuring volatile sulphur compounds in breath have been developed for both research and clinical purposes.

Instrumental Assessment of Halitosis

While there are many reported methods for assessing halitosis, instrumental analysis for the presence of volatile sulfur compounds is recommended because this provides a degree of objective assessment.[27,28]

The first of such instruments, the Halimeter®, was developed in the 1990s as a chairside instrument for measuring volatile sulphur compounds.[29] The readings from this instrument were found to not always correlate well with organoleptic scores due to the presence of other malodorous compounds, such as volatile fatty acids and cadaverine, which could be detected by organoleptic means but not by the Halimeter®. Nonetheless, the development of this instrument opened up new opportunities for research and the development of clinical protocols to measure and monitor treatments for oral malodor.

More recently another device, OralChroma™, has been developed. Rather than measuring total volatile sulphur compounds, it can distinguish and measure the three major volatile sulphur compounds (hydrogen sulfide, methylmercaptan, and dimethyl sulfide) associated with halitosis (see Figure 5). Sample collection is simply achieved by placing a disposable syringe in the mouth with lips sealed for 30 seconds; then the contents are injected into the chromatograph. Analysis takes 8 minutes after which a printout is produced depicting the levels of the three volatile sulfur compounds (see Figure 6). This is particularly useful as it allows for immediate assessment of the source of

Figure 5. OralChroma™ Portable Gas Chromatograph

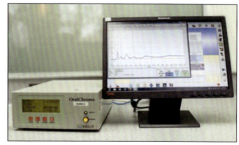

the oral malodor; that is, whether it is likely to be arising from the oral cavity (hydrogen sulfide, methylmercaptan, or both) or elsewhere (dimethyl sulfide).

MANAGEMENT OF HALITOSIS

As previously detailed, thorough investigation and accurate diagnosis are central to the management of halitosis. In general, the initial treatment strategies should be aimed at controlling the factors that are considered to be driving the condition. In the past, this has involved a nonstructured approach of reduction of bacterial load (brushing, flossing, and tongue scraping) and the adjunctive use of chemical agents to freshen the odor.[30] However, more recently, the treatment options for halitosis have been refined according to the various types of halitosis listed in Table 4 and have been divided into six categories.[15,23] A simple matrix has been developed to assist with the decision-making process for the various types of halitosis (see Table 5). Clearly, management of temporary, intraoral, and pseudohalitosis can be undertaken by oral healthcare professionals. However, both extraoral halitosis and halitophobia require the assistance of physicians, psychiatrists, and psychologists.

Table 4. Treatment Options (TO) for Halitosis

TO1. Explanation of halitosis, oral hygiene instruction, and tongue cleaning instructions
TO2. Address any dietary and smoking contributory factors
TO3 Full-mouth prophylaxis and management of any oral conditions likely to be contributing to oral malodor (gingivitis, periodontitis, ulcers, caries, etc.)
TO4. Referral to a medical specialist for further investigations of extraoral sources
TO5. Explanation of examination findings; reinforcement of oral hygiene practices, including tongue cleaning; education on causes of halitosis and reassurance
TO6. Referral to specialist for psychological assistance to understand and deal with condition

Source: J Can Dent Assoc. 200;66(5):257–261.[15]

Therapeutic Interventions

Oral malodor can be suspected if hydrogen sulfide and methylmercaptan are present in elevated

Figure 6. Sample Collection and Analysis for OralChroma™ Assessment
A. Sample of intraoral air is collected in a disposable syringe for 30 seconds. **B.** The contents are injected into the chromatograph. **C.** Analysis takes 8 minutes after which a printout depicts the levels of the three volatile sulfur compounds (hydrogen sulfide, methyl mercaptan, and dimethyl sulfide)

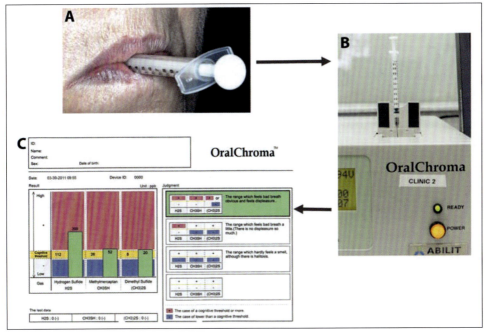

Table 5. Treatment Matrix for Management of Halitosis

Condition	Treatment Options					
	TO1	TO2	TO3	TO4	TO5	TO6
Temporary	X					
Intraoral	X	X	X			
Extraoral	X	X		X		
Pseudo	X	X			X	
Halitophobia	X	X				X

levels. Conversely, an extraoral source of halitosis is usually suspected if dimethyl sulfide readings are high.[20] Once a diagnosis of oral malodor (as distinct from breath malodor) is made, then treatment of the oral condition can commence. Ideally this will be cause related and typically involves a multistep approach. If temporary halitosis is suspected, then an assessment and management of dietary components is essential to eliminate the intake of smelly foods such as garlic, onion, and alcohol. This initial aspect of management should be followed for all five halitosis classifications. In addition, all dental disease, including gingivitis, periodontitis, ulcers, and dental caries, must be diagnosed and effectively managed.

Although periodontal disease (gingivitis and periodontitis) is considered to be a significant cause of oral malodor, surprisingly few studies have fully evaluated the effect of treatment of periodontal disease on halitosis.[31] While some effect on reducing oral malodor following periodontal treatment has been reported, a recent study concluded that both full-mouth disinfection and quadrant root planing resulted in reduced levels of volatile sulfur compounds, but no effect was noted for organoleptic outcomes.[32-34]

The overriding principle for management of intraoral halitosis is reduction of the bacterial burden. An effective and regular oral hygiene regimen involves tooth brushing, interdental cleaning, and regular (twice daily) tongue cleaning using either a toothbrush or tongue scraper (see Figure 7).[35,36] While it is interesting to note that some authors do not recommend tongue scraping due to potential damage to the tongue surface,[15] two systematic reviews evaluating the effectiveness of mechanical

Figure 7. Tongue Scraping
Tongue scraping may be used as an intervention for oral malodor.

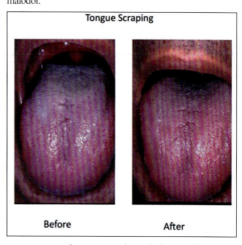

tongue scraping on oral malodor and tongue coating have concluded that tongue scraping results in a small but significant reduction in volatile sulphur compounds.[36,37] Both systematic reviews concluded that the effect may be short lived and of minimal effect for chronic oral malodor and must be carried out on a regular basis to be effective.

Rendering malodorous gases as nonvolatile should also be an aim in the management of oral malodor, which can be achieved through several means. The most common of these is the use of active ingredients in toothpastes and mouthrinses. For the management of intraoral malodor, use of a proven antibacterial toothpaste is recommended. A recent review evaluated studies published to June 2012 investigating the use of toothpastes with various ingredients in the management of oral malodor.[38] A list of ingredients added to toothpastes for oral malodor management and their effectiveness in reducing oral malodor indicators is shown in Table 6. Overall, toothpastes containing antibacterial agents, such as triclosan or metal ions (zinc or stannous), have been most comprehensively studied and show the greatest potential to influence oral malodor.[38] Other agents, such as hydrogen peroxide, essential oils, and flavors, have also been studied and show limited effects in reducing oral malodor.[38]

Table 6. Toothpaste Additives Evaluated for Management of Halitosis

Additive	Reduction in Malodor (%)
Hydrogen peroxide	59
Sodium bicarbonate	29–50
Flavors	24–70
Sodium lauryl sulfate	33–38
Essential oils	37–40
Stannous fluoride	14–59
Zinc ions	35–68
Triclosan	24–88

Source: J Clin Periodontol. 2014;40(5):505–513.[38]

The adjunctive use of antiseptic mouthrinses is essential to a satisfactory outcome in the management of oral malodor.[39,40] While chlorhexidine remains the gold standard for chemical plaque control, its long-term use cannot be recommended. Therefore, formulations with cetylpyridinium chloride or zinc ions have been recommended.[41-43] According to studies, these formulations work by reducing the overall bacterial load and also have a diluting effect on the volatile sulphur compounds responsible for malodor.[41-43] The use of agents containing zinc is particularly interesting as zinc appears to have both an antibacterial effect and an ability to neutralize volatile sulfur compounds.[44] For these reasons, mouthrinses and also toothpastes containing zinc are gaining acceptance as useful adjuncts in the management of oral halitosis.

A recent systematic review evaluated the effectiveness of mouthrinses in the management of oral malodor and reported that mouthrinses containing chlorhexidine (CHX) + cetylpyridinium chloride (CPC) + zinc (Zn) and those containing zinc chloride (ZnCl) + cetylpyridinium chloride (CPC) have the most evidence to support a beneficial outcome.[45] Following application of the Grading of Recommendations Assessment, Development, and Evaluation (GRADE) system,[46] the evidence emerging from this systematic review was graded. Specifically, risk of bias of the individual studies, consistency and precision among the study outcomes, directness of the study results, detection of publication bias, and magnitude of the effect were assessed by the authors. For this assessment, grading was possible for the combination of ingredients CHX + CPC + Zn and ZnCl + CPC mouthwashes. When taken together, the GRADE assessment resulted in the authors concluding that the strength for a recommendation regarding their use in the management of oral malodor was "weak." Another "interesting" mouthrinse is water. Simply by increasing oral hydration, the solubility of volatile sulfur compounds is increased and can lead to some reduction in malodor. For these reasons, it is suggested that frequent water intake can reduce malodor for an hour.[47]

For some time, probiotics have been proposed as a useful adjunct in the management of both intraoral and extraoral halitosis.[48,49] The use of probiotics for oral malodor is based on the bacterial origin of this condition.[3] Thus, controlling the reappearance of bacteria capable of producing oral malodor through the selective introduction of non–odor-producing, commensal bacteria to colonize the oral cavity is an attractive proposal. Early studies demonstrated that by introducing *Streptococcus salivarius* K12 following mechanical periodontal debridement, volatile sulfur compounds could be reduced.[48-51] However, two studies investigating morning bad breath failed to show any effect of probiotic use on volatile sulphur compounds.[52,53] It should be noted that morning bad breath is usually a transient condition and is most likely a different condition than oral malodor. Therefore, to date, the results of studies investigating the use of probiotics as an adjunctive aid for management of oral malodor have been equivocal and are not universally accepted as a proven method to control oral malodor.[49-55]

It is important to recognize that the use of agents that merely mask the offensive smell of oral malodor are generally of limited value. These agents include mouthrinses, sprays, lozenges, and chewing gums. While these products will most likely produce short-term effects, they are not a treatment per se and may delay correct diagnosis.

As stated earlier, it is generally accepted that around 10% of all halitosis cases arise from extraoral sources. An extraoral source of halitosis is usually suspected if dimethyl sulfide readings are high.[20]

In these cases, additional assessment and tests are required. If deemed appropriate, referral to an appropriate physician specializing in the management of nasal, throat, or gastrointestinal abnormalities may be required. The specialist may also recommend blood tests to assess for kidney insufficiency, liver insufficiency or dysfunction, and metabolic diseases. Although good oral hygiene is likely to be of general benefit to the patient suffering from extraoral halitosis, it is unlikely to have any significant impact on this specific condition.

Prevention of Oral Malodor
Surprisingly, there is very little scientific literature published about primary prevention of oral malodor before it develops. Nearly all studies have focused on the treatment and subsequent prevention of recurrence of the problem. Nonetheless, it seems intuitive that prevention of recurrence should be the same as prevention of development. Accordingly, preventive measures for patients should be directed at preventing malodor-forming situations, such as dental and periodontal disease, and the development of tongue coatings. Clearly this will involve (as described above for the management of intraoral malodor) regular dental checkups, as well as good oral hygiene regimens, including toothbrushing, flossing, and tongue scraping, and use of toothpastes and mouthrinses scientifically validated to be effective in the management of oral malodor. Of the few studies published on prevention of oral malodor, one reports that an effective preventive measure for this condition is to continually reinforce to patients the risk of halitosis through an education program utilizing oral malodor as a motivational tool.[56]

CONCLUSIONS
While perhaps not the most glamorous facet of dentistry, management of oral malodor is a fascinating and important aspect of clinical practice and patient care. For many patients, this is a very distressing problem. Through the use of developing aids to detect oral malodor and recognition of the role of certain bacteria in oral malodor, the management of this condition is becoming more predictable.

CASE 1: Intraoral Halitosis (Oral Malodor)

PATIENT OVERVIEW
Gender: Male.
Age: 46 years.
Chief Complaint and Duration: Wife complains he has bad breath. Present for over 12 months.
Oral Hygiene: Brushes once daily with manual toothbrush; does not use dental floss or mouthrinses.
Do Gums Bleed After Brushing/Flossing? Yes.
Bad Taste in Mouth? Yes.
Dry Mouth: Yes; drinks 1 liter of water daily.
Last Prophylaxis: 2 months ago.
Diet: Wife vegetarian, low in dairy foods, otherwise no abnormality detected.
Smoking History: Never a smoker.
Medical History: Slight high blood pressure; no medication for this condition. Otherwise no abnormality detected.

CLINICAL EXAMINATION
Extra-/Intraoral Examination
Oral Hygiene: Fair, poor interproximally.
Bleeding on Probing: All molars.
Periodontal Assessment: Generalized 4- to 5-mm pockets. Minimal radiographic evidence of bone loss. No furcations, no mobility.
Caries: None.
Winkel Tongue Coating: Score 6.
Periodontal Diagnosis: Mild/moderate chronic periodontitis in otherwise healthy 46-year-old male.
Breath Analysis: An OralChroma™ breath analysis was undertaken and the results are shown in Figure 8. Hydrogen sulfide and methylmercaptan levels were high and above the cognitive threshold. The level of dimethyl sulphide was elevated but not above the cognitive threshold.
Halitosis Assessment: Overt oral malodor detected.

TREATMENT PLAN
- Oral hygiene instruction: twice daily brushing, daily flossing.
- Recommend daily tongue scraping.
- Use of therapeutic mouthrinse twice daily.

- Full-mouth subgingival debridement over four visits.
- Reassessment of periodontal condition and breath.

PERIODONTAL OUTCOME

Significant improvement in periodontal tissues was observed with associated good improvement in oral hygiene. No bleeding on probing was detected and pocket depths were not greater than 4 mm. Tongue coating significantly reduced to Winkel score of zero. Halitosis (oral malodor) was no longer detected.

Post-Treatment Breath Analysis

An OralChroma™ breath analysis was undertaken 4 months after completion of the periodontal treatment, and the results are shown in Figure 8. All three gases measured (hydrogen sulphide, methylmercaptan, and dimethyl sulphide) were below the cognitive threshold.

CASE 2: Extraoral Halitosis

PATIENT OVERVIEW

Gender: Female.
Age: 35 years.
Chief Complaint and Duration: Bad breath had been present for several years. Breath fresheners do not seem to help.
Oral Hygiene: Brushes twice daily with manual and electric brush. Daily floss use. Essential oil mouthrinse daily.
Do Gums Bleed after Brushing/Flossing? Yes.
Bad Taste in Mouth? Yes.
Last Prophylaxis: 2 months ago.
Diet: Slightly high in dairy foods, otherwise no

Figure 8. Case 1. Intraoral Halitosis (Oral Malodor)
A. OralChroma™ breath assessment before treatment. B. OralChroma™ breath assessment after treatment. C. Tongue coating before treatment. D. Orthopantomograph taken at initial presentation. E. Tongue coating after treatment.

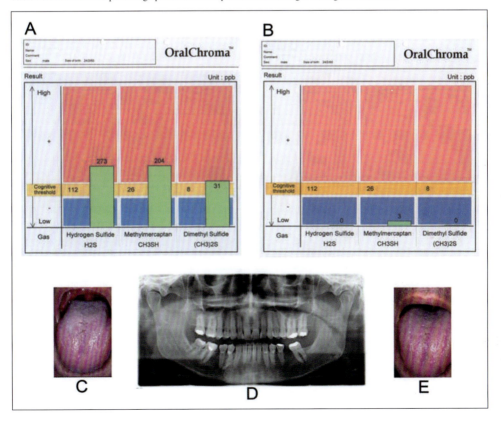

abnormality detected.
Smoking History: Nonsmoker.
Medical History: Tonsillectomy when a child. Hiatus hernia and gastric reflux—taking ranitidine (150 mg twice daily). No abnormality detected.

ORAL EXAMINATION
Extra-/Intraoral Examination
Oral Hygiene: Reasonable but interproximal cleaning could be improved.
Bleeding on Probing: Minimal.
Periodontal Assessment: Minimal pockets (nothing greater than 3 mm). Minimal radiographic evidence of bone loss. No furcations, no mobility.
Caries: None.
Winkel Tongue Coating: Score 0.
Periodontal Diagnosis: Mild gingivitis in an otherwise healthy 35-year-old female.

Breath Analysis: An OralChroma™ breath analysis was undertaken and the results are shown in threshold. The level of dimethyl sulphide was slightly elevated above the cognitive threshold.

Halitosis Assessment: Halitosis was present and most likely of an extraoral source. Possibilities included extraoral malodor associated with hiatus hernia. Although elevated levels of dimethyl sulfide would be consistent with blood-borne halitosis, this is generally a manifestation of serious liver or kidney disease. Individuals afflicted by these conditions usually are aware of their condition and show additional, more diagnostically conclusive symptoms than bad breath.

TREATMENT PLAN
- Oral hygiene instruction: twice-daily brushing, daily flossing.

Figure 9. Case 2. Extraoral Halitosis Associated with Hiatus Hernia
A. OralChroma™ breath assessment before treatment. **B.** OralChroma™ breath assessment after treatment. **C.** Orthopantomograph taken at initial presentation. **D.** Tongue coating after treatment.

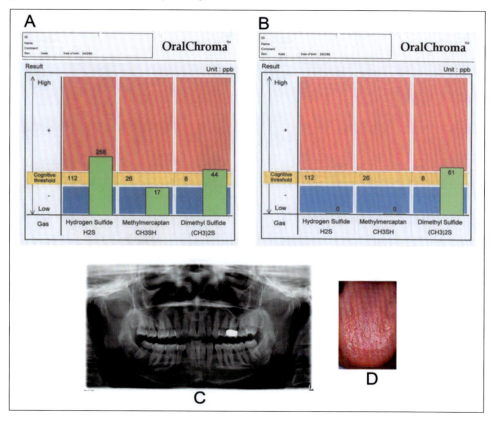

- Recommend daily tongue scraping.
- Use of a therapeutic mouthrinse twice daily.
- Referral for further medical follow up with regard to better management of hiatus hernia, as well as possible source of blood-borne volatile sulfur compounds associated with liver or kidney disease.
- Continue to monitor oral hygiene and halitosis on 6-month basis and provide general full-mouth fine scale and prophylaxis at these visits.

PERIODONTAL OUTCOME

Periodontal condition remained stable. No bleeding on probing was observed, and pocket depths were not greater than 3 mm. Tongue coating significantly remained at Winkel score of zero. Halitosis (oral malodor) still not detected.

Medical Outcome

Hiatus hernia managed by keyhole surgery and appropriate postoperative care. Patient is no longer reporting bad breath.

Post-Treatment Breath Analysis

An OralChroma™ breath analysis was undertaken 12 months after initial consultation, and the results are shown in Figure 9. All three gasses measured (hydrogen sulphide, methylmercaptan, and dimethyl sulphide) were below the cognitive threshold. Halitosis (extraoral malodor) was no longer detected.

SUMMARY OF CASE REPORTS

These two cases illustrate how with correct diagnosis based on clinical and other diagnostic aids, halitosis of both intraoral and extraoral sources can be successfully managed. It is important to remember that the vast majority of halitosis cases have an intraoral source, which can be easily managed by oral health professionals. Extraoral halitosis is uncommon, affecting around 5% to 10% of all halitosis cases. Nonetheless, it is very important to distinguish between intraoral and extraoral halitosis as treatments differ considerably.

Acknowledgment

Parts of this chapter are based on the following publication: Bartold PM. Oral malodor—a review. *Dimensions of Dental Hygiene* (January Issue, 56–61, 2015). Approval for the use of this material has been obtained from the publisher.

REFERENCES

1. Delanghe G, Ghyselen J, Feenstra L, van Steenberghe D. Experiences of a Belgian multidisciplinary breath odour clinic. *Acta Otorhinolaryngol Belg*. 1997;51(1):43–48.
2. Delanghe G, Ghyselen J, van Steenberghe D, Feenstra L. Multidisciplinary breath-odour clinic. *Lancet*. 1997;350(9072):187.
3. Tonzetich J. Production and origin of oral malodor: a review of mechanisms and methods of analysis. *J Periodontol*. 1977;48(1):13–20.
4. Elias MS, Ferriani MD. Historical and social aspects of halitosis. *Rev Lat Am Enfermagem*. 2006;14(5):821–823.
5. Akaji EA, Folaranmi N, Ashiwaju O. Halitosis: a review of the literature on its prevalence, impact and control. *Oral Health Prev Dent*. 2014;12(4):297–304.
6. Söder B, Johansson B, Söder PO. The relation between foetor ex ore, oral hygiene and periodontal disease. *Swed Dent J*. 2000;24(3):73–82.
7. Miyazaki H, Sakao S, Katoh Y, Takehara T. Correlation between volatile sulphur compounds and certain oral health measurements in the general population. *J Periodontol*. 1995;66(8):679–684.
8. Liu XN, Shinada K, Chen XC, Zhang BX, Yaegaki K, Kawaguchi Y. Oral malodor related parameters in the Chinese general population. *J Clin Periodontol*. 2006;33(1):31–36.
9. Nadanovsky P, Carvalho LB, Ponce de Leon A. Oral malodour and its association with age and sex in a general population in Brazil. *Oral Dis*. 2007;13(1):105–109.
10. Zalewska A, Zatoński M, Jabłonka-Strom A, Paradowska A, Kawala B, Litwin A. Halitosis—a common medical and social problem. A review on pathology, diagnosis and treatment. *Acta Gastroenterol Belg*. 2012;75(3):300–309.
11. Nalçaci R, Dülgergil T, Oba AA, Gelgör IE. Prevalence of breath malodour in 7- to 11-year-old children living in Middle Anatolia, Turkey. *Community Dent Health*. 2008;25(3):173–177.
12. Patil PS, Pujar P, Poornima S, Subbareddy VV. Prevalence of oral malodour and its relationship with oral parameters in Indian children aged 7–15 years. *Eur Arch Paediatr Dent*. 2014;15(4):251–258.
13. Villa A, Zollanvari A, Alterovitz G, Cagetti MG, Strohmenger L, Abati S. Prevalence of halitosis in children considering oral hygiene, gender and age. *Int J Dent Hyg*. 2014;12(3):208–212.
14. Miyazaki H, Arao M, Okamura K, et al. Tentative classification of halitosis and its treatment needs (Japanese). *Niigata Dent J*. 1999;32:7–11.
15. Yaegaki K, Coil JM. Examination, classification, and treatment of halitosis; clinical perspectives. *J Can Dent Assoc*. 2000;66(5):257–261.
16. Loesche WJ, Kazor C. Microbiology and treatment of halitosis. *Periodontol 2000*. 2002;28:256–279.
17. Persson S, Edlund MB, Claesson R, Carlsson J. The

formation of hydrogen sulfide and methyl mercaptan by oral bacteria. *Oral Microbiol Immunol.* 1990;5(4):195–201.
18. McNamara TF, Alexander JF, Lee M. The role of microorganisms in the production of oral malodor. *Oral Surg Oral Med Oral Pathol.* 1972;34(1):41–48.
19. Scully C, Greenman J. Halitology (breath odour: aetiopathogenesis and management). *Oral Dis.* 2012;18(4):333–345.
20. Tangerman A, Winkel EG. Volatile sulfur compounds as the cause of bad breath: a review. *Phosphorous Sulfur and Silicon and the Related Elements.* 2013;188:396–402.
21. Tonzetich J, Kestenbaum RC. Odour production by human salivary fractions and plaque. *Arch Oral Biol.* 1969;14(7):815–827.
22. De Boever EH, Loesche WJ. Assessing the contribution of anaerobic microflora of the tongue to oral malodor. *J Am Dent Assoc.* 1995;126(10):1384–1393.
23. Seemann R, Conceicao MD, Filippi A, et al. Halitosis management by the general dental practitioner—results of an international consensus workshop. *J Breath Res.* 2014;8(1):017101. doi: 10.1088/1752 7155/8/1/017101. [Epub Feb 24 2014.]
24. Winkel EG, Roldán S, Van Winkelhoff AJ, Herrera D, Sanz M. Clinical effects of a new mouthrinse containing chlorhexidine, cetylpyridinium chloride and zinc-lactate on oral halitosis. A dual-center, double-blind placebo-controlled study. *J Clin Periodontol.* 2003;30(4):300–306.
25. Rosenberg M, McCulloch CA. Measurement of oral malodor: current methods and future prospects. *J Periodontol.* 1992;63(9):776–782.
26. Greenman J, Duffield J, Spencer P, et al. Study on the organoleptic intensity scale for measuring oral malodor. *J Dent Res.* 2004;83(1):81–85.
27. Dadamio J, Laleman I, De Geest S, et al. Usefulness of a new malodour-compound detection portable device in oral malodour diagnosis. *J Breath Res.* 2013;7(4):046005. doi: 10.1088/1752-7155/7/4/046005. [Epub Nov 1 2013.]
28. Laleman I, Dadamio J, De Geest S, Dekeyser C, Quirynen M. Instrumental assessment of halitosis for the general dental practitioner. *J Breath Res.* 2014;8(1):017103. doi: 10.1088/1752-7155/8/1/017103. [Epub Feb 24 2014.]
29. Rosenberg M, Septon I, Eli I, et al. Halitosis measurement by an industrial sulphide monitor. *J Periodontol.* 1991;62(8):487–489.
30. Yaegaki K, Coil JM, Kamemizu T, Miyazaki H. Tongue brushing and mouth rinsing as basic treatment measures for halitosis. *Int Dent J.* 2002;52(suppl 3):192–196.
31. Soares LG, Tinoco EMB. Prevalence and related parameters of halitosis in general population and periodontal patients. *OA Dentistry.* 2014;2(1):1–7.
32. Pham TA, Ueno M, Zaitsu T, et al. Clinical trial of oral malodor treatment in patients with periodontal diseases. *J Periodontal Res.* 2011;46(6):722–729.
33. Apatzidou DA, Kinane DF. Quadrant root planing versus same-day full-mouth root planing. I. Clinical findings. *J Clin Periodontol.* 2004;31(2):132–140.
34. Soares LG, Castagna L, Weyne SC, Silva DG, Falabella MEV, Tinoco EMB. Effectiveness of full- and partial-mouth disinfection on halitosis in periodontal patients. *J Oral Sci.* 2015;57(1):1–6.
35. van den Broek AM, Feenstra L, de Baat C. A review of the current literature on management of halitosis. *Oral Dis.* 2008;14(1):30–39.
36. Outhouse TL, Al-Alawi R, Fedorowicz Z, Keenan JV. Tongue scraping for treating halitosis. *Cochrane Database Syst Rev.* 2006;2:CD005519.
37. Van der Sleen MI, Slot DE, Van Trijffel E, Winkel EG, Van der Weijden GA. Effectiveness of mechanical tongue cleaning on breath odour and tongue coating: a systematic review. *Int J Dent Hyg.* 2010;8(4):258–268.
38. Dadamio J, Laleman I, Quirynen M. The role of toothpastes in oral malodour management. *Monogr Oral Sci.* 2013;23:45–60.
39. Quirynen M, Zhao H, Soers C, et al. The impact of periodontal therapy and the adjunctive effect of antiseptics on breath odor-related outcome variables: a double-blind randomized study. *J Periodontol.* 2005;76(5):705–712.
40. Quirynen M, Zhao H, van Steenberghe D. Review of the treatment strategies for oral malodour. *Clin Oral Investig.* 2002;6(1):1–10.
41. Young A, Jonski G, Rölla G. Combined effect of zinc ions and cationic antibacterial agents on intraoral volatile sulphur compounds (VSC). *Int Dent J.* 2003;53(4):237–242.
42. Winkel EG, Roldán S, Van Winkelhoff AJ, Herrera D, Sanz M. Clinical effects of a new mouthrinse containing chlorhexidine, cetylpyridinium chloride and zinc-lactate on oral halitosis. A dual-center, double-blind placebo-controlled study. *J Clin Periodontol.* 2003;30(5):300–306.
43. van Steenberghe D, Avontroodt P, Peeters W, et al. Effect of different mouthrinses on morning breath. *J Periodontol.* 2001;72:1183–1191.
44. Dadamio J, Van Tournout M, Teughels W, Dekeyser C, Coucke W, Quirynen M. Efficacy of different mouthrinse formulations in reducing oral malodour: a randomized clinical trial. *J Clin Periodontol.* 2013;40(5):505–513.
45. Slot DE, De Geest S, van der Weijden FA, Quirynen M. Treatment of oral malodour. Medium-term efficacy of mechanical and/or chemical agents: a systematic review. *J Clin Periodontol.* 2015;42(suppl 16):S303–316.
46. Guyatt GH, Oxman AD, Kunz R, et al. GRADE Working Group. Incorporating considerations of resources use into grading recommendations. *BMJ.* 2008;336:1170–1173.
47. Van der Sluijs E, Slot DE, Bakker E, Van der Weijden GA. The effect of water on morning bad breath: a randomized clinical trial. *Int J Dent Hyg.* 2016;14(2):124–134.
48. Burton JP, Chilcott CN, Moore CJ, Speiser G, Tagg JR. A preliminary study of the effect of probiotic

Streptococcus salivarius K12 on oral malodour parameters. *J Appl Microbiol*. 2006;100(4):754–764.

49. Teughels W, Van Essche M, Sliepen I, Quirynen M. Probiotics and oral healthcare. *Periodontol 2000*. 2008;48:111–147.

50. Iwamoto T, Suzuki N, Tanabe K, Takeshita T, Hirofuji T. Effects of probiotic *Lactobacillus salivarius* WB21 on halitosis and oral health: an open-label pilot trial. *Oral Surg Oral Med Oral Pathol Oral Radiol Endod*. 2010;110(2):201–208.

51. Suzuki N, Yoneda M, Tanabe K, et al. *Lactobacillus salivarius* WB21–containing tablets for the treatment of oral malodor: a double-blind, randomized, placebo-controlled crossover trial. *Oral Surg Oral Med Oral Pathol Oral Radiol*. 2014;117(4):462–470.

52. Keller MK, Bardow A, Jensdottir T, Lykkeaa J, Twetman S. Effect of chewing gums containing the probiotic bacterium *Lactobacillus reuteri* on oral malodour. *Acta Odontol Scand*. 2012;70(3):246–250.

53. Sutula J, Coulthwaite LA, Thomas LV, Verran J. The effect of a commercial probiotic drink containing *Lactobacillus casei* strain Shirota on oral health in healthy dentate people. *Microb Ecol Health Dis*. 2013 Oct 29;24. doi: 10.3402/mehd.v24i0.21003.

54. Masdea L, Kulik EM, Hauser-Gerspach I, Ramseier AM, Filippi A, Waltimo T. Antimicrobial activity of *Streptococcus salivarius* K12 on bacteria involved in oral malodour. *Arch Oral Biol*. 2012;57(8):1041–1047.

55. Laleman I, Teughels W. Probiotics in the dental practice: a review. *Quintessence Int*. 2015;46(3):255–264.

56. Ueno M, Shinada K, Zaitsu T, Yokoyama S, Kawaguchi Y. Effects of an oral health education program targeting oral malodor prevention in Japanese senior high school students. *Acta Odontol Scand*. 2012;70(5):426–431.

Chapter 9
Dentin Hypersensitivity
Yiming Li

OVERVIEW OF THE CONDITION
Epidemiology
Dentinal hypersensitivity is commonly known as tooth sensitivity to most patients; it has also been termed cervical hypersensitivity, root hypersensitivity, and cemental hypersensitivity.[1] Dentinal hypersensitivity is one of the most encountered complaints by patients seeking dental treatment.[2] Strassler and coworkers called tooth sensitivity the "common cold of dentistry."[3]

The reported prevalence of dentinal hypersensitivity ranges from 3% to 74%, with an average of 57% among dental patients of different lifestyles and cultures.[2,4-14] Females are affected more than males, with a peak occurrence between 20 and 40 years of age. Women between the ages of 20 and 40 years who have meticulous oral hygiene are most likely to develop dentin hypersensitivity.[15]

In general, canines and premolars are most often affected, and the buccal cervical area is also a commonly affected site.[16] Among patients who received periodontal treatment, the reported prevalence of postoperative dentinal hypersensitivity ranged from 60% to as high as 98%.[5,17,18]

Etiology
Significant efforts have been made to understand the etiology and mechanisms involved in the development of dentinal hypersensitivity. A common key characteristic is the exposed dentin surface. Loss of enamel and root surface denudation result in the exposure of underlying dentinal tubules. It is believed that these exposed dentinal tubules allow various stimuli to disturb the dentinal tubular fluid, which consequently activates the pulpal nerves. This activation is then perceived as pain by the patient. The hydrodynamic theory was first proposed by Kramer in 1955 and later confirmed and developed by Brännström in 1962, who correlated in vivo studies on tooth sensitivity associated with applied pressure, air blasts, and chemical stimuli to in vitro measurements of dentinal fluid shifts in response to these stimuli.[19,20] (See Figure 1.) Results of further research suggest that the pain sensation is caused by the activation of mechanoreceptors in intratubular nerves or in the superficial pulp due to changes of the flow or volume of fluid within dentinal tubules, or both.[18,21] These findings help explain the observation that for sensitivity caused by a tooth wear lesion, symptoms become more difficult to resolve

Figure 1. Brännström's Theory

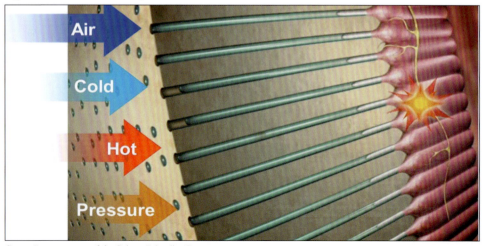

Source: Image courtesy of the Colgate-Palmolive Company.

by normal methods, largely due to more exposed tubules and wider tubule diameter.[22]

Tooth bleaching using peroxide-based materials is also known to cause tooth sensitivity, which may or may not be associated with exposed dentin.[23-25] In most cases, the sensation is mild to moderate and usually transient, dissipating spontaneously without specific treatment.

Risk Factors

Risk factors are primarily those that cause dentin exposure (see Table 1). A number of factors, including gingival recession, periodontal disease, deep tooth cracks, and loss of enamel, cementum, and dentin due to mechanical abrasion, chemical erosion, and chipped or broken cusps, have been identified.[5,18] Gingival recession, resulting from abrasion or periodontal disease, is the primary route through which the underlying dentin becomes exposed, and acid erosion is an important factor in opening exposed dentinal tubules.[2,26,27] Once a patient has exposed dentin with open tubules, any external stimulus can cause discomfort or dentinal hypersensitivity for the patient.

Attrition, abrasion, or erosion causes enamel loss (see Table 2). Attrition is the wear of teeth at sites of direct contact between teeth, which is associated with occlusal function and may be aggravated by habits and bruxism.[28] The latter has been reported to be responsible for pathological tooth wear in 11% of referred tooth wear cases and is a contributing factor in two-thirds of cases of combined etiology.[29]

Abrasion is tooth wear caused by objects other than another tooth, such as toothbrushing and pipe smoking. While a toothbrush itself causes little or no effects on enamel and dentin, certain types of abrasive dentifrices can remove mineral content of enamel, leaving dentinal tubules exposed.[30,31] When combined with erosive agents, toothbrushing is capable of causing enormous enamel and dentin loss.[32] Abfraction occurs as a result of eccentric loading that causes cusp flexure, resulting in compressive and tensile forces in the cervical area of a tooth. Abfraction may potentiate the effects of abrasion and erosion.[33]

Erosion, which can be extrinsic or intrinsic in origin, is considered to be a growing cause of dentin exposure. Extrinsic factors include acidic foods and beverages, chemical exposure, or improper tooth bleaching. There have been reports of significant enamel erosion caused by tooth bleaching products of poor quality.[34] Gastric

Table 1. Frequently Encountered Conditions Associated with Tooth Sensitivity

Primary Origin	Etiological Condition
Tooth	• Dental caries • Erosion, attrition, or abrasion • Chipped or broken tooth • Cracked tooth syndrome • Pulp inflammation • Trauma • Palato-gingival grooves and other anatomical defects
Restoration	• Broken or failing restorations, or both • Marginal leakage • Nanoshrinkage of restorative polymer materials
Periodontal tissues	• Gingival recession • Chronic periodontal disease
Dental procedure	• Tooth whitening • Restoration placement • Scaling and root planing or periodontal surgery

Table 2. Questions for Patients Experiencing Dentin Hypersensitivity

Etiology	Questions
Erosion	• How often do you drink acidic beverages such as soda, citrus juice, wine, etc.? • How often do you drink beverages other than water between meals? • Are you currently experiencing any medical conditions that cause acid reflux?
Abrasion	• What kind of toothpaste do you use at home? • How often do you brush and for how long? • How often do you replace your manual or power brush head? • Do you use light, moderate, or heavy pressure when brushing?
Attrition	• Do you have a history of clenching or grinding your teeth? • Do you currently have a night guard or has one been recommended previously?

fluids are a leading contributing intrinsic factor.

In addition to enamel wear by attrition, abrasion, and erosion, dentinal hypersensitivity can occur from a variety of predisposing factors such as periodontal disease and related treatment, inadequate alveolar bone, or thin biotype.[11,35] Another potential risk factor is dental prophylaxis, a routine and effective procedure for removing dental plaque, calculus, and surface stains. However, the process of scaling and polishing can increase risk, especially in patients with exposed dentin. The unpleasant sensation afterward may temporarily interfere with normal oral hygiene practices and eating and drinking, and may discourage the patient from scheduling regular appointments for preventive care.

It is important to recognize that in many cases, dentinal hypersensitivity may involve multiple risk factors. In addition, the sensation of pain or discomfort is highly subjective and depends on an individual's level of tolerance. Consequently, it can be challenging to identify exact risk factors in certain patients experiencing dentinal hypersensitivity.

Pathogenesis

Dentinal hypersensitivity occurs only with a vital tooth. The following three conditions must be present in order for hypersensitivity to occur (see Figure 2):

1. The dentin must be exposed to the oral cavity.
2. The ends of the exposed dentinal tubules must be open.
3. The dentinal tubule must be open along its entire path from oral cavity to the pulp.

Not all dentinal tubules run the full width of the dentin, and not all tubules possess the mechanoreceptors needed for pain transmission to the brain. As dentin exposure progresses, more tubules become exposed and their diameter increases inversely to the distance from the pulp (see Figure 3). In restorative procedures, removal of smear layers will also result in exposure of dentinal tubules (see Figure 4).

The most widely accepted definition, which was formed by an expert panel of researchers and first published by Holland and colleagues in 1997, states that dentin hypersensitivity is characterized by a short, sharp pain arising from exposed dentin in response to stimuli—typically thermal (hot and cold), evaporative (air blast or inhalation), tactile (touch or pressure), osmotic (sugar, syrup), or chemical (acids)—which cannot be ascribed to any other defects or pathology.[36] The discomfort or pain can be rather unpleasant and bothersome.

Figure 2. Pathogenesis of Dentinal Hypersensitivity

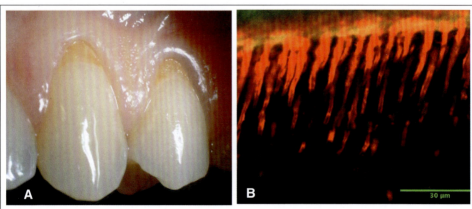

A. Loss of enamel near the gingival margin. B. Dentin tubules extend from dentin surface towards pulp (stained with rhodamine B). Enamel loss commonly occurs as a result of (1) acid erosion due to acidic foods or beverages or stomach regurgitation, and (2) abrasion due to abusive oral hygiene habits. Both conditions often occur simultaneously. Note at the cement-enamel junction, only very minor amounts of enamel need to be lost for dentin exposure to occur.

Figure 3. Odontoblast and Dentinal Tubules

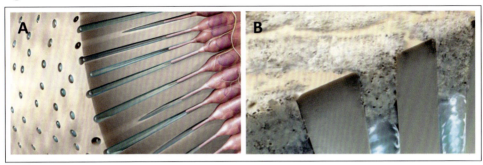

A. Relationship of odontoblasts and the odontoblast processes to nerve fibers. Not all processes are in proximity to a nerve fiber, and not all tubules run the entire width of the dentin. **B.** The seal closes off the tubule ends and prevents dentinal fluid movement and thus stimulation of the mechanoreceptors adjacent to the odontoblasts, eliminating the sensation of dentin hypersensitivity.
Source: Image courtesy of the Colgate-Palmolive Company.

Figure 4. Scanning Electron Micrograph Images

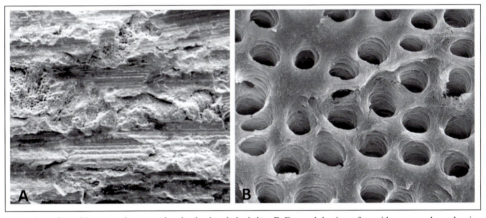

A. Dentin surface with a smear layer covering the dentin tubules below. **B.** Exposed dentin surface with no smear layer showing open ends of dentin tubules. Low-pH foods and beverages and some oral hygiene products can remove the smear layer.

In severe cases, dentin hypersensitivity may have a significant negative impact on an individual's daily life, as it may cause difficulties with eating and drinking, especially hot and cold items, and even interfere with speaking under certain circumstances.[37] Normal hygiene maintenance may also become more difficult, which increases risks of caries, gingivitis, and periodontal problems.

The sensation of dentin hypersensitivity is highly subjective, and its occurrence and severity can be episodic and sporadic. Consequently, it can be challenging to define exact signs and symptoms in certain patients experiencing dentin hypersensitivity.

PATIENT MANAGEMENT AND INTERVENTIONS

Diagnosis

The general approach to the diagnosis of dentinal hypersensitivity includes the following four aspects:

1. Patient history
2. Oral examination
3. Testing of patient response to stimuli
4. Differential diagnosis

When diagnosing dentinal hypersensitivity, it is important to take into consideration the following four specific elements:

1. The nature of the pain

2. The occurrence in areas of exposed dentin
3. An identified stimulus
4. The exclusion of any other possible causes for the pain

Patient History

During review of the patient's history, the individual should be asked whether his or her tooth pain occurs when eating or drinking hot, cold, sweet, or acidic foods or beverages; during toothbrushing; or after a dental procedure. If so, attempts should be made to obtain a specific description of the pain, including onset, severity, and duration. A detailed dietary history and oral hygiene habits, including frequency, duration, and timing of brushing, is helpful for assessing potential risk factors. The patient should be asked to identify the location of the pain, which can help confirm whether dentin exposure is present during the dental examination. When the patient reports undergoing a recent dental procedure, he or she should be questioned about the nature of the procedure to help determine whether the procedure itself or outcomes from the treatment may be possible sources for the pain.

Oral Examination

A comprehensive oral examination is critical for correct diagnosis and differential diagnosis of dentinal hypersensitivity. A thorough examination will also help identify etiological and predisposing factors, particularly with respect to erosion and abrasion, which will be essential for formulating the strategies for intervention and management.

The oral examination should include both the teeth and surrounding gingival tissues, with special attention directed toward exclusion of possible differential diagnoses, including

- Dental or root caries
- Traumatic occlusion
- Fractured restoration
- New restoration for possible postoperative sensitivity
- Marginal integrity of a restoration for possible leakage
- Pulpitis
- Gingival inflammation
- Signs of tooth bleaching
- Atypical odontalgia

Any dentin exposure observed should be characterized by its location, size, and severity. When indicated, radiographs may also be considered.

Testing of Patient Response to Stimuli

A number of clinical tests have been developed for evaluating dentinal hypersensitivity; however, they are all subjective to a certain extent and require patient responses to applied stimuli. As pain sensation is highly dependent on an individual's disposition, its perception may be influenced by psychological factors, past experience, anxiety, ethnic differences, gender, and potential social impacts.

Current clinical methods for detection and diagnosis of dentinal hypersensitivity essentially rely on delivering a mechanical or thermal stimulus to the suspected tooth, and judgment is made based on the patient's response describing the consequential sensation.[11,38-40] The tactile method commonly used in the dental clinic produces mechanical stimuli; it typically involves running a sharp-tipped dental probe on the exposed dentin surface. Such a tactile procedure, though clinically feasible and easy to perform, is difficult to deliver using a consistent, standardized force which may affect the reliability of the response. Specialized electromagnetic devices, such as the Yeaple Electronic Pressure Sensitive Probe (www.yeapleprobe.com), are capable of producing standardized mechanical pressure to the tooth surface. The Yeaple probe delivers pressure in increments of 5 g each progressively until the patient reports the onset of pain; a tooth that sustains pressure of 70 g with no pain is considered nonsensitive.[38,41] The Yeaple probe offers advantages of controllable force delivery and more consistent diagnostic outcomes, but requires the purchase of the device and more clinical time; to date, it has primarily been used in clinical research. (See Figure 5.)

The air blast method is commonly used in dental clinics to produce thermal stimuli for evaluating dentinal hypersensitivity. The tooth to be examined

Figure 5. Yeaple Probe

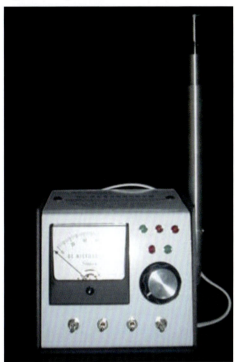

Source: Image courtesy of the Colgate-Palmolive Company.

is isolated by placing fingers over the adjacent teeth; an air blast is then delivered from a standard dental unit air syringe at 60 psi (± 5 psi) and 70°F (± 3°F) directed at the exposed buccal surface of the tooth for 1 second from a distance of approximately 1 cm. (See Figures 6 and 7.) Patient response to the air blast stimulus is assessed using the Schiff Cold Air Sensitivity Scale, as follows:[39]

- 0: Patient did not respond to air stimulus.
- 1: Patient responded to air stimulus but did not request discontinuation of stimulus.
- 2: Patient responded to air stimulus and requested discontinuation or removal of stimulus.
- 3: Patient responded to air stimulus, considered stimulus to be painful, and requested discontinuation of stimulus.

It is important not to deliver the air blast for more than 1 second as the excessive duration may create temperature variations. The air blast method is useful mainly for screening purposes and should be used after the tactile test to eliminate possible residual effects.[33] Several other tests have also been reported for testing dentin hypersensitivity, such as those using electrical, thermoelectric, cold water, or chemical (osmotic) stimulation.[33] However, their clinical application is limited.

The diagnosis of dentin hypersensitivity can be challenging, given the subjectivity of perceived sensation, and because its occurrence and severity can be episodic and sporadic. Conversely, formulation of a correct diagnosis is critical for the development and implementation of an appropriate treatment plan.[42] The dental professional must perform a differential diagnosis to exclude all other dental defects and diseases to which patient symptoms may be attributed as causes of tooth sensitivity.[11,31,33,34]

Differential Diagnosis

Due to difficulties in distinguishing dentinal hypersensitivity from other conditions, it is imperative to rule out active pathological conditions using a variety of diagnostic and evaluation techniques to

Figure 6. The Air Blast Method

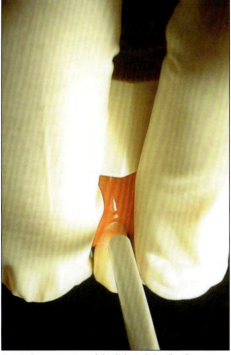

Source: Image courtesy of the Colgate-Palmolive Company.

Figure 7. The Air Blast Method

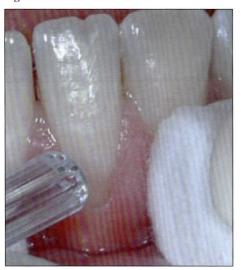

Source: Image courtesy of the Colgate-Palmolive Company.

assess possible causes of dental or pulpal pain.[43] Many conditions share symptoms similar to those of dentinal hypersensitivity. Common confusing conditions include cracked tooth syndrome, caries, traumatic occlusion, fractured restorations, failing or leaking restorations, reversible pulpitis, and developmental defects in which the coronal dentin is not covered by enamel, as well as a recent history of tooth whitening, placement of resin restorations, or periodontal procedures (see Table 1).

Cracked tooth syndrome is unique because it can produce the same symptoms, but with a few notable exceptions. Clinically, it refers to an incomplete fracture of a vital tooth involving dentin; the fracture may or may not reach the pulp.[44,45] Ellis proposed the following definition of the cracked tooth syndrome: "a fracture plane of unknown depth and direction passing through tooth structure that, if not already involving, may progress to communicate with the pulp and/or periodontal ligament."[46] When the crack is more peripheral, it may eventually result in the fracture of a cusp, causing dentin exposure and consequently dentin hypersensitivity. However, in most cases, the crack occurs in posterior teeth often located centrally following the path of the dentinal tubules. When pressure is applied to individual cusps of such a cracked tooth, the separation of the tooth along the line of the crack induces movement of fluid in the dentinal tubules and consequentially the sensation of pain or discomfort.[47] If the crack has reached the pulp and induced pulpitis, the pain often occurs without provocation and may become persistent even after removal of the stimulus. This phenomenon is unique and helps differentiate pulpitis from dentinal hypersensitivity; for the latter, the pain dissipates after the stimulus is removed. Another classical sign of cracked tooth syndrome without pulpitis is that pain arises when biting but ceases after withdrawing the pressure.[45]

In the process of differential diagnosis, radiographic and periodontal assessments, pulp vitality testing, and evaluation of occlusion will provide important information that can help the practitioner rule out alternative causes for the sensitivity. In addition, a follow-up assessment after treatment is needed to ensure that symptoms have subsided, which, if so noted, serves as confirmation of the initial diagnosis. When the patient is fully compliant with treatment but symptoms have not changed, it may be necessary to consider an alternate diagnosis.

Preventive Strategies

Prevention is the most effective and desirable strategy for any potential health issue, including dentinal hypersensitivity. At the time of this writing, there are few evidence-based publications and no systematic reviews about preventive strategies for dentinal hypersensitivity. The primary preventive measures are based on common sense, similar to those advocated for dental erosion.[48] Advice to patients on preventing dentinal hypersensitivity may include the following measures:

- Avoiding erosive or acidic drinks and foods
- Practicing gentle but efficient toothbrushing
- Evaluating brushing technique and providing oral hygiene instructions to help assess use of appropriate brushing patterns, pressure, angulation, and toothbrush placement
- Using a power toothbrush with a built-in pressure sensor that will alert patients when

they are using excessive force
- Rinsing the mouth with water after the intake of soft drinks and fruit juices
- Wearing a night guard as directed for bruxism and clenching

For dental professionals, an obvious preventive measure is to avoid or minimize consequential dentin exposure associated with dental procedures.

Therapeutic Interventions

For established dentinal hypersensitivity, therapeutic interventions may become necessary. A variety of chemicals, products, and measures have been used by professionals in the office. There are two strategic approaches to manage this condition.[11,49] They are

1. inhibition or interference of the transmission of neuronal impulses induced by the stimulus; and
2. occlusion of the dentinal tubules to stop, reduce, or prevent movement of fluid (see Figure 8).

Potassium salts, most commonly potassium nitrate, are the primary agents used to inhibit or interfere with transmission of neural impulses. Potassium nitrate diffuses through the exposed dentinal tubules to the pulp where it affects sensory (A delta) nerves by preventing depolarization. When sensory nerves do not "fire," there is no propagation of the impulse to the brain, thus stopping transmission and pain perception.[50,51] The efficacy of potassium on dentinal hypersensitivity was first observed in cat teeth[52] and then in a study using human premolars scheduled for extraction.[37] Clinical studies have shown toothpastes containing 5% potassium nitrate to be effective in relieving dentinal hypersensitivity symptoms when applied twice daily; however, the effect starts slowly after 2 weeks and provides increasing relief after 8 to 12 weeks of continued use.[11,53]

It is important to instruct the patient to use the toothpaste twice daily for an extended period, as it is the continued use that enables a sufficient concentration of potassium ions to diffuse along the open tubule. Failure to achieve symptom control is most likely a result of poor compliance but may also be due to a misdiagnosis.

Despite the availability of clinical efficacy data, there have been questions and debates about the efficacy of potassium-based desensitizing toothpastes. A Cochrane systematic review and meta-analysis of a subset of six randomized, controlled

Figure 8. Therapeutic Treatment Strategies for Managing Dentinal Hypersensitivity

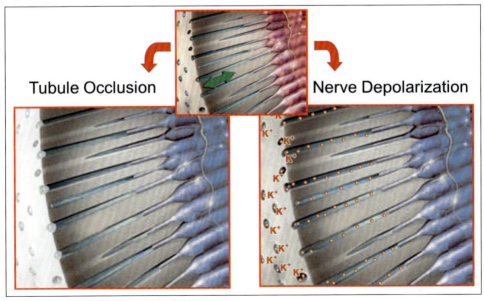

Source: Image courtesy of the Colgate-Palmolive Company.

clinical studies led its authors to conclude that the clinical efficacy of potassium-containing toothpastes in reducing dentin hypersensitivity is equivocal.[51]

To reduce or prevent fluid movement in open dentinal tubules, the most commonly employed technologies include protein precipitants, calcium and phosphate precipitating agents, various crystallizing agents, bonding agents, laser therapy, and surgical grafting of gingival tissue.[11,33] Varnishes and pastes of high fluoride concentration have been reported to be effective in promoting mineral deposition and consequential tubule occlusion leading to symptom relief. However, the evidence supporting fluoride in toothpaste as a desensitizing agent is minimal.

To date, there has been little research into use of lasers for reducing dentinal hypersensitivity.[54,55] Two systematic reviews comparing laser therapy with desensitizing agents suggest that lasers seem to have a slight clinical and immediate advantage over topically applied medicaments.[56,57] Similarly, a systematic review[58] and meta-analysis[59] found no evidence of benefits from treating dentinal hypersensitivity with oxalates beyond a placebo effect and consequently concluded that available evidence did not support the recommendation of using oxalates for treatment, with the possible exception of 3% monohydrogen monopotassium oxalate. The use of professional treatments, such as resin sealers, bonding agents, and gingival surgery, is limited to certain patients due to cost and need for an office visit.

A protein precipitant, casein phosphopeptide (CPP), has been incorporated in oral hygiene products with an intention to reduce dentinal hypersensitivity. CPP is a casein derivative and is capable of stabilizing amorphous calcium phosphate (ACP), which is usually insoluble, in a state forming a CPP-ACP complex.[60] A commercial product containing CPP-ACP has been designed to promote remineralization through deposition of fluoride-containing calcium-phosphate precipitates, which has been suggested for reducing risks of dental caries and dentinal hypersensitivity (MI Paste Plus®, GC America). However, results from published studies are inconsistent.[61-64] A systematic review of the literature concludes that "there is insufficient clinical trial evidence (in quantity, quality, or both) to make a recommendation regarding the long-term effectiveness of casein derivatives, specifically CPP-ACP, in preventing caries in vivo and in treating dentin hypersensitivity or dry mouth."[65] The authors questioned the potential possibility of interactions between fluoride and ACP that may precipitate out as calcium fluoride, rendering both inorganic components ineffective, and expressed their concerns with the 900 ppm fluoride dose in the product, and thus recommended against its use in children younger than 6 years of age.

Approximately 50 years ago, before the widespread adoption of potassium as a desensitizer, strontium chloride was incorporated into toothpaste because it was believed to treat tooth sensitivity by occluding dentinal tubules. More recently, strontium acetate has been used in toothpastes because of its compatibility with fluoride.[66] However, data on the clinical efficacy of strontium-based toothpaste for dentinal hypersensitivity have been inconsistent and equivocal, at best.[11,67-69] A literature review of clinical studies on effects of strontium-based toothpastes used for periods of 4 to 12 weeks determined that many of the double-blind, controlled studies showed no significant benefit for 10% strontium chloride or 8% strontium acetate toothpastes as compared with regular fluoride toothpaste.[70]

More recently, a novel technology using arginine, an amino acid naturally found in saliva, and calcium carbonate has been introduced to control dentinal hypersensitivity.[26,69] The arginine in saliva itself is incapable of providing quick plugging and sealing of open dentinal tubules; however, a new technology delivering arginine and calcium carbonate in dental prophylaxis paste and toothpaste has research that supports its efficacy. The technology of 8% arginine was extensively investigated using atomic force microscopy, confocal laser scanning microscopy, electron spectroscopy, and high-resolution scanning electron microscopy. Results show that the formed sealing plugs are composed of arginine, calcium, phosphate, and carbonate.[70,71] (See Figure 9) Furthermore, hydraulic conductance studies have shown that the strength of these dentin plugs is adequate to withstand normal pulpal pressures and acid challenge, effectively reducing the dentin fluid flow and, consequently, the sensation of tooth sensitivity.[69,70,72,73] Studies have shown that arginine-based desensitizing prophylaxis paste was capable of providing instant sensitivity relief when it was applied to sensitive teeth following prophylaxis; furthermore, this sensitivity relief lasted for at least 28 days after a single application.[41,69,74] The arginine technology has also been successfully used in toothpaste, which contains 8.0% arginine as the active ingredient with calcium carbonate and 1,450 ppm fluoride as sodium monofluorophosphate (MFP) for controlling dentinal hypersensitivity. Clinical trials involving populations in Canada, China, Italy, and the United States all report significant efficacy of this arginine-based toothpaste for reducing dentinal hypersensitivity.[11]

NovaMin™ (GlaxoSmithKline) is a synthetic agent of calcium sodium phosphosilicate that has also been used in prophylaxis paste and toothpaste to promote mineral precipitation to plug exposed dentinal tubules.[75-78] Clinical studies reported efficacy in reducing dentinal hypersensitivity;[79-82] however, a recent clinical study found that the NovaMin toothpaste did not differ significantly from traditional fluoride toothpaste for improving white spot lesions, raising the question of its capability of remineralization or mineral deposition on tooth surfaces.[83]

Patient Management Considerations

For achieving effective and successful patient management, the following actions are recommended:

- *Acquiring necessary knowledge and understanding of dentin hypersensitivity.* Despite the fact that dentinal hypersensitivity is becoming more prevalent in dental practice, determining an appropriate and effective clinical management strategy remains a challenge for dental practitioners. One survey showed that about 50% of practitioners lacked confidence in managing their patients' dentinal hypersensitivity, and only 10% had adequate knowledge of mechanisms of action for toothpastes with potassium nitrate.[84]
- *Conducting a comprehensive examination, diagnosis, and differential diagnosis.* It is imperative to obtain an adequate patient history and perform a careful oral examination for

Figure 9. Arginine Technology Used to Seal Open Dentinal Tubules

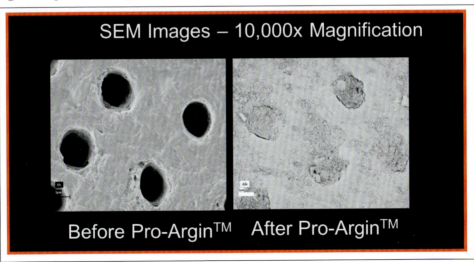

Source: Image courtesy of the Colgate-Palmolive Company.

correct diagnosis and differential diagnosis. Dentinal hypersensitivity is a personal perception of pain or discomfort, and it can be difficult for the patient to describe and a challenge for the practitioner to quantify. The examination using an air blast and tactile method provides semi-objective evidence but may not be able to replicate all types of dentinal hypersensitivity. The Canadian Advisory Board on Dentin Hypersensitivity has concluded that it would be most appropriate to rely on patients' perception of pain following treatment to evaluate efficacy.[84]

- *Removing or modifying predisposing risk factors or causes.* Removal or modification of predisposing risk factors or causes of dentinal hypersensitivity discovered during the patient history and examination should be the first priority. For example, if erosion or abrasion of enamel is detected, efforts should be made to identify and address relevant etiological contributing factors, such as dietary and beverage consumption and oral hygiene practices, prior to implementation of any treatment.
- *Designing and implementing an effective and feasible treatment plan.* The treatment of dentinal hypersensitivity targets reduction of fluid flow in dentinal tubules by plugging the open tubules or by blocking the nerve response to the stimulus, or both. As presented in Tables 3 and 4, a variety of desensitizing products and measures are available for treating dentinal hypersensitivity. In selecting the treatment regimen, considerations must be given to each individual's condition of dentinal hypersensitivity, such as the severity, extent of the teeth affected, identified risk factors, and feasibility of the proposed treatment plan for the patient. In addition, in most cases reversible procedures should be used before nonreversible procedures are considered.
- *Scheduling follow-up after implementing the treatment regimen.* Appropriate follow-up after initial treatment of dentinal hypersensitivity is essential for effective and successful patient management.[84] The follow-up examination and consultation provide a unique opportunity to confirm, or modify if needed, the initial diagnosis and the effectiveness of treatment.
- *Providing individualized education and consultation.* Education and consultation should be an integral part of the patient management

Table 3. Major Products Available for Management of Dentin Hypersensitivity

Desensitizing Product	Mechanism	Onset of Relief*	Duration of Relief*	Application	Product Example†
Potassium nitrate dentifrice	Nerve depolarization	2–8 weeks	Ongoing while used twice daily	Home	Sensodyne Toothpaste Colgate Sensitive Toothpaste
Arginine paste	Tubule occlusion	Immediate	12 weeks after one application	Office	Colgate Pro-Relief Desensitizing Paste
Arginine toothpaste	Tubule occlusion	Immediate when applied as directed	Ongoing while used twice daily	Home	Colgate Sensitive Pro-Relief toothpaste
Arginine mouthwash	Tubule occlusion	2 weeks	Ongoing while used twice daily	Home	Colgate Sensitive Pro-Relief Mouthwash
Amorphous calcium phosphate paste	Tubule occlusion	3–5 minutes	Varies	Office/Home	GC America MI Paste
Amorphous sodium calcium phosphosilicate paste	Tubule occlusion	Immediate	3–4 weeks	Office	NovaMin Paste

*Onset and duration times listed are approximate. Individual patient response varies.
†The product examples listed are not all-inclusive, but rather examples of each type to aid the clinician in selecting the product of their choice. They are for illustrative purpose and do not indicate an endorsement of any particular product by the author.

Table 4. Options for Dentin Hypersensitivity Management

Self-treatment at home	• Toothpaste with an active desensitizing ingredient
	  • Sensodyne Toothpaste, Colgate Sensitive Toothpaste, Crest Pro-Health Sensitive Toothpaste, Colgate Sensitive Pro-Relief Toothpaste
	• Prescription-strength fluoride gel
	  • Colgate Prevident and Gel Kam
	• Prescription-strength fluoride toothpaste
	  • Colgate Prevident, 3M ESPE Control Rx, Clinpro 5000, Fluoridex
	• Amorphous Calcium Phosphate paste
	  • GC America MI Paste or MI Paste Plus with fluoride
	• Mouthrinse with
	  • Listerine Advanced Defense Sensitive
	  • Colgate Sensitive Pro Relief mouthrinse
	• Chewing gum with Recaldent
	  • Trident Extra Care

Professionally applied agents*	• desensitizing ingredient
	  • Preventech Vella, Kolorz Clear Shield, Colgate Prevident and Duraphat varnishes
	• In-office applied arginine–calcium carbonate paste
	  • Colgate Sensitive Pro-Relief paste

Aggressive/ Irreversible treatment	• Restorative materials • Lasers • Periodontal Surgery (gingival grafting or root coverage procedures)

*The products listed are not all-inclusive, but rather a few examples of each type to aid the clinician in selecting the product of their choice. Authors do not have a conflict of interest or endorse any particular product.

plan. The patient's understanding of the problem, proposed corrective measure, and implementation of the treatment regimen will help ensure his or her cooperation and improve compliance to achieve success in managing dentinal hypersensitivity.

CONCLUSION

Dentinal hypersensitivity is a common complaint in dentistry, and in severe cases, it can impair eating, drinking, and even speaking, thus interfering with normal daily life. The unpleasant nature of dentinal hypersensitivity and its high prevalence among the general population have attracted great research interest in understanding etiology and pathogenesis, and have promoted significant advancements in the development of innovative measures for its effective and safe control. Many dental practitioners find it challenging to identify risk factors and conduct diagnosis in certain patients as the sensation of dentinal hypersensitivity is highly subjective and its occurrence and severity can be episodic and sporadic. It is imperative that practitioners be knowledgeable about dentinal hypersensitivity in order to design and implement effective management of the problem. By assessing the patient's history, conducting an oral examination, identifying risk factors, performing correct diagnosis, and designing effective treatment, practitioners can help to ensure adequate patient cooperation and improve compliance with preventive recommendations.

REFERENCES

1. Porto IC, Andrade AK, Montes MA. Diagnosis and treatment of dentinal hypersensitivity. *J Oral Sci.* 2009;51:323–332.
2. Addy M. Dentine hypersensitivity: new perspectives on an old problem. *Int Dent J.* 2002;52(suppl 5):367–375.
3. Strassler HE, Drisko CL, Alexander DC. Dentin hypersensitivity: its interrelationship to gingival recession and acid erosion. *Compend Contin Educ Dent.* 2008;29(5 spec iss):1-9.
4. Al-Wahadni A, Linden GJ. Dentine hypersensitivity in Jordanian dental attenders: a case control study. *J Clin Periodontol.* 2002;29:688–693.
5. Addy M. Etiology and clinical implications of dentine hypersensitivity. *Dent Clin North Am.* 1990;34:503–514.
6. Irwin CR, McCusker P. Prevalence of dentine hypersensitivity in a general dental population. *J Irish Dent Assoc.* 1997;43(1):7–9.
7. Liu HC, Lan WH, Hsieh CC. Prevalence and distribution of cervical dentin hypersensitivity in a population in Taipei, Taiwan. *J Endod.* 1998;24(1):45–47.
8. Rees JS, Addy M. A cross-sectional study of dentine hypersensitivity. *J Clinical Periodontol.* 2002; 29:997–1003.
9. West NX. Dentine hypersensitivity. In: Lussi A. Dental erosion. *Monogr Oral Sci.* 2006;20:173–189.
10. Amarasena N, Spencer J, Ou Y, Brennan D. Dentine hypersensitivity—Australian dentists' perspective. *Aust Dent J.* 2010;55:181–187.
11. Li Y. Dentin hypersensitivity: diagnosis and strategic approaches. *Inside Dentistry.* September 2013 (suppl). Available at: http://cdeworld.com/courses/4674.
12. Shiau HJ. Dentin hypersensitivity. *J Evid Based Dent*

13. Scaramucci T, de Almeida Anfe TE, da Silva Ferreira S, Frias AC, Sobral MAP. Investigation of the prevalence, clinical features, and risk factors of dentin hypersensitivity in a selected Brazilian population. *Clin Oral Investig.* 2014;18:651–657.
14. Haneet RK, Vandana LK. Prevalence of dentinal hypersensitivity and study of associated factors: a cross-sectional study based on the general dental population of Davangere, Karnataka, India. *Int Dent J.* 2015 Nov 19. doi: 10.1111/idj.12206. [Epub ahead of print.]
15. Daniel SJ, Harfst SA, Wilder RS. *Dental Hygiene Concepts, Cases, and Competencies.* 2nd ed. St. Louis, MO: Mosby Elsevier; 2008:623–637.
16. Addy M, Mostafa P, Newcombe RG. Dentine hypersensitivity: the distribution of recession, sensitivity and plaque. *J Dent.* 1987;15:242–248.
17. Drisko CH. Dentine hypersensitivity—dental hygiene and periodontal considerations. *Int Dent J.* 2002;52:385–393.
18. Pashley DH, Tay FR, Haywood VB, Collins MA, Drisko CL. Consensus-based recommendations for the diagnosis and management of dentin hypersensitivity. *Inside Dentistry.* 2008;4(special issue):1–7.
19. Kramer IRH. The relationship between dentine sensitivity and movements in the contents of dentinal tubules. *Br Den J.* 1955; 98:391–392.
20. Brännström M. The elicitation of pain in human dentine and pulp by chemical stimuli. *Arch Oral Biol.* 1962;7:59–62.
21. Matthews B, Vongsavan N. Interactions between neural and hydrodynamic mechanisms in dentine and pulp. *Arch Oral Biol.* 1994;39(suppl):87S–95S.
22. Brännström M. In: Anderson DJ, ed. *Sensory Mechanisms in Dentine.* Oxford, England: Pergamon Press; 1963.
23. Leonard RH Jr, Bentley C, Eagle JC, Garland GE, Knight MC, Phillips C. Nightguard vital bleaching: a long-term study on efficacy, shade retention, side effects, and patients' perceptions. *J Esthet Restor Dent.* 2001;13:357–369.
24. Li Y. The safety of peroxide-containing at-home tooth whiteners. *Compend Contin Educ Dent.* 2003;24:384–389.
25. Li Y. Safety controversies in tooth bleaching. *Dent Clin North Am.* 2011;55:255–263.
26. Cummins D. Dentin hypersensitivity: from diagnosis to a breakthrough therapy for everyday sensitivity relief. *J Clin Dent.* 2009;20(special issue):1–9.
27. Drisko C. Oral hygiene and periodontal considerations in preventing and managing dentine hypersensitivity. *Int Dent J.* 2007;57:399–393.
28. Smith BGN. Toothwear: aetiology and diagnosis. *Dent Update.* 1989;16:204–212.
29. Smith BGN, Knight JK. A comparison of patterns of toothwear with the etiological factors. *Br Dent J.* 1984;157:16–19.
30. Absi EG, Addy M, Adams D. Dentine hypersensitivity—the effect of toothbrushing and dietary compounds on dentine in vitro: an SEM study. *J Oral Rehabil.* 1992;19:101–110.
31. Wolff M. Science behind the sensitivity: science-supported therapy for the effective relief of dentin hypersensitivity. *J Clin Dent.* 2009;20(special issue):23–31.
32. Davis WB, Winter PJ. The effect of abrasion on enamel and dentine after exposure to dietary acids. *Br Dent J.* 1980;148:253–256.
33. Trushkowsky RD, Garcia-Godoy F. Dentin hypersensitivity: differential diagnosis, tests, and etiology. *Compend Contin Educ Dent.* 2014:99–103.
34. Li Y, Greenwall L. Safety issues of tooth whitening using peroxide-based materials. *Br Dent J.* 2013;215:29–34.
35. West NX, Lussi A, Seong J, Hellwig E. Dentin hypersensitivity: pain mechanisms and aetiology of exposed cervical dentin. *Clin Oral Investig.* 2013;17(suppl 1):S9–S19.
36. Holland GR, Narhi MN, Addy M, Gangarosa L, Orchardson R. Guidelines for the design and conduct of clinical trials on dentine hypersensitivity. *J Clin Periodontol.* 1997;24:808–813.
37. Ajcharanukul O, Kraivaphan P, Wanachantararak S, Vongsavan N, Matthews B. Effects of potassium ions on dentine sensitivity in man. *Arch Oral Biol.* 2007;52:632–639.
38. Clark GE, Troullos ES. Designing hypersensitivity studies. *Dent Clin North Am.* 1990;34:531–533.
39. Schiff T, Dotson M, Cohen S, De Vizio W, McCool J, Volpe A. Efficacy of a dentifrice containing potassium nitrate, soluble pyrophosphate, PVM/MA copolymer, and sodium fluoride on dentinal hypersensitivity: a twelve-week clinical study. *J Clin Dent.* 1994;5(special issue):87–92.
40. Gillam DG, Bulman JS, Jackson RJ, Newman HN. Efficacy of a potassium nitrate mouthwash in alleviating cervical dentine. *J Clin Periodontol.* 1996;23:993–997.
41. Li Y, Lee S, Mateo LR, Delgado E, Zhang YB. Comparison of clinical efficacy of three professionally applied pastes on immediate and sustained reduction of dentin hypersensitivity. *Compend Contin Educ Dent.* 2013;34:1–7.
42. Ide M. The differential diagnosis of sensitive teeth. *Dent Update.* 1998;25:462–466.
43. Gernhardt C. How valid and applicable are current diagnostic criteria and assessment methods for dentin hypersensitivity? An overview. *Clin Oral Investig.* 2013;17(suppl 1):S31–S40.
44. Cameron CE. Cracked-tooth syndrome. *J Am Dent Assoc.* 1964;68:405–411.
45. Ehrmann EH, Tyas MT. Cracked tooth syndrome: diagnosis, treatment and correlation between symptoms and post-extraction findings. *Aust Dent J.* 1990;35:105–112.
46. Ellis SG. Incomplete tooth fracture-proposal for a new definition. *Br Dent J.* 2001;190:424–428.

47. Rosen H. Cracked tooth syndrome. *J Prosthet Dent.* 1982;47:36–43.
48. Twetman S. The evidence base for professional and self-care prevention—caries, erosion and sensitivity. *BMC Oral Health.* 2015;15(suppl 1):S4.
49. Mantzourani M, Sharma D. Dentine sensitivity: past, present and future. *J Dent.* 2013;41(suppl 4):S3–S17.
50. Peacock JM, Orchardson R. Action potential conduction block of nerves in vitro by potassium citrate, potassium tartrate and potassium oxalate. *J Clin Periodontol.* 1999; 26:33–37.
51. Poulsen S, Errboe M, Lescay Mevil Y, Glenny AM. Potassium containing toothpastes for dentine hypersensitivity. *Cochrane Database Syst Rev.* 2006;3:CD001476.
52. Markowitz K, Bilotto G, Kim S. Decreasing intradental nerve activity in the cat with potassium and divalent cations. *Arch Oral Biol.* 1991;36:1–7.
53. Nagata T, Ishida H, Shinohara H, et al. Clinical evaluation of a potassium nitrate dentifrice for the treatment of dentinal hypersensitivity. *J Clin Periodontol.* 1994;21: 217–221.
54. Schwarz F, Arweiler N, Georg T, Reich E. Desensitizing effects of an Er:YAG laser on hypersensitive dentine. *J Clin Periodontol.* 2002;29:211–215.
55. Birang R, Poursamimi I, Gutknecht N, Lampert F, Mir M. Comparative evaluation of the effects of Nd:YAG and Er:YAG laser in dentin hypersensitivity treatment. *Lasers Med Sci.* 2007;22:21–24.
56. Sgolastra F, Petrucci A, Severino M, Gatto R, Monaco A. Lasers for the treatment of dentin hypersensitivity: a meta-analysis. *J Dent Res.* 2013;92:492–499.
57. Douglas de Oliveira DW, Oliveira-Ferreira F, Flecha OD, Gonçalves PF. Is surgical root coverage effective for the treatment of cervical dentin hypersensitivity? A systematic review. *J Periodontol.* 2013;84:295–306.
58. Cunha-Cruz J, Stout JR, Heaton LJ, Wataha JC; Northwest PRECEDENT. Dentin hypersensitivity and oxalates: a systematic review. *J Dent Res.* 2011;90:304–310.
59. Poulsen S. Available evidence does not support use of oxalates for dentine hypersensitivity. *Evid Based Dent.* 2011;12:47.
60. Reynolds EC, Cain CJ, Webber FL, et al. Anticariogenicity of calcium phosphate complexes of tryptic casein phosphopeptides in the rat. *J Dent Res.* 1995;74:1272–2379.
61. Reynolds EC. Anticariogenic complexes of amorphous calcium phosphate stabilized by casein phosphopeptides: a review. *Spec Care Dentist.* 1998;18:8–16.
62. Suge T, Ishikawa K, Kawasaki A, et al. Calcium phosphate precipitation method for the treatment of dentin hypersensitivity. *Am J Dent.* 2002;15:220–226.
63. Kowalczyk A, Botuliski B, Jaworska M, et al. Evaluation of the product based on Recaldent technology in the treatment of dentin hypersensitivity. *Adv Med Sci.* 2006;51(suppl 1):40–42.
64. Martinez-Mier EA. Casein phosphopeptide used in toothpaste suggests an efficacy similar to toothpaste containing sodium monofluorophosphate for caries prevention. *J Evid Based Dent Pract.* 2010;10:154–155.
65. Azarpazhooh A, Limeback H. Clinical efficacy of casein derivatives: a systematic review of the literature. *J Am Dent Assoc.* 2008;139:915–924.
66. Markowitz K. The original desensitizers: strontium and potassium salts. *J Clin Dent.* 2009;20(special issue):145–151.
67. Zappa U. Self-applied treatments in the management of dentine hypersensitivity. *Arch Oral Biol.* 1994;39(suppl): 107S–112S.
68. Jackson RJ. Potential treatment modalities for dentine hypersensitivity: home use products. In: Addy M, Embery G, Edgar WM, Orchardson R, eds. *Tooth Wear and Sensitivity: Clinical Advances in Restorative Dentistry.* London, England: Martin Dunitz, 2000;327–338.
69. Cummins D. Recent advances in dentin hypersensitivity: Clinically proven treatments for instant and lasting sensitivity relief. *Am J Dent.* 2010;23(special issue A):3A–13A.
70. Petrou I, Heu R, Stranick M, et al. A breakthrough therapy for dentin hypersensitivity: how dental products containing 8% arginine and calcium carbonate work to deliver effective relief of sensitive teeth. *J Clin Dent.* 2009;20(special issue):23–31.
71. Lavender SA, Petrou I, Heu R, et al. Mode of action studies on a new desensitizing dentifrice containing 8.0% arginine, a high cleaning calcium carbonate system and 1450 ppm fluoride. *Am J Dent.* 2010;23(special issue A):14A–19A.
72. Hamlin D, Williams KP, Delgado E, Zhang YP, DeVizio W, Mateo LR. Clinical evaluation of the efficacy of a desensitizing paste containing 8% arginine and calcium carbonate for the in-office relief of dentin hypersensitivity associated with dental prophylaxis. *Am J Dent.* 2009;22(special issue A):16A–20A.
73. Panagakos F, Schiff T, Guignon A. Dentin hypersensitivity: effective treatment with an in-office desensitizing paste containing 8% arginine and calcium carbonate. *Am J Dent.* 2009;22(special issue A):3A–7A.
74. Kleinberg I. Sensistat. A new saliva-based composition for simple and effective treatment of dentinal sensitivity pain. *Dent Today.* 2002:21:42–47.
75. Earl JS, Leary RK, Muller KH, Langford RM, Greenspan DC. Physical and chemical characterization of dentin surface following treatment with NovaMin technology. *J Clin Dent.* 2011;22:62–67.
76. Layer TM. Development of a fluoridated, daily-use toothpaste containing NovaMin technology for the treatment of dentin hypersensitivity. *J Clin Dent.* 2011;22:59–61.
77. Chen CL, Parolia A, Pau A, Celerino de Moraes Porto IC. Comparative evaluation of the effectiveness of desensitizing agents in dentine tubule occlusion using scanning electron microscopy. *Aust Dent J.* 2015;60:65–72.

78. Jena A, Shashirekha G. Comparison of efficacy of three different desensitizing agents for in-office relief of dentin hypersensitivity: A 4 weeks clinical study. *J Conserv Dent*. 2015;18:389–393.
79. Litkowski L, Greenspan DC. A clinical study of the effect of calcium sodium phosphosilicate on dentin hypersensitivity—proof of principle. *J Clin Dent*. 2010;21:77–81.
80. Salian S, Thakur S, Kulkarni S, LaTorre G. A randomized controlled clinical study evaluating the efficacy of two desensitizing dentifrices. *J Clin Dent*. 2010;21:82–87.
81. Sharma N, Roy S, Kakar A, Greenspan DC, Scott R. A clinical study comparing oral formulations containing 7.5% calcium sodium phosphosilicate (NovaMin), 5% potassium nitrate, and 0.4% stannous fluoride for the management of dentin hypersensitivity. *J Clin Dent*. 2010;21:88–92.
82. Gendreau L, Barlow AP, Mason SC. Overview of the clinical evidence for the use of NovaMin in providing relief from the pain of dentin hypersensitivity. *J Clin Dent*. 2011;22:90–95.
83. Hoffman DA, Clark AE, Rody WJ Jr, McGorray SP, Wheeler TT. A prospective randomized clinical trial into the capacity of a toothpaste containing NovaMin to prevent white spot lesions and gingivitis during orthodontic treatment. *Prog Orthod*. 2015;16:25.
84. Canadian Advisory Board on Dentin Hypersensitivity. Consensus-based recommendations for the diagnosis and management of dentin hypersensitivity. *J Can Dent Assoc*. 2003;69:221–226.

Chapter 10
Dry Mouth

Sharon Compton and Minn Yoon

Part 1: Overview Of Dry Mouth

The importance of saliva in our daily activities of living is often taken for granted. Saliva performs a myriad of functions essential to oral and systemic health and well-being. When the quality or quantity of saliva is altered, it is likely that individuals experience dry mouth. Dry mouth can have a profound impact on both quality of life and oral health status.[1-3] Saliva is pivotal to maintaining overall function of the oral cavity, which can be categorized into three key areas: (1) swallowing, enjoyment, and digestion of food; (2) maintaining and protecting the function and physical structures of the oral cavity; and (3) maintaining the equilibrium of the oral microflora.[4] Patients experiencing dry mouth often show signs of taste disturbances (dysgeusia); difficulties with chewing, swallowing (dysphagia), and speaking (dysarthria);[5] and a range of oral diseases, including ill-fitting dentures,[6] dental caries, oral candidiasis, periodontal disease, halitosis, and burning mouth syndrome.[7] This chapter provides an overview of dry mouth and associated etiologies, and discusses evidence-based prevention and management strategies.

Pathogenesis Of Dry Mouth
What Is Dry Mouth?

Dry mouth is a complex condition. Clinical diagnosis would be straightforward if, in fact, a person's report of dry mouth paralleled his or her physical salivary output. However, much research has shown that the two are not necessarily concurrent.[8] Dry mouth presents in two forms. *Xerostomia* is the subjective self-reported sensation of dry mouth, and *salivary gland hypofunction (SGH)* is the clinically observed condition of lower-than-normal salivary output, which is typically assessed using sialometry. Alterations in the salivary composition further add to the complexity of dry mouth.[9]

The bulk (~90%) of salivary secretion is produced by three bilateral pairs of major salivary glands (parotid, submandibular, and sublingual). The remaining salivary secretion (~10%) is produced in the hundreds of minor salivary glands located throughout the mucosal surfaces of the oral cavity, which are important for lubrication and protection of the oral mucosa due to their mucous secretions. The major and minor salivary glands are made of acinar cells, which are responsible for generating fluid and transporting electrolytes and proteins. Each gland makes a compositionally distinct contribution to the saliva (see Figure 1).

Healthy adults produce between 0.5 and 1.5 L of saliva per day.[10] Salivary secretion occurs in response to autonomic stimulation primarily under the parasympathetic pathway (see Figure 2). Parasympathetic (cholinergic) simulation results in high-volume, watery saliva. Sympathetic (adrenergic) stimulation results in small-volume, highly viscous saliva. When salivary fluid production is decreased by about 50%, a person begins to experience symptoms of dry mouth.[11]

Figure 1. Control of Salivary Secretion

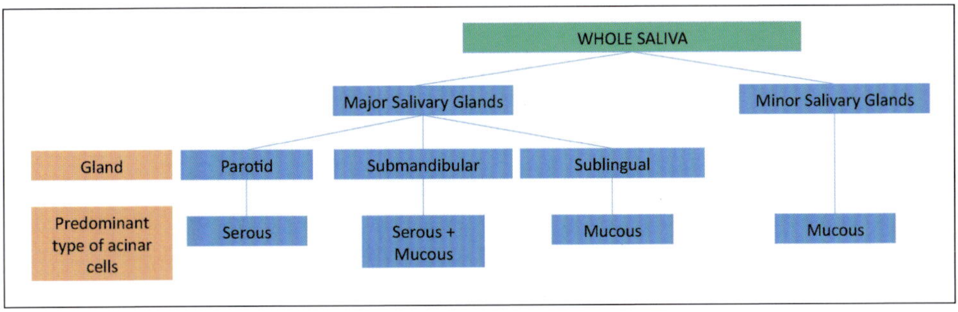

Gland	Parotid	Submandibular	Sublingual	Minor Salivary Glands
Predominant type of acinar cells	Serous	Serous + Mucous	Mucous	Mucous

Whole Saliva → Major Salivary Glands (Parotid, Submandibular, Sublingual) and Minor Salivary Glands

Figure 2. Contributors to Salivary Secretion

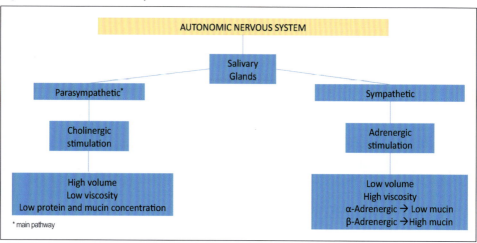

Diagnosis of Dry Mouth
Xerostomia

There are two approaches to assessing the subjective sensation of dry mouth. The first is a single-item approach in which the individual is asked a single question or asked to rate a single statement deriving a global judgment of his or her dry mouth. For example, "Does your mouth usually feel dry?"[12] or "How often does your mouth feel dry? Never, occasionally, frequently or always?"[13] Global items that measure xerostomia have been used extensively[14-17] and can be very useful when the appropriate measure is used. The second approach is a multi-item approach and includes batteries of items[18-20] or summated rating scales.[8,21] A battery is usually a list of questions with a simple yes/no response format that is indexed into categories (e.g., absent, mild, moderate, severe). Although batteries can produce meaningful data for exploring the determinants of xerostomia, the majority of batteries have not been rigorously tested for their psychometric properties.[22] Summated rating scales attempt to address this gap by capturing the respondent health status on a continuum using questions that have demonstrated correlation with the underlying construct (dry mouth). This permits subtle differences in health states to be measured.[22] Multi-item approaches can be validated when used in combination with a global item.

Salivary Gland Hypofunction

Clinical examinations assessing lip dryness, and sticking of instruments to tissues, can inform the presence of SGH;[23] however, such clinical assessments have not been extensively tested. More typically, SGH is measured using salivary flow rates (sialometry). Either unstimulated or stimulated salivary flow rates can be used. (See Table 1 for average whole saliva flow rates.) Stimulated saliva accounts for 80% to 90% of daily production. To measure stimulated saliva, either gustatory (citric acid solution) or masticatory (paraffin wax) stimuli can be administered. Unstimulated salivary flow is collected using one of the following methods:

- *Drain*: Saliva drips off lower lip into a preweighed graduated receptacle over a predetermined time period.
- *Spit:* Saliva accumulated in the floor of the mouth is spit into a preweighed graduated receptacle every 60 seconds for a predetermined time period.
- *Suction*: Saliva is continuously aspirated from the floor of the mouth over a predetermined time period.
- *Swab*: Saliva absorbed by a preweighed swab in the mouth at the orifices of the major glands for a predetermined time period. This method has been shown to be the least valid or reliable.[24]

Table 1. Flow Rates of Whole Saliva

	Normal	Hyposalivation
Unstimulated	0.3–0.5 mL/min	< 0.12–0.16 mL/min
Stimulated	1.0–3.0 mL/min	< 0.5 mL/min

EPIDEMIOLOGY OF DRY MOUTH

Obtaining a representative picture of xerostomia or SGH prevalence is difficult because of methodological discrepancies and variances in diagnostic criteria. Further, xerostomia and SGH are not concurrent, only occurring in approximately one-sixth of those with either condition or 6% of the population.[8] The prevalence of xerostomia is approximately 20% overall,[25] increasing to approximately 30% of the population aged 65 years and older.[26] The population most studied for dry mouth is older adults. A limited number of studies have assessed the prevalence of dry mouth in younger populations.[27] In the older adult population, as health becomes more compromised, a higher prevalence of dry mouth is experienced as compared with the general public.[28] (See Table 2 for prevalence rates.)

Table 2. Prevalence of Xerostomia and Salivary Gland Hypofunction (SGH)

Population	Xerostomia	SGH
General public	5.5–39%	—
Community dwelling	17–40%	15–23%
Institutionalized	20–72%	17–50%

Source: Adapted from Oral Surg Oral Med Oral Pathol Oral Radiol Endod. 2012;114:52–60.[28]

ETIOLOGY OF DRY MOUTH

Age

The deleterious effects of dry mouth are most frequently seen in the older adult population. The paucity of reports on the prevalence of xerostomia and SGH in younger populations creates challenges in distinguishing the true impact of age on dry mouth.[27] A cross-sectional study of stimulated whole saliva from three different age groups found that older adults (> 70 years) did have a significantly decreased flow.[29,30] No differences were found between young (20 to 30 years) and middle-aged (40 to 50 years) adults, but significant differences between the young and old and the middle-aged and old were found.[30] Therefore, much of the literature currently promotes the idea that the prevalence of xerostomia and SGH increases with age but this may be more strongly associated with medication use and health status.

Physiologically, with aging, the number of acinar cells is reduced and replaced by fibrous and fatty tissue, altering the composition of saliva. There is a 30% to 40% decrease in the number of acinar cells within salivary glands between ages 34 and 75+ years.[31] The primary effect of this change is thought to result from disruption of the parasympathetic pathway (see Figure 2).[29] This pathway is also the one most affected by polypharmacy (via anticholinergics).

Medication

One of the most common causes of dry mouth is the use of xerogenic medications. As people age, it is common for them to be taking multiple medications, of which over 1,000 are known to contribute to dry mouth.[32] The primary path of action is through anticholinergic activity, resulting in a reduction of salivary flow. Increasing the number and dosage of anticholinergic drugs being taken (anticholinergic burden) was found to increase the likelihood and severity of dry mouth.[33,34] In a longitudinal study, it was found that the prevalence and incidence of xerostomia was strongly associated with medication exposure.[35] Furthermore, there is a strong correlation between number of diseases, medications, and xerostomia.[36,37]

Systemic Disorders

Many systemic conditions are known to cause or are associated with varying degrees of dry mouth; however, one of the most common autoimmune diseases, Sjögren's syndrome, almost always results in both xerostomia and SGH. In the United States, an estimated 0.4 million to 3.1 million adults are living with Sjögren's syndrome.[38] Disturbances in salivary output arising from this syndrome can cause difficulty chewing or swallowing and increase the risk for oral infections.[39]

Other systemic conditions frequently associated with dry mouth symptoms include diabetes mellitus, infectious diseases (human immunodeficiency and hepatitis C viruses), and neurological disorders, including Parkinson's disease, Alzheimer's disease, and depression[40] (see Table 3). The dry mouth experienced in these situations is often related to medications prescribed for the medical management of these systemic disorders. Lastly, behavioral conditions exhibiting dry mouth symptoms include eating disorders, alcohol abuse, and tobacco use, of which eating disorders are exhibited more often in younger populations. Alcohol and tobacco abuse may be prevalent from young adulthood through older age. In behavioral conditions, dry mouth symptoms should dissipate if the condition is alleviated.

Radiation Therapy

Head and neck cancers are more prevalent in the older population, although reports have shown an increase in younger populations;[41] therefore, dry mouth resulting from radiation therapy may be seen across the broad adult population. (See Chapter 7.) Salivary glands in the head and neck region can be temporarily or permanently damaged as a result of radiation therapy to treat cancer. Pooled data from a systematic review reported a 93% prevalence of xerostomia during radiation therapy, which slightly decreased over time.[42] The impact on whole saliva secretions was also profound, with small improvements in salivary gland function over time.[42] Interestingly, salivary glands may differ in their radiation sensitivity; the parotid glands are highly sensitive, resulting in a decrease of up to 90% after radiation.[43,44] Radiation also can result in taste loss and mucositis, and can affect oral health-related quality of life.[45]

Table 3. Common Systemic Disorders Associated with Dry Mouth

	Specific Condition	Average Age of Onset	Gender and/or GenderRatio
Systemic Change			
Autoimmune and rheumatological disorders	Sjögren's syndrome	Onset at any age, but more common ~50 years	9:1 (F:M)
	Systemic lupus erythematosus	~20–30 years	10:1 (F:M)
	Autoimmune hepatitis	Young adult	F
	Primary biliary cirrhosis	Young adult	F
	Rheumatoid arthritis	~25–45 years	3:1 (F:M)
Endocrine disorders	Type 1 diabetes mellitus (DM)	Childhood	M/F
	Type 2 DM	Middle to older adult	M/F
Neurological disorders	Parkinson's disease	Middle age ~50+ years	M
	Depression	All age groups	M/F
	Alzheimer's disease	Older adult	M/F
Eating disorders	Anorexia nervosa	Adolescent and early adult	F
	Bulimia	Adolescent and early adult	F
Infectious diseases	HIV	Varies	M/F
	Hepatitis C	Adulthood	M
Other			
Other	Sarcoidosis	~20–40 years	F
Behavioral	Tobacco use	Onset in adolescent to early adult years	M/F

Sources: Based on Dry Mouth: A Clinical Guide on Causes, Effects, and Treatments. 2015:7–31.[40]

PART 2: PATIENT MANAGEMENT AND INTERVENTIONS

When considering an approach to patient management and prevention for patients experiencing dry mouth, the clinician must determine whether any salivary gland function remains. If there is some salivary gland function, the next step would be to determine the underlying cause of dry mouth. The dominant contributors to dry mouth are medications, systemic or behavioral conditions, and radiation therapy. Once the clinician determines the underlying cause, a management strategy can be devised. The management strategy may include changing the contributing factors or preventing the intensification of the dry mouth condition, or both. This section addresses the three main areas of care for patients with dry mouth, namely (1) preventive strategies, (2) therapeutic interventions, and (3) patient management strategies.

PREVENTIVE STRATEGIES
Preventive Strategies in Dry Mouth Resulting from Radiation Therapy

Until the more recent widespread use of intensity-modulated radiation therapy (IMRT), patients treated for head and neck cancer (HNC) with radiation therapy experienced severe damage to the salivary glands, which often resulted in permanent dry mouth. When patients are about to undergo radiation therapy for HNC treatment, a few preventive strategies exist that may limit or decrease the likelihood of extreme postradiation dry mouth. The strategies include IMRT, three-dimensional (3D) conformal radiation therapy, and submandibular gland transfer surgical procedures.[46,47] An overarching process as a preventive strategy with HNC patients is for the dental practitioner to work with the patient's oncology care team in order to advocate for gland sparing or gland transfer techniques for the patient's cancer care.

Intensity-Modulated Radiation Therapy or 3D Conformal Radiation Therapy

In the past 10 years, IMRT use for HNC has increased considerably in the United States,[48] United Kingdom,[49,50] and Canada.[51] IMRT and 3D conformal radiation therapy techniques are able to more specifically target the delivery of radiation to the affected area and consequently have produced results that decrease the destructive impact on salivary glands.[42,46] Studies have shown that IMRT and 3D conformal radiation therapies were able to better preserve salivary gland function in comparison to conventional radiation therapy processes that were not able to deliver radiation therapy to the tissues in a focused and specific manner.[32,42] Better results in decreasing dry mouth have been reported with use of IMRT versus 3D conformal radiation therapy.[47,52,53]

Salivary Gland Transfer

A substantial preventive approach for reducing the risk of developing radiation-induced dry mouth is the salivary gland transfer (SGT) procedure described and implemented in 2000, and known as the Seikaly Jha procedure (SJP).[46,53,54] In an appropriate patient, this surgical procedure preserves the submandibular gland by moving it away from the intended path of radiation, thereby eliminating or minimizing detrimental effects to the salivary gland. Studies show very encouraging results related to minimizing dry mouth when the SJP is used in HNC patients.[53,55] In both a systematic review and meta-analysis, subjects who had received the SJP maintained their stimulated and unstimulated salivary flow rates at near-normal levels pre–cancer treatment.[53] Furthermore, over time, post-treatment, the subjects who received SJP continued to report improvement in salivary flow rates.[53]

Preventive Strategies in Dry Mouth Resulting from Medications

In the case of medication-induced dry mouth, prevention strategies include consulting with medical practitioners to review the patient's medications and assessing whether alterations could be made in medication number, dose or formulation, and type. There is minimal evidence to support any relief of symptoms from altering medications, and the process is very much a time-consuming, trial-and-error approach.[32] Although studies have shown that taking multiple medications or different doses, formulations, or brands of drug can result in more or less xerostomic effects, situations in which any aspect of a person's medication regimen can be altered are limited, and the evidence is minimal to support its effectiveness for decreasing dry mouth.[56]

Preventive Strategies in Dry Mouth Resulting from Systemic or Behavioral Conditions

In patients whose dry mouth is the result of a systemic change, there is little to nothing that can be done preventively to change the condition. Once the diagnosis has been made, the process focuses on therapies and management protocol, as appropriate. If the condition contributing to dry mouth is systemic, such as an eating disorder or alcohol abuse, the patient should be referred to an appropriate health practitioner to provide support, treatment, and a management program. In situations of dry mouth resulting from behavioral conditions, the dry mouth should resolve and normal salivary function return if the behavior is greatly modified or eliminated.

THERAPEUTIC INTERVENTIONS

When considering therapeutic approaches to alleviating the effects of dry mouth in any of these three dominant contributing situations, the clinician should determine if the salivary glands have any remaining function.[56] The following sections describe therapeutic interventions for patients with and without salivary gland function. Although a 2011 Cochrane review found no strong evidence to support any topical therapies for stimulating or substituting saliva,[57] patients have reported responding to topical therapies and receiving some relief from dry mouth symptoms.[58] The therapeutic interventions are included here so clinicians will be versed in the various topical therapy options patients may want to discuss.

Salivary Glands Remain Functioning

When some salivary flow remains, two groups of therapeutic interventions can be considered for patients with dry mouth: (1) saliva stimulants (sialagogues), and (2) saliva substitutes.

Saliva Stimulants

Saliva stimulants commonly used and readily available include chewing gum, oral lozenges, topical or systemic pilocarpine, acupuncture, and electrostimulation.[59] Studies of each of these forms of stimulants have demonstrated some efficacy for managing the symptoms of dry mouth; however, available evidence is weak, and no specific intervention has any strong evidence to support its efficacy for relieving dry mouth.[57,59,60] The dental practitioner must assess the individual's condition and consider the etiology, as well as patient acceptance, willingness to try, and level of compliance, as all will influence the degree of effectiveness and relief experienced by patients for any of these interventions.

Chewing Agents. Chewing gums have shown effectiveness in stimulating salivary flow; however, the patient must continue the chewing action as the relief of dry mouth symptoms comes from the chewing function.[57,61] Studies have not shown whether chewing gums are more or less effective than any salivary substitute, but patients have reported a preference for chewing agents over salivary substitutes.[57] To preserve and protect the dentition, the chewing gum should be sugar-free or sweetened with xylitol or sorbitol.[32]

Lozenges. Similar to chewing gums, lozenges have produced some relief of symptoms while the agent is being consumed and possibly for a short time after it dissolves; however, long-term relief is not apparent with any lozenge. Additionally, the lozenges should be sugar-free or sweetened with a sugar substitute to protect the dentition from caries. Lozenge use may be more appealing than chewing gum to older adults, both as a more socially acceptable action and because their use avoids possible discomfort of chewing associated with arthritis or wearing of dentures.[32]

Prescription Medications. Pilocarpine, in both topical and systemic forms, has shown some effectiveness in relieving the effects of dry mouth. This agent is a muscarinic receptor agonist and stimulates the secretion of saliva; however, a common side effect is stimulation of sweat glands, resulting in excessive sweating by users. Pilocarpine is contraindicated in people with asthma, acute iritis, and certain types of glaucoma, and patients should be closely monitored if they have cardiovascular or pulmonary diseases.[62] Dental professionals should consult with the patient's physician before prescribing pilocarpine to ensure compatibility with concurrent systemic conditions and medication use. Pilocarpine has been most effective in people who have some remaining salivary gland function and salivary flow; however, patients do report improvement in the subjective sensation of dry mouth.[32] The positive effects cease when pilocarpine is discontinued; therefore, continued use is necessary for ongoing relief of symptoms.[32]

Topical preparations of pilocarpine include lozenges, sprays, and mouthwashes. Studies have shown the most effective form of topical pilocarpine is the lozenge, in both the 5 mg[59] and 10 mg formulations. Systemic preparations are in the form of tablets.

Cevimeline is a muscarinic acetylcholine receptor agonist that has a longer half-life and duration of action than pilocarpine, and has also been shown to have fewer adverse effects on cardiovascular and respiratory conditions. Cevimeline is approved by the U.S. Food and Drug Administration for use in people with Sjögren's syndrome and for treatment of radiation therapy-induced salivary hypofunction.[59,63]

Nonpharmacological Interventions for Salivary Stimulation. Other processes being researched or used to stimulate salivary flow with some demonstrated positive effect on reducing dry mouth symptoms are acupuncture and electrostimulation. Studies of acupuncture as a therapy to stimulate salivary flow reported varied outcomes for effectiveness, and it is clear that more research is needed to determine if acupuncture is an effective therapy for dry mouth. In studies showing some positive effect, the patients had some remaining salivary gland function.[32,59,64,65]

Electrostimulation is a newer technique being studied to stimulate salivary flow.[59] An intraoral electrostimulating appliance, which was studied in a multicenter, randomized control trial, was found to reduce dry mouth symptoms and stimulate salivary flow.[66,67] However, a Cochrane review published in 2013 concluded that there was limited evidence to determine the effectiveness of electrostimulation; therefore, more research studies are needed before making any recommendations for therapeutic use.[65]

Saliva Substitutes

Saliva substitutes contain lubricating macromolecules as a substitute for salivary glycoproteins, whereas stimulants increase the salivary flow rate resulting in an increasing level of protein secreted per minute.[59] The salivary substitute should be neutral pH and should contain fluoride to aid in protecting the dentition. Patients must be cautioned about using any products with higher acidity due to the damaging effect on the dentition. Different agents have been developed in the form of gels, lubricants, sprays, and lozenges.[32,64] A short list of products and home remedies is provided in Table 4. Most of the substances used for moisturizing or coating the tissues need to be applied many times during the day, which may limit patient compliance. Therefore, some form of a sugar-free or sugar-substitute lozenge may be best for providing relief of dry mouth symptoms, as it is easy to use and may be more acceptable in work or social settings.

Sprays. Sprays may be effective for some people. The product is sprayed into the mouth, coating the oral tissues in an attempt to provide moisture and lubrication. Sprays must also be used frequently, and therefore must be kept on hand for ease of use, both of which may limit compliance.
Rinses. Rinses with antimicrobial and caries-preventive properties should be recommended for their action of decreasing the oral bacterial load and for reducing the incidence of new carious

Table 4. Saliva Substitutes

Active Agent	Product Name	Product Form
Over-the-Counter Products		
Mucin	Saliva Orthana®	Spray
Hydroxy methylcellulose–based gels	Biotene Oral Balance®	Gel, rinse, spray, toothpaste
	BioXtra®	Gel, rinse, toothpaste
Electrolytes in carboxymethylcellulose	Optimoist (contains citric acid)	Spray
Home Remedies		
Olive oil[68,69]	Many varieties	
Water	—	—
Hydroxy methylcellulose; glycerin	K-Y® Jelly	Gel

Content derived from Pedersen 2015[40]

lesions. With regard to their lubricating or moistening action, rinses have not been successful in providing patients relief from their symptoms. As with other topical products, it has been the authors' experience that a cool rinsing action may provide some immediate soothing effect, but the effect is not sustained after rinsing is stopped.

Saliva substitutes are limited by the short-term relief provided; however, one must weigh the benefits of *some relief* versus *no relief* when someone is suffering the impact of dry mouth. Some relief could positively improve quality of life.

PATIENT MANAGEMENT CONSIDERATIONS

Patient management of a person reporting dry mouth must begin with a thorough assessment. If the assessment identifies contributing factors that can be changed, the dental practitioner can make these appropriate suggestions and monitor accordingly. If contributing factors cannot be altered in any way, the clinician must focus on supportive therapy to prevent any worsening of the dry mouth and to ensure preventive protocols are in place to address potential oral and dental manifestations. Clinicians should assess the degree of dry mouth, identify the etiology, educate the patient, and develop an individualized prevention program for the patient. This program should include strategies for caries control, risk reduction for onset and recurrence of oral infections, appropriate denture care (if applicable), and limiting the extent and severity of mucositis.

The diagnostic process conducted by a dental practitioner should include the following components (adapted from Narhi and colleagues[68]):

• Documented history and description of the symptoms being experienced
• Thorough medical history with review of medications
• Clinical oral and dental examination
• Salivary flow measurements

After the diagnostic information has been gathered, the clinician can determine a management program in consultation with the patient. There is no strong evidence to clearly delineate support for any of the salivary stimulants or substitutes; however, studies have shown varying levels of relief with use of different products or combinations of products.[58] Therefore, it is imperative to work individually with each patient to devise a management plan. It is very likely that many therapeutic agents will not bring relief, so if the patient reports no change in symptoms after a set trial period, another agent should be attempted in an ongoing process.[70] Patients need to clearly understand that many management strategies will be attempted on a trial basis, as they may become easily discouraged. It is important for clinicians to work together with their patients to determine and devise the best possible management program for symptom relief, improved function, and quality of life.

Additionally, patients need to be advised on the

following professional recommendations and home remedies that in some cases have provided relief of symptoms for some periods of time. They include (1) increasing hydration with water;[70] (2) using a room humidifier;[70] (3) avoiding coffee, alcohol, and any other dehydrating beverages;[61,70] (4) avoiding or preferably quitting tobacco use;[61,70] (5) avoiding oral irritants such as spicy, sour, and acidic foods and sweetened beverages;[70] (6) practicing optimal oral hygiene;[70] (7) using fluoride products;[70] and (8) maintaining regular care with a professional dental office (dentist, dental hygienist).[70]

During the clinical examination, the dentist or dental hygienist must assess for new carious lesions and treat accordingly. If the patient has dentures, the denture and the oral tissues need to be examined as the likelihood of oral candidiasis increases with dry mouth. Furthermore, since saliva is vitally important to the fit and stability of dentures, patients need to understand how their denture fit may increasingly decline to the point of not being able to wear dentures if salivary flow is extremely compromised. In addition to the treatments for these oral and dental issues, patients need to be clearly informed and supported to follow a strict oral hygiene protocol; however, even with optimal oral hygiene, it may not be possible to prevent some oral conditions from deteriorating. Saliva has many important functions in the oral cavity and without it, oral status is compromised.

Some specific recommendations to maintain oral health include (1) use of home and professionally applied fluoride therapies, (2) following dietary recommendations to decrease sugar intake, and (3) increasing the number of professional office visits for monitoring and maintenance. Patients with dentures should be advised to wear dentures only during the day, to clean dentures daily, and to soak dentures overnight in an appropriate solution. Rinsing twice daily with an antiseptic mouthrinse has been shown to be beneficial for edentulous patients to reduce the bacterial load and to prevent denture stomatitis.[71,72]

Lastly, it is imperative that dentists and dental hygienists work collaboratively with other healthcare providers to determine the most effective strategies for managing patients suffering with dry mouth.

Therapeutic Interventions Specific to Radiation-Induced Dry Mouth

There is new and ongoing research on therapeutic interventions to address damage to the salivary glands after radiation therapy and the severe dry mouth associated with Sjögren's syndrome.[42,73-75] Some of these therapeutic interventions include stem cell therapy, gene therapy, and hyperbaric oxygen therapy.

Stem Cell Research

Research investigating the use of mesenchymal stem cells to regenerate salivary production and decrease dry mouth has shown some promise. However, a systematic review published in 2014 reported a lack of conclusive evidence and called for future research to substantiate the possibilities of this therapy to regenerate salivary glands and restore salivary flow.[74]

Gene Therapy

Results are favorable from a human clinical trial involving salivary gland gene transfer to repair damaged salivary glands after radiation therapy. It is expected that this research will initiate further efforts to determine whether gene transfer may be an effective therapy to aid in relief from dry mouth after radiation therapy to the salivary glands.[75]

Hyperbaric Oxygen Therapy

Hyperbaric oxygen therapy delivers oxygen to irradiated tissues. A recent study of hyperbaric oxygen showed a decrease in dry mouth symptoms resulting from radiation therapy; however, this was a small pilot study and further research is recommended to assess the effectiveness of these interventions.[73] Similarly, a 2010 systematic review reported a decrease in dry mouth symptoms after varying regimens of hyperbaric oxygen treatment; however, the results were reported with high caution noting the potential of many confounding variables that could have influenced the positive results.[42]

CASE 1: Patient with Systemic Lupus Erythematosus and Sjögren's Syndrome

PATIENT OVERVIEW

Ms. Dianna B. is a 53-year-old woman who is presently not working and receiving a disability allowance. Both the patient and her sister were diagnosed with systemic lupus erythematosus in their early 20s. Subsequently, Dianna developed Sjögren's syndrome and Raynaud phenomenon. She also has fibromyalgia, asthma, osteoporosis, and osteoarthritis.

For many years, Dianna has managed to live with the sores and cuts inside her mouth, accepting that they are side effects of her condition. Approximately 25 years after her diagnosis, she visited the dental hygiene clinic at a university-based educational training program. During this visit, she was referred to an oral pathologist at the same clinic due to her extensive oral candidiasis. Dianna mentioned she had extremely dry eyes and had been using pilocarpine for saliva stimulation, but she felt the medication was no longer providing relief for her dry mouth symptoms. The oral pathologist has diagnosed Dianna with xerostomia and salivary gland hyposalivation (SGH) and begins to work with her to manage the symptoms of her condition.

Chief Complaint: Dianna notes irritation and pain from frequent sores and cuts in her mouth and the continual oral dryness that she understands is a "part of her lupus."

Medical History: Dianna was diagnosed with systemic lupus erythematosus, Sjögren's syndrome, fibromyalgia, asthma, osteoporosis, and osteoarthritis. Her current medications (see Table 5) and other supplements (see Table 6) are recorded. It is noted that Dianna is allergic to penicillin, sulfa drugs, venlafaxine, duloxetine, and latex.

Risk Factor Assessment: Sjögren's syndrome has a known side effect of dry mouth as well as dryness of other tissues (e.g., eyes). Dianna takes several medications that are known to be xerogenic.

CLINICAL EXAMINATION

The initial clinical examination by the oral pathologist reveals the following:

Extraoral: Masseteric hyperplasia
Intraoral: Central erythematous denuded patch on the dorsal aspect of the tongue; white striations

Table 5. Case 1—Patient Medications

Agent	Dosage/Frequency
Pregabalin	75 mg, twice daily (BID)
Methotrexate	2.5 mg, 6 tablets weekly
Folic acid	5 mg, weekly (on Tuesday)
Hydroxychloroquine	200 mg, BID
Prednisone	5 mg, daily
Nifedipine	30 mg, daily
Clopidogrel bisulfate	75 mg, 1 tablet at night
Pilocarpine	5 mg, 6 tablets daily
Domperidone	10 mg, BID
Ondansetron	4 mg, 3× daily (TID)
Pantoprazole	40 mg, 1 tablet in morning
Celecoxib	200 mg, BID
Risedronate	150 mg, once monthly (on the 10th)
Montelukast sodium	10 mg, 1 tablet at night
Fluticasone furoate	7.5 mg, 2 sprays BID
Formoterol fumarate inhaler	200 mg, 2 puffs BID (may increase to 4× daily [QID])
Cyclosporine 0.05% (ophthalmic)	1 drop in each eye BID
Estradiol	10 mcg, 1 vaginally twice weekly
Clotrimazole 1.07%	2 mL, up to 5 times daily
Chlorhexidine 0.2%	As once-daily rinse
Neutral 1.1% sodium fluoride	For use in trays once daily
Ipratropium inhaler	1–2 sprays in each nostril BID–QID

Table 6. Case 1—Patient Supplements

Supplement	Dosage/Frequency
Glucosamine sulfate	750 mg, BID
Women's multivitamin	1 tablet daily
B-100 complex	1 tablet daily
Omega-3	900 mg, 1 capsule daily
Vitamin C	1,000 mg, 1 tablet daily
Niacin	500 mg, 1 tablet daily
Calcium carbonate	500 mg, TID
Vitamin D	1,000 IU, 1 tablet daily

with a red background on both the hard and soft palates; minimal saliva pooling in the floor of the mouth.

Diagnostic Tests and Results: No specific diagnostic tests for the dry mouth.

Diagnosis: Xerostomia and SGH resulting from Sjögren's syndrome and multiple medications.

Risk Reduction: The oral pathologist prescribes chlorhexidine 0.2% rinse and clotrimazole suspension (10 mg/mL) with a re-evaluation scheduled for 6 weeks. He discusses having custom fluoride trays fabricated for daily fluoride treatments at home with 0.2% neutral sodium fluoride gel. The patient is also advised to use PreviDent® 5000 for further caries prevention (see Table 7).

OUTCOMES

Five weeks later, Dianna returns for her follow-up appointment with the oral pathologist. She reports using the chlorhexidine rinse regularly but not the clotrimazole suspension. She also reports that her dry mouth has worsened (see Figure 3).

The extraoral examination shows continued masseteric hyperplasia and angular cheilitis. Intraorally, dry mouth is still evident, and white patches on the soft palate that can be wiped off are present. The clinical appearance is consistent with candidiasis, and fluconazole is recommended. Given the potential interactions of fluconazole with Dianna's multiple medications, a physician consultation is needed.

Figure 3. Case 1—Dry Tongue

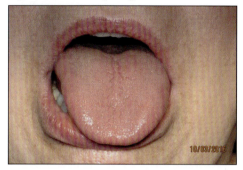

Figure 4. Case 1—Custom Fluoride Trays

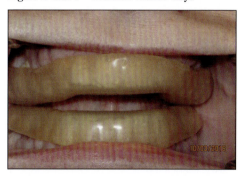

Table 7. Case 1—Risk Reduction for Oral Dryness

Preventive Interventions
- Custom trays for home fluoride application with 1.1% neutral sodium fluoride
- Regular fluoride varnish for all remaining natural teeth
- PreviDent® 5000

Therapeutic Interventions
- Pilocarpine tablets, 5 mg
- Chlorhexidine rinse 0.2%
- Clotrimazole, 10-mg lozenges; dissolve 1 in mouth 3–4 times daily
- Clotrimazole suspension, 10 mg/mL (blend of 900 mg clotrimazole powder with 2 tubes Oral Balance moisturizing gel); swab mouth 4 times daily.
- Nystatin (100,000 units/gram) apply thin film to commissures of mouth
- Fluconazole (100mg tablets)

Lifestyle Recommendations
- Hydration with water

CHAPTER 10 Dry Mouth

Figure 5. Case 1–Radiographs

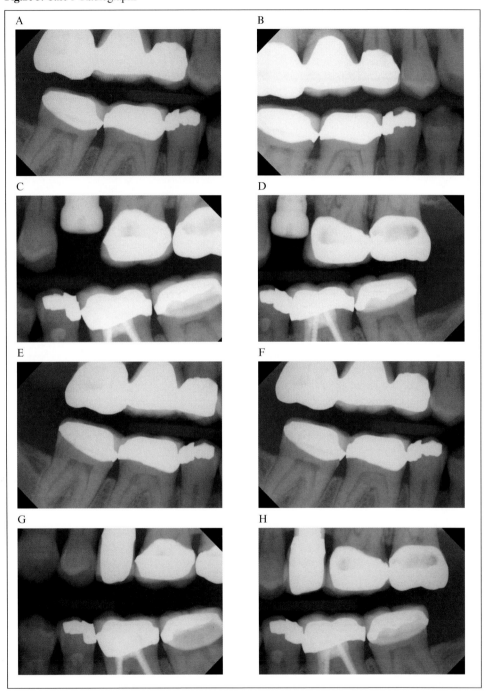

A. Right molar radiograph, 2013. B. Right premolar radiograph, 2013. C. Left premolar radiograph, 2013. D. Left molar radiograph, 2013. E. Right molar radiograph, 2014. F. Right premolar radiograph, 2014. G. Left premolar radiograph, 2014. H. Left molar radiograph, 2014.

Six weeks later, Dianna returns for a follow-up appointment. At this appointment she explains that her home care regimen consists of the following: (1) using the fluoride custom trays for 10 to 15 minutes per day (see Figure 4), (2) regular chlorhexidine rinsing, (3) PreviDent® 5000 for tooth brushing, (4) irregular use of clotrimazole suspension, and (5) nystatin ointment as needed for angular cheilitis. The fungal infection on her palate is markedly diminished with only a few light white areas.

FUTURE CONSIDERATIONS

A recall maintenance schedule with visits to the oral pathology clinic is set for every 3 months; however, depending on the oral condition at the time of the recall visit, there may be follow-up visits of a shorter duration (often 2 to 4 weeks). Over a span of 4 years, Dianna has 16 appointments with the oral pathologist and others in the dental hygiene clinic for routine dental hygiene maintenance. At the dental hygiene appointments, she receives fluoride varnish application for any of her remaining natural teeth for caries prevention. Dianna is diligent with her own home care and it has been noted many times by the dental clinicians that she has excellent oral hygiene. Radiographs show no new caries from June 2013 through June 2014 (see Figure 5A–5H).

Dianna also experiences many outbreaks of dryness at the corners of her mouth and uses prescribed nystatin for the angular cheilitis. At one of her appointments in 2013, the oral pathologist prescribes clotrimazole lozenges, which Dianna reports provided some relief from dry mouth symptoms.

Since Dianna began treatment 4 years ago at the oral pathology clinic, she has expressed how her life has changed dramatically. She does not have as many sores in her mouth and is diligent in following the home care protocol (see Figure 6). Additionally, Dianna has become very informed about dry mouth and monitors the introduction of any new products on the market, often bringing them to the clinician's attention at her recall visits.

Figure 6. Case 1—Healthy Gingival Tissues

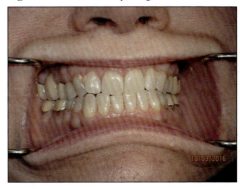

CASE 2: Patient with History of Head and Neck Cancer Radiation Therapy

PATIENT OVERVIEW

Mr. Roy G. is a 65-year-old man who worked for the past 40 years in the construction business. He was a heavy smoker and had severe periodontitis that required him to have a maxillary clearance approximately 10 years ago at age 55. He has a partially dentate mandible. After receiving his cancer diagnosis and having successfully undergone a combination of surgery and radiation therapy, Roy has now been referred to a prosthodontic office by an oral surgeon. The referral includes a request from the radiation oncologist that the patient have hyperbaric oxygen treatment and a fixed hybrid prosthesis due to the higher risk for osteoradionecrosis from trauma to the mandibular bone as a result of the treatment interventions.

Chief Complaint: Roy complains of extreme dry mouth and that his complete upper denture is not fitting well.

Medical History: Seven years ago Roy first noticed some discomfort when he swallowed. He dismissed the symptom as a sore throat due to a cold or flu and did a warm salt water gargle twice a day for approximately 2 weeks. He thought that his throat felt better. However, over the next several months he noticed that he frequently choked on his food and drink, which caused him to cough. His wife and coworkers also inquired whether he was still feeling "under the weather" as he sounded "different." He went to see his family physician who prescribed an antibiotic. Over the next month Roy noticed no improvement to his condition. His sore throat seemed to have returned, and the discomfort was now a dull pain accompanied by an earache. He returned to his physician, who referred him to an ear, nose, and throat specialist. During his appointment with the specialist, a biopsy was taken which revealed squamous cell cancer at the base of the tongue and throat. He received surgery and radiation therapy. His salivary glands were not shielded during his radiation therapy. Roy's current medications are listed in Table 8.

Risk Factor Assessment: Due to the amount and location of radiation, Roy suffers from radiation-induced xerostomia.

CLINICAL EXAMINATION

The clinical examination conducted by the prosthodontist notes that there is severe decay and periodontal involvement of the mandibular teeth, which are fracturing at the gingival margin (see Figure 7A–D). The saliva is noted as thick and ropey.

Diagnostic Tests and Results: A pretreatment panoramic radiograph was taken (see Figure 8). No specific diagnostic tests for categorizing the dry mouth condition were performed.

Diagnosis: Radiation-induced xerostomia.

Risk Reduction: It is recommended that Roy have a hybrid fixed lower denture and implant-supported complete upper denture. Biotene® mouthrinse and a moisture spray are recommended to manage his dry mouth.

Table 8. Case 2—Patient Medications

Agent	Dosage/Frequency
Bisoprolol	10 mg BID
Hydrochlorothiazide	25 mg daily
Quinapril	40 mg daily
Aspirin	81 mg daily

OUTCOMES

Roy reports that he is comfortable with his new dentures (see Figure 9A–C). He feels that he is functioning well with the dentures. However, the

Figure 7. Case 2—Pretreatment Photographs

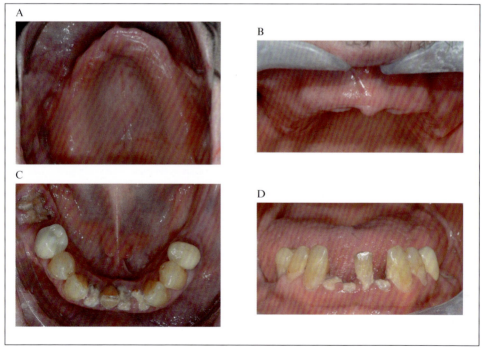

A, B. Maxillary photographs, pretreatment. C, D. Mandibular photographs, pretreatment.

Figure 8. Case 2—Panoramic Radiograph Pretreatment

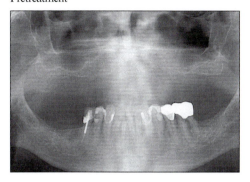

Figure 9. Case 2—Implant Fixtures

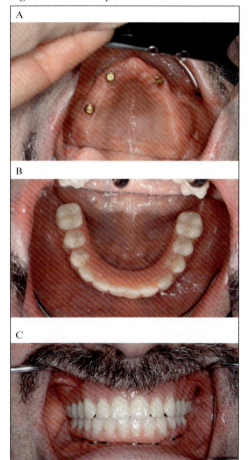

A. Maxillary implant fixtures. B. Implant-supported mandibular complete denture. C. Maxillary denture and fixed hybrid mandibular denture.

Biotene® mouthrinse and moisture spray are only providing limited relief. He has tried to constantly sip water for additional relief, but struggles with dry mouth overnight.

FUTURE CONSIDERATIONS

Further recommendations to relieve the xerostomia include the use of XyliMelts®, which are recommended to help with overnight dry mouth. Frequent follow-up appointments are suggested to monitor Roy's dental implants and his dry mouth.

REFERENCES

1. Hopcraft MS, Tan C. Xerostomia: an update for clinicians. *Aust Dental J.* 2010;55:238–244.
2. Naito M, Yuasa H, Nomura Y, et al. Oral health status and health-related quality of life: a systematic review. *J Oral Sci.* 2006;48:1–7.
3. Cassolato SF, Turnbull RS. Xerostomia: clinical aspects and treatment. *Gerodontology.* 2003;20:64–77.
4. Amerongen A, Veerman E. Saliva–the defender of the oral cavity. *Oral Dis.* 2002;8:12–22.
5. Villa A, Nordio F, Gohel A. A risk prediction model for xerostomia: a retrospective cohort study. *Gerodontology.* 2015 Nov 17. [Epub ahead of print.]
6. Turner M, Jahangiri L, Ship JA. Hyposalivation, xerostomia and the complete denture: a systematic review. *J Am Dental Assoc.* 2008;139:146–150.
7. Rouleau TS, Shychuk AJ, Kayastha J, et al. A retrospective, cohort study of the prevalence and risk factors of oral burning in patients with dry mouth. *Oral Surg Oral Med Oral Pathol Oral Radiol Endod.* 2011;111:720–725.
8. Thomson WM, Chalmers JM, Spencer AJ, et al. The occurrence of xerostomia and salivary gland hypofunction in a population-based sample of older South Australians. *Spec Care Dentist.* 1999;19:20–23.
9. Nederfors T. Xerostomia and hyposalivation. *Adv Dent Res.* 2000;14:48–56.
10. Humphrey SP, Williamson RT. A review of saliva: normal composition, flow, and function. *J Prosthet Dent.* 2001;85:162–169.
11. Dawes C. Physiological factors affecting salivary flow rate, oral sugar clearance, and the sensation of dry mouth in man. *J Dent Res.* 1987;66(spec no):648–653.
12. Nederfors T, Isaksson R, Mörnstad H, et al. Prevalence of perceived symptoms of dry mouth in an adult Swedish population—relation to age, sex, and pharmacotherapy. *Community Dent Oral Epidemiol.* 1997;25:211–216.
13. Thomson WM, Brown RH, Williams SM. Medication and perception of dry mouth in a population of institutionalised elderly people. *N Z Med J.* 1993;106(957):219–221.
14. Fox PC, Busch KA, Baum BJ. Subjective reports of xerostomia and objective measures of salivary gland perform-

ance. *J Am Dent Assoc.* 1987;115:581–584.
15. Fure S, Zickert I. Salivary conditions and cariogenic microorganisms in 55, 65, and 75 year old Swedish individuals. *Eur J Oral Sci.* 1990;98:197–210.
16. Närhi TO. Prevalence of subjective feelings of dry mouth in the elderly. *J Dent Res.* 1994;73:20–25.
17. Locker D. Subjective reports of oral dryness in an older adult population. *Community Dent Oral Epidemiol.* 1993;21:165–168.
18. Locker D. Dental status, xerostomia, and the oral health related quality of life of an elderly institutionalized population. *Spec Care Dentist.* 2003;23:86–93.
19. Osailan SM, Pramanik R, Shirlaw P, et al. Clinical assessment of oral dryness: development of a scoring system related to salivary flow and mucosal wetness. *Oral Surg Oral Med Oral Pathol Oral Radiol Endod.* 2012;114:597–603.
20. Pai S, Ghezzi EM, Ship JA. Development of a visual analogue scale questionnaire for subjective assessment of salivary dysfunction. *Oral Surg Oral Med Oral Pathol Oral Radiol Endod.* 2001;91:311–316.
21. Thomson WM, Chalmers JM, Spencer AJ, et al. The xerostomia inventory: a multi-item approach to measuring dry mouth. *Community Dent Health.* 1999;16:12–17.
22. Thomson WM. Subjective aspects of dry mouth. In: Carpenter G, ed. *Dry Mouth: A Clinical Guide on Causes, Effects, and Treatments.* New York, NY: Springer-Verlag; 2015:103–115.
23. Navazesh M, Christensen C, Brightman V. Clinical criteria for the diagnosis of salivary gland hypofunction. *J Dent Res.* 1992;71:1363–1369.
24. Navazesh M, Christensen C. A comparison of whole mouth resting and stimulated salivary measurement procedures. *J Dent Res.* 1982;61:1158–1162.
25. Thomson WM. Issues in the epidemiological investigation of dry mouth. *Gerodontology.* 2005;22:65–76.
26. Ship JA, Pillemer SR, Baum BJ. Xerostomia and the geriatric patient. *J Am Geriatr Soc.* 2002;50:535–543.
27. Orellana MF, Lagravere MO, Boychuk DG, et al. Prevalence of xerostomia in population-based samples: a systematic review. *J Public Health Dent.* 2006;66:152–158.
28. Liu B, Dion MR, Jurasic MM, et al. Xerostomia and salivary hypofunction in vulnerable elders: prevalence and etiology. *Oral Surg Oral Med Oral Pathol Oral Radiol Endod.* 2012;114:52–60.
29. Nagler RM, Hershkovich O. Relationships between age, drugs, oral sensorial complaints, and salivary profile. *Arch Oral Biol.* 2005;50:7–16.
30. Smith CH, Boland B, Daureeawoo Y, et al. Effect of aging on stimulated salivary flow in adults. *J Am Geriatr Soc.* 2013;61:805–808.
31. Navazesh M. Salivary gland hypofunction in elderly patients. *J Calif Dent Assoc.* 1994;22:62–68.
32. Han P, Suarez-Durall P, Mulligan R. Dry mouth: a critical topic for older adult patients. *J Prosthodont Res.* 2015;59:6–19.
33. Chew ML, Mulsant BH, Pollock BG, et al. Anticholinergic activity of 107 medications commonly used by older adults. *J Am Geriatr Soc.* 2008;56:1333–1341.
34. Desoutter A, Soudain-Pineau M, Munsch F, et al. Xerostomia and medication: A cross-sectional study in long-term geriatric wards. *J Nutr Health Aging.* 2012;16:575–579.
35. Murray Thomson W, Chalmers JM, John Spencer A, et al. A longitudinal study of medication exposure and xerostomia among older people. *Gerodontology.* 2006;23:205–213.
36. Smidt D, Torpet LA, Nauntofte B, et al. Associations between oral and ocular dryness, labial and whole salivary flow rates, systemic diseases and medications in a sample of older people. *Community Dent Oral Epidemiol.* 2011;39:276–288.
37. Pajukoski H, Meurman JH, Halonen P, et al. Prevalence of subjective dry mouth and burning mouth in hospitalized elderly patients and outpatients in relation to saliva, medication, and systemic diseases. *Oral Surg Oral Med Oral Pathol Oral Radiol Endod.* 2001;92:641–649.
38. Helmick CG, Felson DT, Lawrence RC, et al. Estimates of the prevalence of arthritis and other rheumatic conditions in the United States: Part I. *Arthritis Rheum.* 2008;58:15–25.
39. Mavragani CP, Moutsopoulos HM. Sjögren's syndrome. *Can Med Assoc J.* 2014;186:E579–E586.
40. Pedersen AML. Diseases causing oral dryness. In: Carpenter G, ed. *Dry Mouth: A Clinical Guide on Causes, Effects, and Treatments.* New York, NY: Springer-Verlag; 2015:7–31.
41. Chaturvedi AK, Engels EA, Pfeiffer RM, et al. Human papillomavirus and rising oropharyngeal cancer incidence in the United States. *J Clin Oncol.* 2011;29:4294–4301.
42. Jensen SB, Pedersen AM, Vissink A, et al. A systematic review of salivary gland hypofunction and xerostomia induced by cancer therapies: prevalence, severity, and impact on quality of life. *Support Care Cancer.* 2010;18:1039–1060.
43. Wijers OB, Levendag PC, Braaksma MMJ, et al. Patients with head and neck cancer cured by radiation therapy: a survey of the dry mouth syndrome in long-term survivors. *Head Neck.* 2002;24:737–747.
44. Eisbruch A, Ship JA, Kim HM, Ten Haken RK. Partial irradiation of the parotid gland. *Semin Radiat Oncol.* 2001;11:234–239.
45. Kielbassa AM, Hinkelbein W, Hellwig E, et al. Radiation-related damage to dentition. *Lancet Oncol.* 2006;7:326–335.
46. Seikaly H, Jha N, Harris JR, et al. Long-term outcomes of submandibular gland transfer for prevention of postradiation xerostomia. *Arch Otolaryngol Head Neck Surg.* 2004;130:956–961.
47. Zhang B, Mo Z, Du W, et al. Intensity-modulated radiation therapy versus 2D-RT or 3D-CRT for the treatment of nasopharyngeal carcinoma: a systematic review and meta-analysis. *Oral Oncol.* 2015 Aug 18. PMID: 26296274.
48. Mell LK, Mehrotra AK, Mundt AJ. Intensity modulated radiation therapy use in the US, 2004. *Cancer.* 2005;104:1296–1303.
49. Mayles W. Survey of the availability and use of advanced radiotherapy technology in the UK. *Clin Oncol.* 2010;22:636–642.

50. Mayles W, Cooper T, Mackay R, et al. Progress with intensity-modulated radiotherapy implementation in the UK. *Clin Oncol*. 2012;24:543–544.
51. AlDuhaiby EZ, Breen S, Bissonnette J-P, et al. A national survey of the availability of intensity-modulated radiation therapy and stereotactic radiosurgery in Canada. *Radiat Oncol*. 2012;7:18.
52. Klein J, Livergant J, Ringash J. Health related quality of life in head and neck cancer treated with radiation therapy with or without chemotherapy: a systematic review. *Oral Oncol*. 2014;50:254–262.
53. Sood AJ, Fox NF, O'Connell BP, et al. Salivary gland transfer to prevent radiation-induced xerostomia: a systematic review and meta-analysis. *Oral Oncol*. 2014;50:77–83.
54. Jha N, Seikaly H, McGaw T, et al. Submandibular salivary gland transfer prevents radiation-induced xerostomia. *Int J Radiat Oncol Biol Phys*. 2000;46:7–11.
55. Rieger J, Seikaly H, Jha N, et al. Submandibular gland transfer for prevention of xerostomia after radiation therapy: swallowing outcomes. *Arch Otolaryngol Head Neck Surg*. 2005;131:140–145.
56. Villa A, Wolff A, Aframian D, et al. World Workshop on Oral Medicine VI: a systematic review of medication-induced salivary gland dysfunction: prevalence, diagnosis, and treatment. *Clin Oral Investig*. 2015;19:1563–1580.
57. Furness S, Worthington HV, Bryan G, et al. Interventions for the management of dry mouth: topical therapies. *Cochrane Database Syst Rev*. 2011(12):CD008934.
58. Davies A, Bagg J, Laverty D, et al. Salivary gland dysfunction (dry mouth) in patients with cancer: a consensus statement. *Eur J Cancer Care (Engl)*. 2010;19:172–177.
59. Lovelace TL, Fox NF, Sood AJ, et al. Management of radiotherapy-induced salivary hypofunction and consequent xerostomia in patients with oral or head and neck cancer: meta-analysis and literature review. *Oral Surg Oral Med Oral Pathol Oral Radiol Endod*. 2014;117:595–607.
60. Wolff A, Fox PC, Porter S, et al. Established and novel approaches for the management of hyposalivation and xerostomia. *Curr Pharm Des*. 2012;18:5515–5521.
61. Visvanathan V, Nix P. Managing the patient presenting with xerostomia: a review. *Int J Clin Pract*. 2010;64:404–407.
62. Dirix P, Nuyts S, Van den Bogaert W. Radiation-induced xerostomia in patients with head and neck cancer: a literature review. *Cancer*. 2006;107:2525–2534.
63. Spolarich AE. Risk management strategies for reducing oral adverse drug events. *J Evid Based Dent Pract*. 2014;(14 suppl):87–94.
64. Hanchanale S, Adkinson L, Daniel S, et al. Systematic literature review: xerostomia in advanced cancer patients. *Support Care Cancer*. 2015;23:881–888.
65. Furness S, Bryan G, McMillan R, et al. Interventions for the management of dry mouth: non-pharmacological interventions. *Cochrane Database Syst Rev*. 2013;(8):CD009603.
66. Strietzel FP, Lafaurie GI, Mendoza GR, et al. Efficacy and safety of an intraoral electrostimulation device for xerostomia relief: a multicenter, randomized trial. *Arthritis Rheum*. 2011;63:180–190.
67. Strietzel FP, Martin-Granizo R, Fedele S, et al. Electrostimulating device in the management of xerostomia. *Oral Dis*. 2007;13:206–213.
68. Narhi TO, Meurman JH, Ainamo A. Xerostomia and hyposalivation—causes, consequences, and treatment in the elderly. *Drugs Aging*. 1999;15:103–116.
69. Dost F, Farah CS. Stimulating the discussion on saliva substitutes: a clinical perspective. *Aust Dent J*. 2013;58:11–17.
70. Napenas JJ, Brennan MT, Fox PC. Diagnosis and treatment of xerostomia (dry mouth). *Odontology*. 2009;97:76–83.
71. DePaola L, Minah G, Leupold R, et al. The effect of antiseptic mouthrinses on oral microbial flora and denture stomatitis. *Clin Prevent Dent*. 1985;8:3–8.
72. DePaola LG, Minah GE, Elias SA, et al. Clinical and microbial evaluation of treatment regimens to reduce denture stomatitis. *Int J Prosthodont*. 1990;3:369–374.
73. Forner L, Hyldegaard O, von Brockdorff AS, et al. Does hyperbaric oxygen treatment have the potential to increase salivary flow rate and reduce xerostomia in previously irradiated head and neck cancer patients? A pilot study. *Oral Oncol*. 2011;47:546–551.
74. Jensen DH, Oliveri RS, Trojahn Kølle SF, et al. Mesenchymal stem cell therapy for salivary gland dysfunction and xerostomia: a systematic review of preclinical studies. *Oral Surg Oral Med Oral Pathol Oral Radiol Endod*. 2014;117:335–342.
75. Baum BJ, Alevizos I, Chiorini JA, et al. Advances in salivary gland gene therapy—oral and systemic implications. *Expert Opin Biol Ther*. 2015;15:1443–1454.

Chapter 11

Orofacial Injuries

Zameera Fida

OVERVIEW OF OROFACIAL INJURIES

Orofacial injuries are commonly encountered by dental professionals. The general/pediatric dentist or oral and maxillofacial surgeon, with an assistant or hygienist, may manage the acute needs of a patient.[1] The endodontist, periodontist, prosthodontist, and orthodontist comprise a secondary team that assists in providing long-term care. These injuries most often present in the form of traumatic dental injuries (TDIs) in which a patient's quality of life may decrease.

This chapter aims to provide an overview of orofacial injuries, specifically TDIs, including the epidemiology, acute management, and prevention of such injuries. Prevention in this context consists of anticipatory guidance for identifying and modifying risk factors, using interceptive orthodontics and correcting habits when there is potential for malocclusion to contribute to risk, preventing treatment delays, and preventing long-term adverse outcomes after injury has been sustained.

EPIDEMIOLOGY

The incidence and prevalence of TDIs have been reviewed extensively in the literature.[2-4] While the oral region of the body comprises 1% of the total body area, this area accounts for 5% of all body injuries.[3] Approximately one-third of all preschool-aged children, one-quarter of all school-aged children, and one-third of all adults have suffered trauma to their dentition.[3] This is consistent with an often cited prospective study completed in 1972, which demonstrated that 30% of children experienced trauma in their primary dentition and 22% in their permanent dentition.[5]

A review of emergency department visits in the United States for children younger than 18 years of age found an annual rate of 32 dental injuries per 100,000 population from 1990 to 2003. In the primary dentition, half of all injuries were a result of falls on home structures (e.g., steps, tables, beds). In the mixed dentition, almost half were associated with bicycles. In the permanent dentition, sports were the leading cause, with baseball and basketball associated with the highest number of injuries.[6]

TDIs occur more frequently in the maxilla, and the central incisors are affected more than the lateral incisors, as demonstrated in Figure 1A–C, showing a complicated fracture of the maxillary

Figure 1. Complicated Fracture in a 10-Year-Old Girl

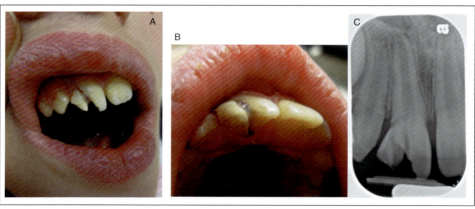

A. Frontal view: traumatic pulp exposure and crown fracture can be appreciated. **B.** Occlusal view. **C.** Periapical radiograph showing immature root formation and complicated crown-root fracture.
Source: Courtesy of Dr. Zameera Fida.

right central incisor in a 10-year-old girl. Other examples of TDIs affecting the maxilla are shown in Figures 2 and 3.

TDIs are classified as either luxation or fracture-type injuries. Luxation injuries include concussion, subluxation, lateral luxation, extrusion, intrusion, and avulsion injuries. Fractures are classified as uncomplicated or complicated crown or root fracture, or combined crown-root fracture. An uncomplicated crown fracture has no pulp involvement (previously known as Ellis class I and II injuries). Complicated crown fractures involve the enamel, dentin, and pulp tissue. Crown and root fractures may occur in isolation or in combination. Luxation or fracture-type injuries may also occur in isolation or in combination with each other. In the primary dentition, luxation or displacement injuries predominate. In the permanent dentition, fractures are more often seen.[2]

A 2012 study of TDIs to permanent teeth found that crown fractures without pulp involvement were the most common injury (35%), followed by dental concussion (24%) and subluxations (22%).[4] In addition, one-third of injuries were a combination of fracture and luxation injuries, which may complicate management; as the number of injuries increases, the risk for pulpal necrosis increases. The frequency of injury type varied by age groups. As age increased, the following injuries decreased: crown fracture without pulp exposure, and concussion. As age increased, the following injuries also increased: crown-root fracture, root fracture, and lateral luxation.[4] These patterns indicate that the older a patient is when injured, the more complex will be the resulting TDI.

SEQUELAE ON THE PRIMARY AND PERMANENT DENTITION

Although injuries to the orofacial structures are often not life threatening, the resulting pain, psychological effects, and economic implications may be significant. The sequelae of injury may leave a lasting mark on the patient. A socioeconomic burden is placed on the patient and family that is difficult to quantify. Direct and indirect costs with which a dentist should be familiar play a role when obtaining informed consent for treatment. One study found that parents are willing to pay over $2,000 in cash to save an incisor.[7] This becomes a burden on lower income families, uninsured patients, and minorities. In Sweden, the estimated cost in US dollars is $3.3 to $4.4 million per million individuals per year in those aged 0 to 19 years.[8] In Denmark, the annual cost of treatment of TDIs in US dollars ranges between $2 and $5 million per million inhabitants per year, irrespective of age.[8]

Injuries to the primary dentition may result in discolorations, premature root resorption, ankyloses, developmental defects on the succedaneous teeth, or eruption disturbances to both the

Figure 2. Complicated Fracture of Left Maxillary Incisor

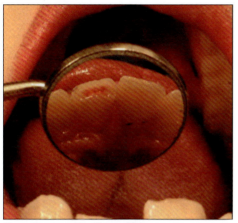

Source: Courtesy of Dr. Zameera Fida.

Figure 3. Palatal Displacement of Primary Maxillary Incisors Resulting in Traumatic Occlusion

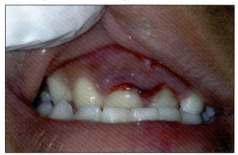

Source: Courtesy of Dr. Zameera Fida.

Figure 4. Grey Discoloration on Primary Maxillary Right Central Incisor as a Result of Necrosis

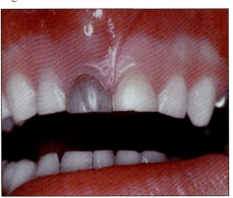

Source: Courtesy of Dr. Howard Needleman

Figure 5. Radiograph to Accompany Figure 4

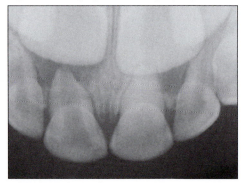

Source: Courtesy of Dr. Howard Needleman

primary and permanent dentition[9] (see Figures 4 and 5). After a permanent tooth sustains an injury, there is concern for pulp changes such as necrosis, pulp canal mineralization and internal resorption, and appropriate periodontal ligament healing (see Figure 6).

The quality of life of patients who have sustained TDIs has been examined in the literature, and findings are mixed. Among pediatric patients, esthetics and quality of life are often cited as more of a concern for the parents than the child.[9] However, other studies demonstrate that younger children may report lower quality of life scores.[10,11] More research is required in this area.

RISK FACTORS

A recent review of the literature highlighted the alarming increase in risk factors for TDI.[8] The author attributed this trend to an increased interest in the causes and underlying complexity of TDI. This paper reported the following risk factors: increased overjet and protrusion, "deprived areas," risk-taking children, children being bullied, emotionally stressful conditions, obesity, attention deficit hyperactivity disorder, learning difficulties, physical limitations, and inappropriate use of

Figure 6. Inflammatory Root Resorption Postluxation of Maxillary Left Central Incisor

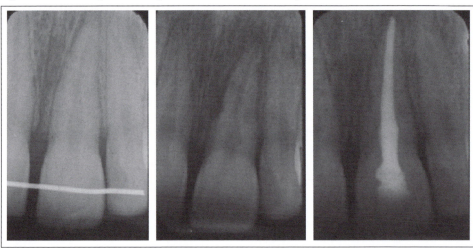

The pathological process was arrested with pulpectomy, calcium hydroxide, and subsequent gutta percha fill.
Source: Courtesy of Dr. Howard Needleman

teeth. A newer cause is oral piercing. Amateur athletes suffer TDIs more than professional athletes. Falls and collisions mask intentional TDIs, such as physical abuse, assault, and torture.

Oral piercing is associated with pain, infection, scar, tooth fracture, metal hypersensitivity reactions, localized periodontal disease, speech impairment, and nerve damage. Unregulated piercing parlors may also be a source for disease transmission.[12]

Age is a common risk factor for TDI. The incidence peaks around 2 years of age in the primary dentition as toddlers start to explore the world around them. In the permanent dentition, TDI peaks around age 9, which may be an indication of dental development and flaring of the incisors in the so called "ugly duckling stage."[3] These factors are a reflection of the varied activity levels across the lifespan. Higher risk activities may change as a patient ages and develops personal interests.

Gender as a risk factor for TDI varies among studies. Historically, males tended to experience more TDIs than females; however, new studies demonstrate that the risk is equalizing.[3] What appears to be more important are the experiences that may contribute to an increased risk of TDI. For example, an increased risk has been found in those of higher socioeconomic status due to access to more high-risk sports.[13] Alternatively, TDI has been associated with lower socioeconomic status, which may be a result of less supervision or access to preventive gear.[14,15] Lack of a traditional nuclear family also increases risk for TDI.[14,16]

Evaluating the occlusion and growth patterns of patients is very important. An increased overjet with protrusion, a short upper lip, incompetent lips, and mouth breathing are cited as predisposing factors for TDI[17] (see Figure 7). In the primary dentition, patients who have an overjet greater than 3 mm and an anterior open bite demonstrated a higher prevalence for TDI as compared with those having a normal occlusion.[18] An anterior open bite was defined as the lack of vertical overlap of any incisor in the occlusal position. In the permanent dentition, patients are four times more likely to have trauma to the maxillary incisors with a class II skeletal pattern as compared with a class I pattern. In addition, an

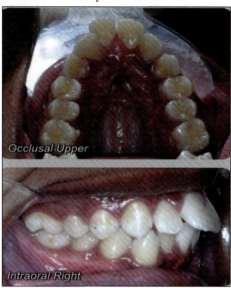

Figure 7. Teenaged Patient with Increased Overjet and Flared Maxillary Incisors

Source: Courtesy of Dr. Mesou Lai.

overjet greater than 3.5 mm is associated with increased TDI as compared with less overjet. If a cephalometric analysis is being completed, patients with a decreased Frankfort Mandibular-Plane Angle (FMPA) have greater odds of trauma to the maxillary incisors than with an average FMPA.[19]

Injuries to the orofacial region may also be a result of intentional trauma from abuse, assault, or other types of violence. Child abuse involves trauma to the head and associated areas in 50% of physically abused children.[20] Bruises are the most common injury identified. The severely abused young child may present with injury of the upper lip and maxillary labial frenum.[20] Facial fractures are relatively uncommon in children, but may occur in physical assault.

The elderly may be at increased risk for physical abuse that may manifest as injuries to the head and neck. Elder abuse can be classified into five types: physical, psychological or verbal, sexual, financial exploitation, and neglect. Approximately 10% of the elderly in the United States are abused in some manner. Women are more likely than men to be victims. Risk factors include living with a larger number of household members other than a spouse, lower income, being isolated, and having a lack of social support. With the exception of dementia, specific diseases have not been identified as increasing risk for abuse.[21]

Another risk factor for orofacial injury is silent trauma, which is a well-known complication of general anesthesia during endotracheal intubation and extubation. Although the incidence reported in the literature is very low, varying from 0.01% to 0.1%, preexisting dental and periodontal damage are risk factors. Silent trauma may occur in a broad range of surgical specialties.[22] Prompt assessment by a dental specialist is required upon occurrence.

Finally, the lack of a dental home may increase the risk for orofacial injuries. In this circumstance, a patient may not have access to appropriate preventive care, as defined earlier (i.e., anticipatory guidance for identifying and modifying risk factors, using interceptive orthodontics and correcting habits when there is potential for malocclusion to contribute to risk, preventing treatment delays, and preventing long-term adverse outcomes after injury has been sustained).

MANAGEMENT OF OROFACIAL INJURIES

A growing body of literature supports the management of traumatic dental injuries. The International Association of Dental Traumatology (IADT) most recently updated its guidelines for treatment in 2012.[23-25] In addition, the interactive website created by the IADT provides a real-time resource for clinicians.[26] Interested dental care providers are able to join the IADT and have access to *Dental Traumatology*, which is a Medline-indexed scientific journal and the official publication of the IADT. It provides the latest research in the field of traumatology. More research is needed in the area of management of TDI as it is difficult to perform randomized clinical studies with traumatic injuries. The research that has been completed in animal models may be difficult to extrapolate or not applicable to humans. One important factor to consider is preventing delay in treatment. For this reason, preparation is critical when addressing TDI (see Figure 8 and Table 1).

Figure 8. Example of a Trauma Bin

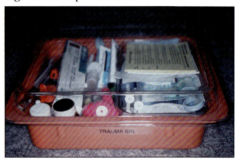

Source: Courtesy of Dr. Howard Needleman.

Treatment may differ between primary and permanent teeth as the health of the developing permanent dentition plays a role in decision making when primary teeth are injured.[27] The ability to recognize what constitutes an injury requiring acute, emergent care is key and will be discussed in

Table 1. Sample Contents of a Trauma Bin

Examination	Anesthetic	Splinting Material	Pulp Treatment	Miscellaneous
Gauze	Topical lidocaine	Acid etch	Anterior rubber dam clamp	Suture material
Cotton rolls		Bond		Ice pack
Slow- and high-vacuum suction	**Restorative Material**	Flowable composite	Rubber dam	Over-the-counter pain control medications
Air/water syringe tip	High- and low-speed handpieces	Fishing line as alternative to orthodontic wire	Endodontic files and broaches	Nitrous oxide nasal hood
Mirror	Burs		Irrigation liquid	
Explorer	Glass ionomer liner	Flexible orthodontic wire	Calcium hydroxide, formocresol, MTA	Periodontal dressing
Periodontal probe	Topical lidocaine			Topical fluoride
Endo-Ice®				Chlorhexidine
	Extraction Forceps			
	Upper, lower			

the subsequent paragraphs. The following factors affect the treatment considerations for each patient: medical history, developmental age, need for behavioral guidance adjuncts, financial considerations, psychological or guilt issues, and anatomical and occlusal factors. In addition, the dentist's training and prior experiences will shape the encounter.

While acute care is ideal, this may not always be possible on a population level due to logistics or economics. A review of the literature in 2002 grouped treatment needs as acute (within a few hours), subacute (within the first 24 hours), or delayed (after the first 24 hours).[28] The 2012 IADT guidelines provide updated treatment recommendations; however, the groupings offer helpful categories if limited resources are available. The following recommendations were made:[28]

- Uncomplicated fractures—subacute or delayed treatment
- Complicated crown fracture
  - Pulp cap or partial pulpotomy—subacute or delayed treatment
  - Cervical pulpotomy—subacute approach as there is a significant relationship between pulp necrosis and treatment delay of more than 24 hours; no longer indicated if a more favorable prognosis for partial or pulp cap is considered
- Crown-root fracture—subacute or delayed treatment if a mature root
  - Most cases of mature root formation will require complete pulp extirpation
- Root fracture—acute or subacute treatment as only a radiographic examination can verify the diagnosis
- Fracture of alveolar process—existing research has bias; however, it is reasonable to assume an acute treatment approach
- Concussion and subluxation—no relation, as there is usually lack of treatment and, therefore, lack of data
- Extrusion and lateral luxation—uncertain; but to remedy clinical symptoms such as traumatic occlusion, an acute or subacute approach
- Intrusion—subacute approach at the time of this writing; the 2012 IADT guidelines offer more detailed recommendations
- Avulsion
  - Acute approach to replant the tooth
  - Subacute if the tooth has been replanted and requires splinting
- Trauma to primary teeth—subacute or delayed unless there are occlusal problems due to tooth displacement, then an acute approach is warranted

Given concerns for intentional versus accidental trauma, legal battles over fault, and monitoring of traumatized teeth over time, it is important to take a detailed history, perform a thorough examination, and document all findings in a consistent manner (see Figures 9, 10, and 11 for examples). Lack of standardized documentation has been associated with misdiagnosis of TDIs.[29] The chief complaint; medical and dental history; extraoral, intraoral, and radiographic findings; and vitality testing should be documented[30] (see Table 2). The goal of treatment when a TDI is present is to alleviate acute pain. In addition, minimizing trauma to the permanent dentition in the case of primary tooth injury is paramount. When the permanent dentition is injured, the goal is to maintain the vitality of the pulp and periodontal ligament cells.

PATIENT MANAGEMENT AND INTERVENTIONS TO PREVENT OROFACIAL INJURIES

The prevention of TDIs by increasing access to dental care or to a dental home, advising colleagues and patients about silent trauma, and managing occlusion are all within our purview as dentists to modify. Additionally, providing anticipatory guidance during routine visits to educate patients about risk factors is essential. There appears to be little agreement about whether TDIs are, in fact, preventable as the traditional view is that they are unavoidable.[8] However, there is agreement that improved education efforts may have the best effects.[8,31]

A 2013 evidence-based review on prevention of TDIs showed that there are gaps in our knowledge base about prevention. The dental healthcare team should focus on educating children, adolescents, and caregivers about the importance of prevention using the Internet and applications ("apps") aimed at prevention and response to dental injury. The author notes that studies on how to approach this education are also lacking.[31] Promoting mouthguard use and other protective equipment has become the standard of care. The statistics related to injury are worth emphasizing: Children and adolescents who have sustained TDIs are almost five times more likely to be injured again as compared with their uninjured counterparts.[32] If a child is younger than 9 years of age at the time an initial TDI is sustained, the same individual is eight times more likely to sustain another injury as compared with a child who was 12 years of age or older when the first injury occurred.[33]

Another review commented on the use of social programming to decrease the risk of orofacial injuries. These efforts included targeting older schoolboys from disadvantaged backgrounds,

Figure 9. Enamel-Dentin Fracture with Tooth Fragment

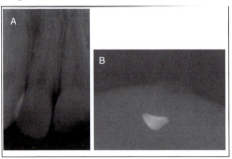

A. Radiograph of the maxillary right incisor in an uncomplicated enamel-dentin fracture. **B.** The adjacent image shows a soft tissue radiograph of the lower lip with the embedded fractured tooth piece.
Source: Courtesy of Dr. Howard Needleman.

Figure 10. Tooth Fragment Embedded in Tongue

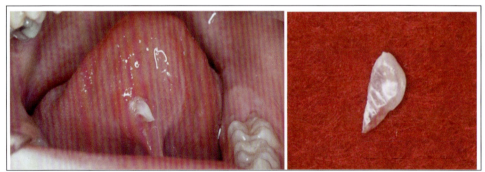

Source: Courtesy of Dr. Howard Needleman.

Figure 11. Special Needs Patient with BB Gun Pellet Embedded in Soft Tissues

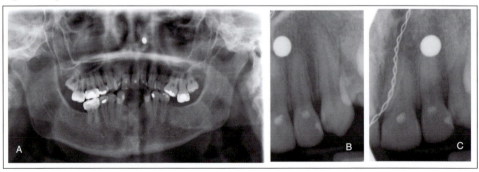

A. The panoramic image demonstrates the round, well circumscribed, radiopaque area near the nose. **B, C.** The periapical images were exposed to determine if the object was located more anteriorly or posteriorly. The object was located at the base of the left nostril.
Source: Courtesy of Dr. Zameera Fida.

Table 2. Example of a Trauma Record

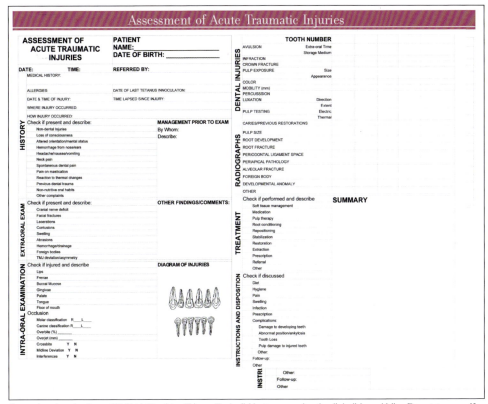

Source: American Academy of Pediatric Dentistry, Chicago, IL. Available at www.aapd.org/media/policies_guidelines/R_acutetrauma.pdf.

improving public social policies, and the WHO Healthy Cities program.[8] The WHO program defines a healthy city as one that continually creates and improves the physical and social environment and expands community resources for enabling mutual support among populations.[8]

In the United States, regulation of head and face protection is not standardized across the 50 states. Bike helmet legislation is state dependent, and not all states have laws that require helmet use. The Centers for Disease Control and Prevention estimated in 1994 that universal helmet use would prevent 151,400 nonfatal bicycle-related head injuries per year.[34] The National Federation of State High School Association (www.nfhs.org) mandates mouth protectors in football, ice hockey, lacrosse, and field hockey;[35] in Massachusetts, mouth protectors are also required in wrestling (www.miaa.net).

Mouth Protectors

When addressing how to prevent orofacial injuries, the conversation usually centers around the use of mouthguards. However, extraoral devices, such as helmets or face masks, may also be used. Although the methodology for research on mouthguards and injury prevention varies widely, studies show that mouthguards offer significant protection against orofacial injuries. A meta-analysis revealed that orofacial injury is 1.6 to 1.9 times higher when a mouthguard is not worn.[36] Few studies report on compliance, however, and there is insufficient evidence to determine whether mouthguards offer protection against concussion injury. More work of good methodological quality is needed.[36] The bulk of the literature focuses on physical properties of materials rather than the true effectiveness of protection, and studies that investigate use of mouthguards in real time are lacking due to ethical concerns.

Three types of mouthguards are in use. The first is a stock appliance that is the least expensive option. This appliance is held in place by clenching the teeth together. It is available in only a few sizes. Patients may find that it obstructs speech and breathing and, therefore, may decide not to wear it. The second is a mouth-formed, or "boil and bite," type appliance (see Figure 12). This is an inexpensive and disposable alternative to purchasing a custom-made mouthguard. This appliance is heated and adapted for a better fit, which can be done by a dentist in-office during a clinic visit. It may be a good option for the mixed dentition or during orthodontic therapy.

The custom-made appliance has two versions: (1) a single layer, which is a vacuum-formed appliance (see Figure 13), and (2) laminate of multiple layers (see Figure 14). Again, more research in the area of mouthguard laminating is needed. Computer models have been studied, but there is a lack of standardization in these models and the findings may not be translated into clinical practice.[36]

The more common materials used in mouthguard fabrication are polyvinylacetate-polyethylene or ethylene vinyl acetate (EVA) copolymer, polyvinylchloride, latex rubber, acrylic resin, and polyurethane. EVA copolymers are the most popular because of their ease of use in custom fabrication. Polyvinylchloride has been criticized for presumed links with certain chronic conditions. EVA appears to be the most studied material. Studies have demonstrated that an increase in EVA increases the shock-absorbing capability, but after 4 to 5 mm of thickness, there is little additional improvement. The inclusion of systematic air cells in EVA copolymers also improves shock absorbency.[36]

A 2007 review on mouthguard use addressed the physical properties of mouthguards and their effectiveness in prevention of injuries.[36] Many variables influence the effectiveness of the mouthguard: material, thickness, manner of fabrication, area of coverage over teeth and gingiva, characteristics of the protected tissue (teeth, bone, gingiva), and direction or force and nature of impact. The physical properties of mouthguards (shock-absorbing capability, hardness, stiffness, tear strength, tensile strength, and water absorption) are measured differently in different studies. The shock, hardness, and stiffness indicate protective capability. The tensile and tear strength indicate durability, as the appliance will likely be bitten and chewed by the user. Water absorption suggests stability in the aqueous environment of the mouth, and a high water absorption indicates the appliance is likely to retain saliva and oral bacteria.[36]

Figure 12. Examples of Mouth-Formed, "Boil and Bite" Mouthguards

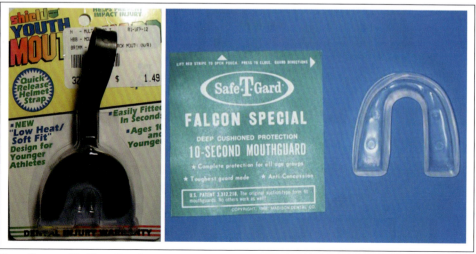

Source: Courtesy of Dr. Howard Needleman.

Figure 13. Single-Layer Custom-Made Mouthguard.

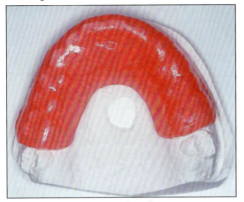

Source: Courtesy of Dr. Howard Needleman.

Figure 14. Custom-Made Laminate Mouthguard

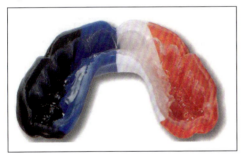

Source: Courtesy of Dr. Howard Needleman.

The following recommendations on mouthguard construction have been made:[36]
- A custom-made appliance of EVA results in less tooth deflection and fewer fractured teeth than a "boil and bite" type appliance.
- Custom-made laminate appliances may include a stainless steel arch or foil in an inner layer to assist in distributing forces, but this may cause additional injury if the appliance is broken. Further investigation is needed here.
- Mouthguards may lose their thickness during fabrication, so the final thickness should be measured and controlled.
- Use of a large occlusal surface area is recommended to decrease mandibular distortion and possibility of mandibular fracture. This also results in a faster decay rate of the impact, which suggests more dispersion of the impact forces.
- Material in use should be moderately stiff or hard. If it is too hard, then high forces may be transmitted to underlying tissues. If it is too soft, then the appliance itself may compress and deliver forces to a small area of tissue.
- The object causing the impact should be considered in mouthguard fabrication (hard or soft).
- The patient-specific oral characteristics should also be considered in mouthguard fabrication. These include
  - the occlusal surface available to distribute forces. A softer material with good shock-absorbing capability should be used here.
  - the position and periodontal support around incisors, as they are exposed to forces that can be concentrated in a small area. A material with moderate stiffness and shock-absorbing capability should be used to assist in redistributing forces and absorbing shock.
  - the gingiva is a soft tissue capable of absorbing force and may need a stiffer material to assist in force redistribution.

The literature is limited regarding whether mouthguards can decrease the rate of brain concussion. The studies that advocated this were completed in the 1960s.[31] A recent review concludes there is no strong evidence for protection of brain injuries and that manufacturers may make unsubstantiated claims.[37] Face masks also have limited evidence regarding prevention of injuries. It has been speculated that spinal injuries may be increased when young adults use face masks as they may take unwarranted risks from a false sense of security.[38] Nevertheless, the American Dental Association encourages dentists to educate their patients on risk of oral injury in sports, fabricate properly fitted mouthguards, and provide appropriate guidance on mouthguard types, costs, and benefits.[39] Mouthguard use is recommended anytime there is a risk for orofacial injury.[36]

Interceptive Orthodontics

As issues related to occlusion may increase the risk

for orofacial injuries, it is reasonable to consider whether orthodontic treatment may decrease this risk. An increased overjet, short upper lip, and incompetent lips are known predisposing factors. This occlusal pattern may be the result of a dental or skeletal issue.

Nonnutritive habits—such as pacifier or digit sucking, tongue thrust swallow, and abnormal tongue position—that are of sufficient frequency, duration, and intensity may be associated with increased overjet, reduced overbite, posterior crossbite, or long facial height.[40] Nonnutritive habits are normal in infants and young children. Dentoalveolar changes resulting from sucking habits may persist after the habit stops. Part of the anticipatory guidance of early dental visits should be to encourage parents to help children stop these habits by the age of 36 months.[40]

Management of an oral habit should be considered if there is an adverse effect on dentofacial development. Treatment must be appropriate for the child's development and ability to cooperate.[40] Treatment modalities include patient–parent counseling, behavior modification, myofunctional therapy, appliance therapy, or referral to other providers, such as orthodontists or speech therapists. Appliance therapy should only be considered if the child wants to stop the habit and would benefit from a reminder.[40]

The research to pursue orthodontic appliance therapy as a modality to decrease overjet has only been completed in children. A 2003 clinical trial showed no difference in the incidence of trauma if an overjet of greater than 7 mm was treated early with phase 1 orthodontic therapy.[41] However, a Cochrane review in 2013 provided evidence suggesting that early orthodontic treatment (phase 1) for children younger than 16 years of age with prominent upper incisors is more effective in reducing the incidence of incisal trauma than providing one course of orthodontic treatment when the child is in early adolescence. This review also noted that there appears to be no other advantage for providing early phase 1 treatment as compared with a single phase of treatment in adolescence.[42]

INTENTIONAL ABUSE

Dentists are able to prevent orofacial injuries by recognizing patterns that are indicative of intentional trauma. The goal is to prevent further injury by bringing appropriate services to the patient or family. In the United States, dental professionals are considered mandated reporters in cases of suspected head and neck abuse. If one suspects intentional abuse, the following questions should be considered:[20]

- Is the injury consistent with the history?
- Is there a history of or signs of repeated trauma?
- Are there cutaneous manifestations that strongly suggest abuse?
- Does the parent, patient, or caretaker exhibit unusual behaviors that may indicate abuse?
- Is there any evidence of neglect or poor supervision of the patient—specifically, a child or elderly patient?

An increasing body of literature has been published on abuse in the elderly population. A recent review demonstrated that studies have uncovered high rates of interpersonal violence and aggression toward older adults, in particular by other residents in long-term care facilities, rather than by staff in these facilities.[21] In general, the victims of elder abuse have some functional impairment and are in poor physical health.[21] Studies to identify risk factors for becoming a perpetrator in elder abuse are limited. However, limited evidence shows that perpetrators are more likely to be adult children or spouses of the elder; to be male; to have histories that include substance abuse, mental health issues, and trouble with police; to be socially isolated; to be unemployed; or to experience financial problems or major stress.[21]

The importance of recognizing victims of abuse cannot be overstated. These patients may be isolated and their interactions with healthcare providers may be rare.[21] The dental care team has an opportunity to recognize warning signs and make referrals to the appropriate specialists for care.

CASE 1: Patient with Malocclusion Caused by Thumbsucking Habit

PATIENT OVERVIEW
The patient is an 8-year-old Hispanic girl.
Chief Complaint: Her mother wants to find out what can be done about her thumbsucking habit.
Medical History: Noncontributory.
Risk Factor Assessment: Patient sucks her thumb for more than 30 minutes per day. She has an anterior open bite, and increased overjet.

CLINICAL EXAMINATION
Figure 15 shows findings on initial examination.
Diagnostic Test and Results: Determination of whether patient is ready to stop habit; periapical radiographs (see Clinical Examination).
Diagnosis: Class I malocclusion with anterior open bite; excessive overjet due to a nonnutritive habit.

RISK REDUCTION
A habit-breaking appliance resulted in some spontaneous self-correction.

OUTCOMES
Patient showed improved position of maxillary incisors. Habit has ceased.

FUTURE CONSIDERATIONS
Comprehensive orthodontic treatment is recommended to further improve dental malocclusion.

CASE 2: Patient with a Sports-Related TDI

PATIENT OVERVIEW
The patient is a 15-year-old Caucasian boy.

Figure 15. Case 1—Initial Presentation

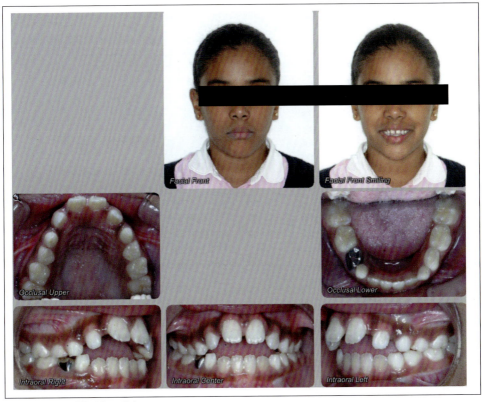

Source: Courtesy of Dr. Mesou Lai.

Chief Complaint: Injury during a basketball game.
Medical History: Noncontributory.
Risk Factor Assessment: High-risk sports participation.

CLINICAL EXAMINATION

Figure 16 shows physical and radiographic findings on initial examination.

Diagnostic Test and Results: Determination of mobility; vitality testing; periapical radiographs. The maxillary right lateral and central incisor are mobile, but stabilized with the existing orthodontic wire. There is palpation and percussion sensitivity. Thermal testing was not completed. The radiograph shows an increased periodontal ligament space without any indication of root fracture.

Diagnosis: Extrusive luxation injury to maxillary right lateral and central incisors.

RISK REDUCTION

Placement of orthodontic appliances acted like a mouthguard. It can be seen that the extent of the injury would have been much worse if the appliances were not in place.

FUTURE CONSIDERATIONS

Monitor for pulp and periodontal healing of maxillary right lateral and central incisors.

Figure 16. Case 2—Initial Presentation

REFERENCES

1. Needleman H, Stucenski K, Forbes, P, Chen Q, Stack AM. Emergency departments' resources and physicians' knowledge of management of traumatic dental injuries. *Dental Traumatol.* 2013;29:272–279.
2. Andersson L. Epidemiology of traumatic dental injuries. *Pediatr Dent.* 2013;35:102–105.
3. Glendor U. Epidemiology of traumatic dental injuries—a 12 year review of the literature. *Dent Traumatol.* 2008;24:603–611.
4. Lauridsen E. Pattern of traumatic dental injuries in the permanent dentition among children, adolescents, and adults. *Dent Traumatol.* 2012;28:358–363.
5. Andreasen JO, Ravn JJ. Epidemiology of traumatic dental injuries to primary and permanent teeth in a Danish population sample. *Int J Oral Surg.* 1972;1:235–239.
6. Stewart GB, Shields BJ, Fields S, Comstock RD, Smith GA. Consumer products and activities associated with dental injuries to children treated in United States emergency departments, 1990–2003. *Dent Traumatol.* 2009;25:399–405.
7. Nguyen PM, Kenny DJ, Barrett EJ. Socio-economic burden of permanent incisor replantation on children and parents. *Dent Traumatol.* 2004;20:123–133.
8. Glendor U. Aetiology and risk factors related to traumatic dental injuries—a review of the literature. *Dent Traumatol.* 2009;25:19–31.
9. Holan G, Needleman H. Premature loss of primary anterior teeth due to trauma—potential short- and long-term sequelae. *Dent Traumatol.* 2013;30:100–106.
10. Berger TD, Kenny DJ, Casas MJ, Barrett EJ, Lawrence HP. Effects of severe dentoalveolar trauma on the quality-of-life of children and parents. *Dent Traumatol.* 2009;24:462–469.

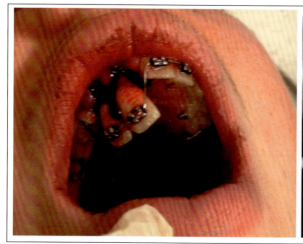
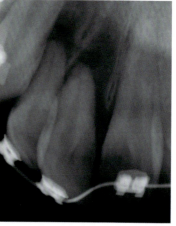

Source: Courtesy of Dr. Zameera Fida.

11. Traebert J, Lacerda JT, Foster Page LA, Thomson WM, Bortoluzzi MC. Impact of traumatic dental injuries on the quality of life of schoolchildren. *Dent Traumatol.* 2012;28:423–428.
12. Council on Clinical Affairs, American Academy of Pediatric Dentistry. Policy on intraoral/perioral piercing and oral jewelry/accessories, revised 2011. Available at: http://www.aapd.org/media/Policies_Guidelines/P_Pierce.pdf. Accessed March 30, 2016.
13. Marcenes W, Zabot NE, Traebert J. Socio-economic correlates of traumatic injuries to the permanent incisors in schoolchildren aged 12 years in Blumenau, Brazil. *Dent Traumatol.* 2001;17:222–226.
14. Lalloo R. Risk factors for major injuries to the face and teeth. *Dent Traumatol.* 2003;19:12–14.
15. Jorge KO, Moysés SJ, Ferreira e Ferreira E, Ramos-Jorge ML, de Aranjo Zarzar PM. Prevalence and factors associated to dental trauma in infants 1-3 years of age. *Dent Traumatol.* 2009;25:185–189.
16. Nicolau B, Marcenes W, Sheiham A. Prevalence, causes and correlates of traumatic dental injuries among 13-year-olds in Brazil. *Dent Traumatol.* 2001;17:213–217.
17. Güngör HC. Management of crown-related fractures in children: an update review. *Dent Traumatol.* 2014;30: 88–99.
18. Bonini GC, Bönecker M, Braga MM, Mendes FM. Combined effect of anterior malocclusion and inadequate lip coverage on dental trauma in primary teeth. *Dent Traumatol.* 2012;28:437–440.
19. Bozabadi-Farahani A, Bozabadi-Farahani A, Eslamipour F. An investigation into the association between facial profile and maxillary incisor trauma, a clinical non-radiographic study. *Dent Traumatol.* 2010;26:403–408.
20. Needleman HL. Orofacial trauma in child abuse: types, prevalence, management and the dental profession's involvement. *Pediatr Dent.* 1986;8:(special issue 1): 71–80.
21. Lach MS, Pillemer KA. Elder abuse. *N Engl J Med.* 2015; 373:1947–1956.
22. Adolphs N, Kessler B, von Heymann C, et al. Dentoalveolar injury related to general anesthesia: a 14 years review and a statement from the surgical point of view based on a retrospective analysis of the documentation of a university hospital. *Dent Traumatol.* 2011;27:10–14.
23. Diangelis AJ, Andreasen JO, Ebeleseder KA, et al. International Association of Dental Traumatology guidelines for the management of traumatic dental injuries. I. Fractures and luxations of permanent teeth. *Dent Traumatol.* 2012;28:2–12.
24. Andersson L, Andreasen JO, Day P, et al. International Association of Dental Traumatology guidelines for the management of traumatic dental injuries. II. Avulsion of permanent teeth. *Dent Traumatol.* 2012;28:88–96.
25. Malmgren B, Andreasen JO, Flores MT, et al. International Association of Dental Traumatology guidelines for the management of traumatic dental injuries. III. Injuries in the primary dentition. *Dent Traumatol.* 2012;28:174–182.
26. University Hospital of Copenhagen. The dental trauma guide, updated 2014. Available at: http://www.dental-traumaguide.org._Accessed April 18, 2016.
27. Needleman HL. The art and science of managing traumatic injuries to primary teeth. *Dent Traumatol.* 2011;27:295–299.
28. Andreasen JO, Andreasen FM, Skeie A, Hjørting-Hansen E, Schwartz O. Effect of treatment delay upon pulp and periodontal healing of traumatic dental injuries—a review article. *Dent Traumatol.* 2002;18:116–128.
29. Andreasen FM, Kahler B. Diagnosis of acute dental trauma: the importance of standardized documentation: a review. *Dent Traumatol.* 2015;31:340–349.
30. American Academy of Pediatric Dentistry. Assessment of acute traumatic injuries. Available from: http://www.aapd.org/media/Policies_Guidelines/R_AcuteTrauma.pdf. Accessed March 30, 2016.
31. Sigurdsson A. Evidence-based review of prevention of dental injuries. *Pediatr Dent.* 2013;35;184–190.
32. Ramos-Jorge ML, Peres MA, Traebert J, et al. Incidence of dental trauma among adolescents: a prospective cohort study. *Dent Traumatol.* 2008;24:159–163.
33. Glendor U, Koucheki B, Halling A. Risk evaluation and type of treatment of multiple dental trauma episodes to permanent teeth. *Endod Dent Traumatol.* 2000;16: 205–210.
34. Centers for Disease Control and Prevention. Injury control recommendations: Bicycle helmets. 1995;44(RR-1);1–18. Available at: http://www.cdc.gov/mmwr/preview/mmwrhtml/00036941.htm. Accessed March 30, 2016.
35. American Academy of Pediatric Dentistry. Policy on prevention of sports-related orofacial injuries, revised 2013. Available from: http://www.aapd.org/media/Policies_Guidelines/P_Sports.pdf. Accessed March 30, 2016.
36. Knapik JJ, Marshall SW, Lee RB, et al. Mouthguards in sports activities: history, physical properties and injury prevention effectiveness. *Sports Med.* 2007;37(2):117–144.
37. Benson BW, Hamilton GM, Meeuwisse WH, et al. Is protective equipment useful in preventing concussion? A systematic review of the literature. *Br J Sports Med.* 2009;43(suppl 1):i56–67.
38. Murray TM, Livingston LA. Hockey helmets, face masks, and injurious behavior. *Pediatrics.* 1995;95: 419–421.
39. ADA Council on Access, Prevention and Interprofessional Relations, ADA Council on Scientific Affairs. Using mouthguards to reduce the incidence and severity of sports-related oral injuries. *J Am Dent Assoc.* 2006;137:1712–1720.
40. Clinical Affairs Committee–Developing Dentition Subcommittee. Guideline on management of the developing dentin and occlusion in pediatric dentistry. Available from: http://www.aapd.org/media/Policies_Guidelines/

G_DevelopDentition.pdf. Accessed March 30, 2016.
41. Koroluk LD, Tulloch JF, Phillips C. Incisor trauma and early treatment for Class II Division 1 malocclusion. *Am J Orthod Dentofacial Orthop.* 2003;123:117–126.
42. Thiruvenkatachari B, Harrison JE, Worthington HV, O'Brien KD. Orthodontic treatment for prominent upper front teeth (Class II malocclusion) in children. *Cochrane Database Syst Rev.* 2013;(11):CD003452.

ADDITIONAL READINGS

A. Andreasen JO, Andreasen FM and Andersson, L. *Textbook and Color Atlas of Traumatic Injuries to the Teeth.* 4th ed. Munksgaard, Cogenhagen: 2007.

B. *Dental Traumatology*—Official publication of the International Association of Dental Traumatology and Academy of Sports Medicine (http://interscience.wiley.com/journal/dt).

Chapter 12
Prevention in the Context of Oral–Systemic Health

Philip M. Preshaw

Since the late 1980s, there has been a steady accumulation of scientific evidence linking poor oral health (specifically the presence of periodontitis) with a number of systemic diseases, notably diabetes and cardiovascular disease. Potential links between adverse pregnancy outcomes and presence of maternal periodontitis have also been extensively investigated. While many of the individual studies that have evaluated links between oral health and systemic health have been relatively small and of short duration, sufficient numbers have now been published to enable systematic reviews and meta-analyses to be performed. These permit researchers to combine data from different studies to create much larger datasets and therefore allow analyses to be performed with increased statistical power.

These studies have led to a resurgence of interest into the links between periodontal health and general health. Given the huge increases in prevalence rates of noncommunicable diseases (such as diabetes and cardiovascular disease) currently being observed in many populations around the world, in parallel with increases in obesity, the importance of optimizing oral health and preventing development or progression of periodontal disease is likely to become increasingly relevant. Dental professionals will find they have an increasingly important role to play in the overall health management of their patients. This represents a paradigm shift in the way the dental profession has operated in recent times. For many years, the dental profession has been functioning quite distinctly from the broader medical profession, to the detriment of our patients. This separation of medicine and dentistry became particularly evident in the latter half of the twentieth century, driven partly by differences in clinical care pathways and remuneration systems between the medical and dental professions, and partly also by technical advances in dental surgical and restorative techniques and materials that were used exclusively by the dental profession to treat (i.e., repair) the consequences of diseases such as dental caries. However, in the twenty-first century, we now recognize the importance of moving away from a restorative/reparative paradigm that focused on restoring damaged, diseased, or missing teeth toward a disease prevention paradigm within the context of overall systemic health.

While it may appear that the expansion in the numbers of studies investigating oral–systemic links is a relatively recent phenomenon, the concept is not new. Indeed, in the late 1800s, following the publication of Robert Koch's germ theory of disease, a number of authors were linking oral diseases with a wide range of systemic diseases and disorders.[1] In broad terms, it was believed that microorganisms from the mouth would translocate to other regions of the body, thereby causing disease at those distant locations. Thus, Miller, in his 1891 publication, considered a wide range of systemic disorders to be caused by bacteria from the teeth and mouth (see Table 1).[2]

Table 1. Systemic Diseases and Conditions Attributable to Oral Bacteria

Actinomycosis
Diphtheria
Encephalitis
Meningitis
Noma
Osteomyelitis
Pneumonia
Pyemia
Septicemia
Sinusitis
Syphilis
Tonsillitis
Tuberculosis

Source: Based on *Dental Cosmos.* 1891;33:689–713.[2]

Numerous publications and prominent speakers of that time expounded upon and developed this theme, leading to the concept of "focal infection," which stated that infections and disease could be caused by the dissemination of bacteria or bacterial products from a focus of infection at one location in the body to another site in the body via the circulatory or lymphatic systems.[3] The primary foci of infection were considered to be the teeth, tonsils, and sinuses, and this concept was particularly attractive for explaining the cause of various diseases for which there was, at that time, no other known etiology. This led to patients undergoing procedures such as dental clearances and tonsillectomies as a management strategy for systemic diseases, procedures that clearly would not be indicated today according to our modern understanding of various disease etiologies.

Fortunately, the more rigorous application of scientific methods in the early parts of the twentieth century began to reverse this trend. For example, a study of different treatments for rheumatoid arthritis (tonsillectomy, dental clearance, and no treatment) found no benefit from the surgical interventions, with the authors questioning the validity of the focal infection theory.[4] A 1940 editorial in the *Journal of the American Medical Association* vigorously discredited the concept of focal infection, bringing this era of clinical and research activity to an end.[5] Although this was appropriate, given that the focal infection theory was not supported by scientific or clinical evidence, one consequence was that for the next 50 years or so, medicine and dentistry went their separate ways.

The study that rekindled interest in the links between oral health and systemic disease in more recent times was a case-control study of patients who had experienced acute myocardial infarction, published in 1989.[6] Poor oral health, as assessed using a dental index that was calculated based on the numbers of caries lesions, missing teeth, periapical lesions, probing depths, and presence of pericoronitis, was found to be significantly associated with acute myocardial infarction, independent of other cardiac risk factors that included age, social class, smoking, serum lipid concentrations, and presence of diabetes. Since then, numerous studies have investigated links between oral health and a range of systemic conditions; this chapter considers current knowledge in this area.

KEY CONSIDERATIONS

The term *periodontal disease* refers to a range of conditions that affect the supporting structures of the teeth, including the gingiva, connective tissue and alveolar bone. *Gingivitis* refers to inflammation that affects the gingiva only, whereas *periodontitis* refers to inflammation that also affects the periodontal ligament and alveolar bone, leading to breakdown of the attachment between the teeth and the bone, alveolar bone resorption, and ultimately tooth mobility and tooth loss (see Chapter 5). Our understanding of periodontal pathogenesis has evolved over the years: in the mid-twentieth century, periodontitis was considered to be ubiquitous, with dental plaque being the sole etiological factor. However, our modern concept of disease pathogenesis focuses on the role of inflammation as a response to the subgingival microbiota in driving periodontal tissue breakdown, and hence, the development of clinical signs and symptoms of disease. Thus, we consider that the subgingival microbiota initiates and perpetuates the chronic inflammatory response in the gingival and periodontal tissues, yet it is the inflammation that is primarily responsible for the tissue destruction that characterizes disease. There are variations in disease susceptibility between different individuals, likely derived from variations in the inflammatory response profile, which in turn is influenced by a wide variety of genetic, epigenetic, microbial, and environmental factors.[7] The common end point is the tissue damage that dental professionals recognize clinically as periodontitis.

The inflammatory response in the gingival and periodontal tissues is characterized by infiltration of the tissues by circulating host defense cells (neutrophils, monocytes/macrophages, and lymphocytes), together with increasing concentrations of inflammatory mediators such as cytokines, prostaglandins, and matrix metalloproteinases (MMPs). Key cytokines include interleukin-1β (IL-1β), IL-6, tumor necrosis factor-α (TNF-α),

T-cell regulatory cytokines, chemokines (such as IL-12 and IL-18), and cytokines that mediate bone metabolism, such as receptor activator of NF-κB ligand (RANKL) and osteoprotegerin (OPG). Cytokines do not function in isolation, but interact functionally in complex networks in the periodontium, with regulatory control exerted at a number of levels and involving infiltrating immune cells as well as resident cells in the periodontium.[8] Periodontitis can be regarded as a complex chronic disease in which the inflammation is ineffective in eliminating the initiating pathogens, the persistence of which leads to chronic inflammation and concomitant progressive tissue destruction.[9]

In broad terms, there are two main potential pathways in which the microbiota-induced inflammation in the periodontal tissues may have an impact on overall health.[10] One mechanism is via translocation of bacteria and bacterial products across the pocket or junctional epithelium into the circulation, leading to bacteremia and systemic inflammatory responses. It is noteworthy that the surface area of inflamed and ulcerated pocket epithelium in a patient with generalized periodontitis has been estimated as being approximately 20 cm^2, presenting clear opportunity for passage of bacteria and their products into the circulation.[11] The second mechanism is via passage of inflammatory mediators produced locally in the periodontal tissues into the circulation, leading to increased systemic inflammation and acute phase responses from the liver. Both pathways are likely to play a role in the links between periodontal and systemic diseases, and the precise mechanisms are the focus of considerable research efforts currently. Whereas many systemic diseases and conditions have been linked to periodontitis, those that have been the subject of most research activity are diabetes, cardiovascular disease, and adverse pregnancy outcomes.

PERIODONTAL DISEASE AND DIABETES

In considering all the systemic diseases that have been associated with periodontal disease, the strongest evidence exists for the links between periodontal disease and diabetes. A large number of epidemiological studies and population-based surveys have confirmed that the risk of periodontitis is significantly increased in people with diabetes, with the level of glycemic control being a key factor in determining risk. It has been estimated that people with poorly controlled diabetes have an approximately threefold increased risk of periodontitis compared with those who do not have diabetes.[12] In the US National Health and Nutrition Examination Survey III (NHANES III), patients with glycated hemoglobin (HbA1c) greater than 9% (> 75 mmol/mol) had a significantly higher prevalence of severe periodontitis compared with those who did not have diabetes (odds ratio [OR]: 2.90; 95% confidence interval [CI]: 1.40–6.03) after controlling for age, smoking, gender, and ethnicity.[13] Most studies of the epidemiological links between the two conditions have tended to focus on type 2 diabetes, because historically, type 2 diabetes and chronic periodontitis tended to present in patients in their 40s and 50s. The risk of periodontitis is increased in type 1 diabetes also, with the level of glycemic control appearing to be the key factor in determining risk. Therefore, all people with diabetes should be considered to be at increased risk of periodontitis, particularly if they have poor glycemic control.[14]

The pathogenesis of periodontal disease is characterized by the development of chronic (i.e., persisting) and dysregulated inflammatory responses in the periodontal tissues as a defense mechanism against the subgingival microbiota, which results in the tissue damage that we identify clinically as disease. Key inflammatory mediators were listed earlier and have been extensively reviewed elsewhere.[8] Dysregulated immune responses also contribute to the pathogenesis of type 1 and type 2 diabetes, and are associated with hyperglycemia, hyperlipidemia, and other metabolic and physiological changes. Hyperglycemia drives the formation of advanced glycation end products (AGEs), a process in which nonenzymatic glycation of structural proteins of the body (including collagens) leads to altered cellular function and proinflammatory effects involving interactions between AGEs and the receptor for advanced glycation end products (RAGE), resulting in activation of proinflammatory genes. As a result of increased numbers of RAGE ligands in diabetes (because of hyperglycemia), this receptor is considered to have a causative role in many of the complications of diabetes. Elevated circulating levels of cytokines, such as IL-6 and TNF-α, are found in diabetes, and increased serum levels of IL-6 and C-reactive protein (CRP) have been linked to future occurrence of type 2 diabetes.[15-17] Inflammation is of central importance to the pathogenesis of both periodontitis and diabetes, and mechanistically links the pathogenesis of both conditions. This area has been extensively reviewed: IL-1β, TNF-α, IL-6, OPG, and RANKL mediate periodontitis in patients with diabetes, with the AGE-RAGE axis also being an important pathway of periodontal tissue destruction in people with diabetes.[18]

Inflammation clearly drives the increased susceptibility to periodontitis that is observed in people with diabetes, similar to many of the complications of diabetes. There is also evidence that periodontal inflammation has a negative impact on glycemic control and complications of diabetes, thus suggesting a potential benefit of periodontal disease prevention and treatment on the diabetic state. The potential negative impact of periodontitis on diabetes outcomes was initially described in studies in which severe periodontitis was associated with increased risk of poorer glycemic control (defined as HbA1c ≥ 9%, or 75 mmol/mol) in individuals from the Gila River Indian community, a population with a very high prevalence of periodontitis, who were monitored longitudinally over 2 years.[19] Further studies in the same population identified that the presence of severe periodontitis was associated with a more than twofold increased risk of development of nephropathy (macroalbuminuria and end-stage renal disease) in individuals with diabetes compared with diabetic individuals who did not have severe periodontitis, after adjusting for potential confounders such as age, sex, smoking, diabetes duration, and body mass index.[20] In a long-term study of Pima Indians with type 2 diabetes in which the impact of periodontitis on cardiovascular disease mortality was assessed, the presence of severe periodontitis was a statistically significant predictor of deaths from ischemic heart diseases and diabetic nephropathy, and, after adjusting for known risk factors (age, sex, smoking, diabetes duration, body mass index, HbA1c macroalbuminuria, cholesterol, hypertension), subjects with severe periodontitis and diabetes had a three times increased risk of cardiorenal mortality (ischemic heart disease and diabetic nephropathy combined) compared with those who did not have severe periodontitis.[21]

The impact of periodontitis on HbA1c levels in individuals who did not have diabetes has been studied in a 5-year longitudinal follow-up study.[22] After adjustment for risk factors (age, sex, smoking, family history of diabetes, obesity), those individuals who had the most advanced periodontitis at study commencement experienced a five times greater increase in HbA1c over the 5-year study period (ΔHbA1c = 0.11%) compared with those who had no periodontitis at baseline (ΔHbA1c = 0.02%), suggesting that severe periodontitis possibly increases risk for incidence of diabetes. In a cross-sectional study of periodontitis and prediabetes (defined according to American Diabetes Association criteria for impaired fasting glucose and impaired glucose tolerance), presence of severe periodontitis was associated with a 93% increase in the odds of having impaired glucose tolerance, after adjusting for confounders, suggesting a role for periodontitis in the etiology of impaired glycemic regulation and risk for development of diabetes.[23]

In a systematic review of studies that have evaluated the effects of periodontal disease on diabetes control, complications, and incident diabetes, it was concluded that, although few studies have addressed this topic, current evidence suggests that compared with individuals who are periodontally healthy, those who have poor periodontal health and no diabetes have a greater risk of developing diabetes, and those who have poor periodontal health and diabetes have a greater risk for developing diabetes complications and developing poorer glycemic control.[24] If these findings are confirmed by larger scale definitive studies in different population groups, the observation that periodontitis may be a risk factor for development of diabetes and its complications would have profound implications for overall diabetes care with recognition of the importance of prevention and treatment of periodontal diseases as part of routine diabetes management.

The impact of periodontal treatment on glycemic control in patients with diabetes has been extensively studied. A number of systematic reviews have been conducted to combine the data from individual studies, and the main findings are presented in Table 2. Generally, there is evidence that in the short term (3 to 4 months) following periodontal treatment in patients with diabetes, there is a reduction in HbA1c of around 0.3 to 0.4 percentage points. This is a clinically relevant reduction, similar to that achieved by the addition of second-line drug therapies in the management of diabetes. However, this benefit appears to be lost in the studies that continued up to 6 months. This might suggest that a benefit of periodontal treatment on glycemic control may persist for a relatively short period of time after treatment. With regard to the studies that followed patients for up to 6 months, it must also be noted that the number of studies that could be included in the meta-analyses was low, due to variations in treatment modalities, with a small sample size and significant heterogeneity across studies. Clearly, the longer term impact of periodontal treatment on diabetes control warrants further investigation in adequately powered and well-designed studies. However, the inference from the 3-month data presented in Table 2 is quite clear—that periodontal treatment can have a positive impact on glycemic control, with measureable and clinically relevant reductions in HbA1c following nonsurgical periodontal therapy.

The mechanism of any impact of periodontal treatment on improvements in glycemic control is not fully understood at present, but could result from reduced systemic inflammation (e.g., reductions in the levels of circulating IL-6 and TNF-α) as a result of resolution of periodontal inflammation.

Table 2. Meta-Analyses That Have Investigated the Effect of Periodontal Treatment on Glycemic Control in People with Type 2 Diabetes

Author, Year	Number of Studies	Number of Subjects	HbA1c Change (Percentage Points)	95% CI	P
Janket et al., 2005[25]	5	268	-0.66%	-2.2 to 0.9	NS
Darre et al., 2008[26]	9	485	-0.46%	-0.82 to -0.11	0.01
Teeuw et al., 2010[27]	5	180	-0.40%	-0.77 to -0.04	0.03
Simpson et al., 2010[28] (Cochrane Review)	3	244	-0.40%	-0.78 to -0.01	0.04
Sgolastra et al., 2013[29]	5	315	-0.65%	-0.88 to -0.43	< 0.05
Engebretson and Kocher, 2013[30]	9	775	-0.36%	-0.54 to -0.19	<0.0001
Liew et al., 2013[31]	6	422	-0.41%	-0.73 to -0.09	0.013
Wang et al., 2014[32] 3 months post-treatment	10	1,135	-0.36%	-0.52 to -0.19	< 0.0001
Wang et al., 2014[32] 6 months post-treatment	4	754	-0.30%	-0.69 to 0.09	NS
Simpson et al., 2015[33] (Cochrane Review) 3–4 months post-treatment	14	1,499	-0.29%	-0.48 to -0.10	0.003
Simpson et al., 2015[33] (Cochrane Review) 6 months post-treatment	5	826	-0.02%	-0.20 to 0.16	NS

CI, confidence interval; HbA1c, glycated hemoglobin.
Source: Adapted and updated from *J Evid Based Dent Prac.* 2014;14:127–132.[34]

Both of these cytokines induce the production of acute phase proteins, including CRP, and evidence indicates that these cytokines can impair insulin signaling.[35-37] Reduction of periodontal inflammation could thus lead to reductions in systemic inflammation, with a potential benefit of improved glycemic control. However, more research is necessary to test this hypothesis. Whereas elevated CRP levels are a consistent finding in patients with periodontitis compared with healthy controls,[38] evidence that has consistently demonstrated elevated circulating cytokine levels in patients with periodontitis compared with controls is lacking.[18] Further research in this area is required, but clearly optimizing oral and periodontal health is an important aspect of contributing to good general health, and prevention and treatment of periodontitis should form part of the overall healthcare management of all patients, including those with diabetes.

PERIODONTAL DISEASE AND CARDIOVASCULAR DISEASE

Cardiovascular diseases include conditions such as coronary heart disease (myocardial infarction, angina); peripheral artery disease; and cerebrovascular disease (stroke, transient ischemic attack). Bacteria, including those from the oral cavity, have been implicated in the etiology of cardiovascular diseases, and it is clear that periodontal bacteria can enter the circulation, particularly following any form of trauma to the gingival tissues (such as following toothbrushing, chewing, flossing, and dental procedures), causing a bacteremia.[39] Transient bacteremias involving periodontal bacteria appear, therefore, to be a regular occurrence. There is also clear evidence that periodontal bacteria can be found in atheromatous tissues, and species such as *Porphyromonas gingivalis* and *Aggregatibacter actinomycetemcomitans* have been demonstrated to live in atheromas.[40] In a review of the literature, evidence was identified to support a process by which periodontal bacteria enter the circulation and disseminate to systemic vascular tissues, where they can live in sites affected by atheromas. Periodontal bacteria can also invade affected cell types in vitro and induce atherosclerosis in animal models of disease.[40] The bacteria activate host inflammatory responses at these distant sites, and the host immune–inflammatory response favors atheroma formation, maturation, and exacerbation.[41] Although it is difficult to differentiate the direct role of bacteria from the resultant inflammatory response, taken collectively these findings support the concept that periodontal bacteria can contribute to atherosclerosis.

Epidemiological studies have reported an increased risk for cardiovascular disease in patients with periodontal disease compared with those who do not have periodontal disease. In a systematic review of cohort and case-control studies on the association between periodontal disease and cardiovascular disease, it was identified that incidence (i.e., new cases) of cardiovascular disease (specifically incident coronary heart disease, cerebrovascular disease, and peripheral artery disease) is higher in patients who had periodontal disease or more advanced periodontal disease compared with patients who did not have periodontal disease or had better periodontal status, independent of many cardiovascular disease risk factors.[42] In other words, periodontal disease was found to impart a statistically significant excess risk for incident cardiovascular disease, independent of other risk factors. The level of excess risk varied across populations and was greater in cerebrovascular disease than coronary heart disease, in males, and in younger individuals. There was no evidence for an association between periodontal disease and incident cardiovascular disease in patients older than 65 years.

Clearly, many potential confounding variables can affect associations between periodontal disease and cardiovascular disease. The studies that were included in the systematic review routinely controlled for smoking, and excess risk for cardiovascular disease in patients with periodontal disease was also reported in never-smokers in a number of the studies. Excess risk associated with periodontitis was also reported in studies that controlled for diabetes as a confounder. It is quite possible that the association between periodontal disease and cardiovascular disease could be affected by as yet unrecognized confounders, such as shared proinflammatory phenotypes that result from common genetically controlled pathways of inflammation that influence the nature of the host inflammatory responses to bacterial challenge. The importance of inflammation in the pathogenesis of cardiovascular disease is well established, and several mechanisms have been reported by which periodontal bacteria may cause increased inflammatory responses associated with atheroma lesions.[43] More research is required in this area, particularly prospective clinical trials and studies to identify causal relationships as opposed to associations.

A number of intervention studies have been conducted to evaluate the effect of periodontal treatment on cardiovascular disease. Many are association studies, for example, a population-based national survey identified that as patient-reported frequency of toothbrushing increased, prevalence of hypertension decreased, after adjusting for confounders such as presence of periodontitis, age, sex, smoking, body fat, alcohol consumption, exercise, education, and income.[44] When considering intervention studies, periodontal treatment has been reported to induce a short-term acute inflammatory response (characterized by increases in systemic inflammatory markers such as CRP, IL-6, TNF-α, and endothelial dysfunction),[45] followed by progressive reductions in systemic inflammation and improvements in endothelial function.[46] A systematic review concluded that there is moderate evidence for a reduction in systemic inflammation following periodontal treatment as evidenced by reductions in serum CRP levels and improvements in endothelial function.[46] Both of these parameters (elevated CRP and impaired endothelial function) have been associated with risk for cardiovascular disease. The review also identified moderate evidence that periodontal treatment has no effect on lipid profiles and serum IL-6 levels, and limited evidence that periodontal treatment results in reductions of other biomarkers for cardiovascular disease (markers of inflammation, coagulation, and biomarkers of endothelial cell activation), as well as limited evidence that periodontal treatment reduces arterial blood pressure.[46] Clearly, intervention studies are indicated to investigate the impact of periodontal treatment on primary prevention of cardiovascular disease (i.e., prevention of first ischemic event) and secondary prevention of cardiovascular disease (i.e., prevention of subsequent ischemic events), although these are very challenging to design and implement.

To summarize, there is consistent and strong epidemiological evidence that periodontal disease imparts an excess risk for cardiovascular disease, after controlling for the impact of other risk factors. From a mechanistic perspective, the impact of periodontitis on cardiovascular diseases is biologically plausible, relating to periodontal bacteria gaining access to the circulation and, both directly and indirectly (by inducing systemic inflammation), affecting the pathogenesis of atheroma formation. Although intervention and animal studies report reductions in the levels of specific inflammatory biomarkers that are associated with cardiovascular disease risk following periodontal treatment, more research is required in this area to investigate the impact of prevention and treatment of periodontal diseases on primary and secondary prevention of cardiovascular diseases.[41]

PERIODONTAL DISEASE AND ADVERSE PREGNANCY OUTCOMES

Pregnancy is a physiological process that usually proceeds normally but sometimes has adverse outcomes, including low birthweight (defined as < 2,500 g), preterm birth (defined as < 37 weeks of gestation), and other complications such as growth restriction, preeclampsia, miscarriage, and stillbirth. Adverse pregnancy outcomes are associated with several risk factors, including environmental exposures (e.g., smoking), medical conditions and treatments, genetic susceptibility, and individual behavioral and psychosocial factors. Adverse pregnancy outcomes are thought to mainly originate from ascending infections from the vagina or cervix, or from hematogenous (i.e., blood-borne) spread from known or unknown nongenital sources of infection. The presence of periodontitis in the mother represents a potential source of microorganisms that are known to enter the circulation and thus may have both direct and indirect effects on the developing fetal–placental unit.[47]

A systematic review of epidemiological studies concluded that maternal periodontitis is significantly, but modestly, associated with low birthweight and preterm birth.[48] However, the strength of the associations was influenced by factors such as the case definition employed in individual studies to describe whether or not a participant had periodontitis. Indeed, studies that used a categorical assessment of the presence of periodontitis (e.g., based on a case definition defined dichotomously according to the presence of variable numbers of teeth and sites with specific probing depth or attachment loss thresholds) were more likely to report significant positive associations between maternal periodontitis and adverse pregnancy outcomes than studies (including some conducted in the same populations) that used continuous variables (e.g., mean probing depths) as the outcome measure for periodontitis in the statistical analyses. Further limitations in the studies that have been conducted include highly variable study designs, differing case definitions for periodontitis, and inadequate and varying management of potential confounders such as socioeconomic status, race and ethnicity, and smoking. Other potential exposures that may affect risk for adverse pregnancy outcomes include maternal age and weight, weight gain during pregnancy, behavioral factors (e.g., alcohol consumption, nutrition, exercise, and stress), and medical conditions (e.g., diabetes).

Regarding the possible mechanistic links between maternal periodontitis and adverse pregnancy outcomes, two major pathways have been proposed that could trigger an immune–inflammatory response in the fetal–placental unit. These include

1. A direct pathway by which periodontal or oral bacteria and bacterial products enter the circulation in the oral cavity and reach the fetal–placental unit by means of the circulation, or alternatively, oral bacteria reach the fetal–placental unit by an ascending route through the genitourinary tract.
2. An indirect pathway by which inflammatory mediators (e.g., prostaglandin E_2, TNF-α) produced locally in the periodontal tissues enter the circulation and affect the fetal–placental unit, or microbial products or inflammatory mediators enter the circulation from the periodontal tissues and circulate to the liver, resulting in acute-phase protein responses (e.g., production of CRP) and release of cytokines such as IL-6, which then affect the fetal–placental unit.

The evidence from animal and human studies is strongest to support the direct pathway, in which hematogenous spread of periodontal bacteria and their products leads to effects on the fetal–placental unit. These include various outcomes that are dependent on the nature and the timing of the exposure. For example, lower exposures may lead to increased risk of prematurity by causing hypercontractility of the uterus, cervical dilation, and loss of membrane integrity. Higher exposures potentially could lead to abortion, miscarriage, and stillbirth.[49]

Given the associations that have been reported between maternal periodontitis and adverse pregnancy outcomes, several clinical trials have been conducted in which periodontal treatment has been provided to pregnant mothers and outcomes have been assessed. These studies have consistently reported that periodontal therapy (root surface debridement) is safe to perform during pregnancy and results in improved periodontal status in the pregnant women, but there is no clear or consistent evidence of any impact of the periodontal therapy in reducing overall rates of low birthweight or preterm birth.[50] Nonetheless, the positive outcomes reported in some clinical trials suggest that specific patient populations may benefit more from periodontal treatment than other populations. More research is required to investigate this area further, but clearly prevention and treatment of periodontal conditions in pregnant women is important for optimizing oral health, just as it is in nonpregnant individuals.[47]

APPLICATION TO CLINICAL PRACTICE

Dental clinicians have long been aware that prevention of disease is better than cure. We have had a tendency, however, to focus specifically on the mouth, and our role in preventing and treating oral and dental diseases has naturally been placed primarily within the context of the oral cavity. We would all agree, also, that good oral health is integral to good general health and life quality, and that optimizing oral health and preventing oral disease should be a part of overall healthcare management strategies.[51]

Now we have a further extension of this concept; namely, that the prevention and treatment of periodontal disease may have a benefit on the general health and systemic disease states of our patients. This opens up the potential for the dental team to play a broader role in the overall general health management of our patients. For example, the importance of optimized oral hygiene in the prevention of systemic disease has been demonstrated in the context of hospital-acquired pneumonias in institutionalized elderly and nursing home residents,[52] and the use of oral antiseptics has been shown to significantly reduce the risk of ventilator-associated pneumonia.[53] Clearly, improvements in oral hygiene achieved by routine preventive strategies for periodontal disease are important in the prevention of pneumonia in susceptible populations, emphasizing the importance of oral and dental care as part of overall medical management.

It is noteworthy that there are similarities between the management strategies required for successful treatment of periodontitis and those for other chronic diseases such as diabetes and cardiovascular diseases. For example, the management of diabetes requires lifestyle changes by the patient, achieved by a process of patient education about aspects such as exercise, diet, and use of medications, as well as self-management and self-monitoring. A key concept is that patients must take responsibility (assisted by their medical clinicians in this task) for the management of their diabetes if successful outcomes are to be achieved. These principles are instantly recognizable to dental clinicians who manage patients with periodontitis. Lifestyle changes by periodontal patients are similarly important, such as optimizing oral hygiene, compliance with the periodontal maintenance care plan, and smoking cessation, all achieved by patient education and regular and repeated interactions with dental clinicians. Structured educational programs exist for the management of diabetes,[54,55] and similar initiatives have also been reported for the management of periodontitis.[56,57] The unifying concept behind these educational programs is the emphasis on developing self-efficacy for managing disease, achieved by patient education to effect lifelong behavior change, supported by the clinical team as they progress toward this goal (see Chapter 2).

Patient education and self-efficacy are fundamental to the management of chronic diseases such as diabetes and periodontitis, and it is certainly the case that dental clinicians are adept at influencing behavior change in their patients. Given the evidence of links between periodontal disease and systemic diseases such as diabetes, as well as the potential systemic health benefits following periodontal treatment that have been observed, it is likely that decisions about preventive strategies and oral disease management will be influenced by the dental clinician's knowledge of the patient's general health status. The rising tide of obesity and increasing prevalence of diabetes in populations throughout the world, coupled with the already high prevalence of periodontal diseases, make this topic highly relevant to both dental and medical professionals. Dental professionals will have an increasingly important role to play in overall healthcare management, alongside our medical colleagues, in preventing and managing periodontitis (and other oral conditions) so as to have a positive impact on general health status and life quality. As dental professionals, we can now recognize that we have important contributions to make in improving the overall health care of our patients.

The results of a recent study conducted in the United States exemplify the roles that dental professionals may have in the future. The researchers evaluated 239 dental patients with risk factors for diabetes who were screened in a dental clinic; of these, 101 were identified as having HbA1c greater than 5.7%, or 39 mmol/mol.[58] These individuals were then randomized to two groups. Participants in the first group were told about their diabetes risk factors and blood test results and advised to see a physician; those in the second group were given a detailed explanation of the findings together with a written report for the physician, and were then followed up. Whereas no significant differences in outcomes between the two groups were recorded at 6 months after the intervention, 84% of all the patients reported having seen a physician and 49% reported at least one positive lifestyle change as a result of the intervention in the dental clinic.

In a study conducted in various dental clinical settings, including general dental practices in the UK, 166 patients were screened for diabetes risk.[59] All patients were given written advice on healthy lifestyles by the dental team, and those at moderate or high risk for diabetes were referred to their medical practitioner for further investigation, resulting in 30% of the moderate-risk and 20% of the high-risk patients visiting their medical professional. The patients welcomed the opportunity to discuss their general health in the dental practice, and the dental clinicians also enjoyed the additional training and skills that they acquired. Whereas the main challenge was the time taken for the diabetes assessment (adding approximately 20 minutes to each dental appointment), this study suggests that people at risk of developing type 2 diabetes can be identified in primary, community, and secondary dental care settings. The use of blood collected from the gingival crevice for the purpose of measuring HbA1c has also been evaluated, and researchers identified a very high degree of correlation between HbA1c values derived from gingival crevice blood and those derived from standard fingerstick blood samples.[60] This finding suggests that the dental team, with appropriate equipment and training, could use gingival crevicular fluid blood collected at the time of routine dental appointments to screen for presence of diabetes.

The prevention and treatment of periodontal disease is fundamentally important in patients with diabetes, not only because of the increased risk for periodontitis in patients with diabetes (particularly if glycemic control is poor), but also because of the potential negative impacts of periodontitis on glycemic control and diabetes complications. Patients with diabetes should therefore be informed about their increased risk for periodontitis. It should also be explained that the presence of periodontitis may make glycemic control more difficult, and may increase the risk for other diabetes complications such as cardiovascular disease and kidney disease.[61] Patients with diabetes should receive an appropriate periodontal examination and if periodontitis is diagnosed, it should be properly managed. Other potential oral complications of diabetes should also be evaluated, such as dry mouth, burning mouth, and candidal infections. People with diabetes who do not have periodontitis should receive appropriate preventive care, including optimized oral hygiene and professional mechanical plaque removal as required, and regular monitoring of periodontal status. Patients who do not have a diagnosis of diabetes, but who present with other obvious risk factors for diabetes together with signs of periodontitis should be informed about their risk of having diabetes and referred to their medical physician for assessment, with the results of a chairside HbA1c test, if available, provided.[61]

As described earlier, the presence of periodontitis has also been associated with increased risk for incident cardiovascular disease after controlling for known cardiovascular risk factors. Clearly, it is important to treat periodontal disease to improve oral health and prevent progression of disease, and the association with cardiovascular disease further underscores the importance of primary and secondary prevention of periodontal disease. Given the consistent epidemiological evidence that periodontitis imparts increased risk for cardiovascular disease, it is important for the dental clinician to be aware of this evidence and to communicate it to patients when necessary. In particular, patients with periodontitis who also have other risk factors for cardiovascular disease (e.g., smoking, hypertension, overweight, obesity) should be made aware of shared disease risks and advised to see their medical practitioner. Modifiable risk factors associated with both conditions (e.g., smoking) should routinely be addressed in the dental setting, and patients should be encouraged to take action to manage these risks (e.g., through referral to smoking cessation services).[41]

Procedures to improve periodontal health are safe during pregnancy, and these procedures are usually effective in improving and maintaining oral and periodontal health.[48] In accordance with routine clinical practice, elective procedures should be avoided in the first trimester of pregnancy to avoid stress to the fetus and generally should be undertaken in the second trimester. Preventive treatment regimens are important during pregnancy, and recommendations have been published regarding preventive care in pregnant women with varying periodontal disease presentations.[47] Thus, for women with a healthy periodontium, health education about preventing periodontal diseases is important for their own health and that of their children. This includes explanation of transient changes to the gingival tissues during pregnancy (such as increased bleeding and possible gingival enlargement as a result of increased vascularity of the tissues), as well as advice and instruction in oral hygiene techniques. For pregnant women with gingivitis, the same health promotion measures should be undertaken, together with professional intervention to treat the gingivitis to reduce the bacterial load and reduce inflammation. For those with periodontitis, in addition to the same health promotion advice, nonsurgical periodontal therapy should be provided to disrupt and reduce the subgingival biofilm and to reduce inflammation. The current lack of evidence to indicate that treatment of maternal periodontitis has a beneficial effect on reducing adverse pregnancy outcomes[50] suggests that such preventive and therapeutic regimens during pregnancy have their primary efficacy in treating periodontal disease and reducing periodontal disease progression rather than having an effect on the outcomes of the pregnancy.

CONCLUSIONS

This chapter has reviewed the evidence for the linkage between periodontal disease and systemic diseases such as diabetes and cardiovascular disease, and also adverse pregnancy outcomes. The plausibility of the biological links between periodontitis and diabetes and cardiovascular disease is based on the finding that periodontal inflammation that develops in response to the challenge from the subgingival microbiota contributes to the cumulative systemic inflammatory burden in the host.[24] Furthermore, blood-borne spread of periodontal bacteria and their products can have effects throughout the body, contributing to systemic inflammation and risk for disease.

Associations between a number of different systemic diseases and periodontitis have been reported in the periodontal literature. Some of the systemic conditions that have been associated with periodontitis include chronic obstructive pulmonary disease, pneumonia, osteoporosis, chronic kidney disease, rheumatoid arthritis, cognitive impairment, obesity, metabolic syndrome, and cancer, and the interested reader is referred to texts that have dealt with these topics in greater detail.[62] However, it is recognized that research into possible associations between periodontitis and many systemic conditions has been hampered by the inherent difficulties in controlling for common risk factors or confounders such as smoking and socioeconomic status. Furthermore, by necessity of cost and practicality, most studies have been of relatively short duration and have relied on surrogate disease markers to assess outcomes. Further problems, such as inconsistent use of case definitions for periodontitis, have hampered our efforts to advance knowledge in this area.[63]

Research into the links between periodontal disease and various systemic diseases will therefore continue. Clearly, it is important to prevent and treat periodontal disease for the oral health and quality of life benefits that such treatments are known to achieve. Prevention of periodontal diseases requires the combined efforts of the patient in achieving effective oral hygiene and reducing risk factors with those of the clinician in providing professionally delivered therapies for mechanical plaque removal and root surface debridement. Repeated and individually tailored oral hygiene instruction is fundamental to achieving gingival and periodontal health, together with professionally delivered mechanical plaque removal both supra- and subgingivally to disrupt and reduce the biofilm and remove hard deposits.[64] As our understanding of the mechanisms that underpin the links between periodontal disease and systemic conditions improves, and if causality is clearly demonstrated, then a new paradigm for care will be warranted, with closer collaboration between medical and dental healthcare providers and new standards for prevention and management of systemic diseases such as diabetes.[24] Periodontal diseases are largely preventable, and the prevention and treatment of periodontitis is warranted not only to establish and optimize oral health, but potentially to have positive effects on general health and well-being and quality of life.

REFERENCES

1. Williams RC. Understanding and managing periodontal diseases: a notable past, a promising future. *J Periodontol.* 2008;79:1552–1559.
2. Miller WD. The human mouth as a focus of infection. *Dental Cosmos.* 1891;33:689–713.
3. Billings FA. Chronic focal infections and their etiologic relations to arthritis and nephritis. *Arch Int Med.* 1912;9:484–498.
4. Cecil RL, Angevine DM. Clinical and experimental observations on focal infection, with an analysis of 200 cases of rheumatoid arthritis. *Ann Intern Med.* 1938;12:577–584.
5. Reimann HA, Havens WP. Focal infection and systemic disease: a critical appraisal. *JAMA.* 1940;114:1–6.
6. Mattila KJ, Nieminen MS, Valtonen VV, et al. Association between dental health and acute myocardial infarction. *BMJ.* 1989;298:779–781.
7. Kinane DF, Preshaw PM, Loos BG. Host-response: understanding the cellular and molecular mechanisms of host-microbial interactions-consensus of the Seventh European Workshop on Periodontology. *J Clin Periodontol.* 2011;38(suppl 11):44–48.
8. Preshaw PM, Taylor JJ. How has research into cytokine interactions and their role in driving immune responses impacted our understanding of periodontitis? *J Clin Periodontol.* 2011;38(suppl 11):60–84.
9. Chapple ILC. Periodontal diagnosis and treatment—where does the future lie? *Periodontol 2000.* 2009;51:9–24.
10. Williams RC, Barnett AH, Claffey N, et al. The potential impact of periodontal disease on general health: a consensus view. *Curr Med Res Opin.* 2008;24:1635–1643.
11. Hujoel PP, White BA, Garcia RI, et al. The dentogingival epithelial surface area revisited. *J Periodontal Res.* 2001;36:48–55.
12. Mealey BL, Ocampo GL. Diabetes mellitus and periodontal disease. *Periodontol 2000.* 2007;44:127–153.
13. Tsai C, Hayes C, Taylor GW. Glycemic control of type 2 diabetes and severe periodontal disease in the US adult population. *Community Dent Oral Epidemiol.* 2002;30:182–192.
14. Preshaw PM, Bissett SM. Periodontitis: oral complication of diabetes. *Endocrinol Metab Clin North Am.* 2013;42:849–867.
15. Brownlee M. The pathobiology of diabetic complications: a unifying mechanism. *Diabetes.* 2005;54:1615–1625.
16. Dandona P, Aljada A, Bandyopadhyay A. Inflammation: the link between insulin resistance, obesity and diabetes. *Trends Immunol.* 2004;25:4–7.
17. Schmidt MI, Duncan BB, Sharrett AR, et al. Markers of inflammation and prediction of diabetes mellitus in adults (Atherosclerosis Risk in Communities study): a cohort study. *Lancet.* 1999;353:1649–1652.
18. Taylor JJ, Preshaw PM, Lalla E. A review of the evidence for pathogenic mechanisms that may link periodontitis and diabetes. *J Clin Periodontol.* 2013;40(suppl. 14):S113–S134.
19. Taylor GW, Burt BA, Becker MP, et al. Severe periodontitis and risk for poor glycemic control in patients with non-insulin-dependent diabetes mellitus. *J Periodontol.* 1996;67:1085–1093.
20. Shultis WA, Weil EJ, Looker HC, et al. Effect of periodontitis on overt nephropathy and end-stage renal disease in type 2 diabetes. *Diabetes Care.* 2007;30:306–311.
21. Saremi A, Nelson RG, Tulloch-Reid M, et al. Periodontal disease and mortality in type 2 diabetes. *Diabetes Care.* 2005;28:27–32.
22. Demmer RT, Desvarieux M, Holtfreter B, et al. Periodontal status and A1C change: longitudinal results from the study of health in Pomerania (SHIP). *Diabetes Care.* 2010;33:1037–1043.
23. Arora N, Papapanou PN, Rosenbaum M, et al. Periodontal infection, impaired fasting glucose and impaired glucose tolerance: results from the Continuous National Health and Nutrition Examination Survey 2009–2010. *J Clin Periodontol.* 2014;41:643–652.
24. Borgnakke WS, Ylostalo PV, Taylor GW, et al. Effect of periodontal disease on diabetes: systematic review of epidemiologic observational evidence. *J Clin Periodontol.* 2013;40(suppl. 14):S135–S152.
25. Janket SJ, Wightman A, Baird AE, et al. Does periodontal treatment improve glycemic control in diabetic patients? A meta-analysis of intervention studies. *J Dent Res.* 2005;84:1154–1159.

26. Darre L, Vergnes JN, Gourdy P, et al. Efficacy of periodontal treatment on glycaemic control in diabetic patients: A meta-analysis of interventional studies. *Diabetes Metab*. 2008;34:497–506.
27. Teeuw WJ, Gerdes VEA, Loos BG. Effect of periodontal treatment on glycemic control of diabetic patients: a systematic review and meta-analysis. *Diabetes Care*. 2010;33:421–427.
28. Simpson TC, Needleman I, Wild SH, et al. Treatment of periodontal disease for glycaemic control in people with diabetes. *Cochrane Database Syst Rev*. 2010;(5):CD004714. doi: 10.1002/14651858.CD004714.pub2.
29. Sgolastra F, Severino M, Pietropaoli D, et al. Effectiveness of periodontal treatment to improve metabolic control in patients with chronic periodontitis and type 2 diabetes: a meta-analysis of randomized clinical trials. *J Periodontol*. 2013;84:958–973.
30. Engebretson S, Kocher T. Evidence that periodontal treatment improves diabetes outcomes: a systematic review and meta-analysis. *J Clin Periodontol*. 2013;40(suppl 14):S153–S163.
31. Liew AK, Punnanithinont N, Lee YC, et al. Effect of non-surgical periodontal treatment on HbA1c: a meta-analysis of randomized controlled trials. *Aust Dent J*. 2013;58:350–357.
32. Wang X, Han X, Guo X, et al. The effect of periodontal treatment on hemoglobin a1c levels of diabetic patients: a systematic review and meta-analysis. *PLoS One*. 2014;9:e108412. doi: 10.1371/journal.pone.0108412.
33. Simpson TC, Weldon JC, Worthington HV, et al. Treatment of periodontal disease for glycaemic control in people with diabetes mellitus. *Cochrane Database Syst Rev*. 2015;(11):CD004714. doi: 10.1002/14651858.CD004714.pub3.
34. Borgnakke WS, Chapple ILC, Genco RJ, et al. The multi-center randomized controlled trial (RCT) published by the Journal of the American Medical Association (JAMA) on the effect of periodontal therapy on glycated hemoglobin (HbA1c) has fundamental problems. *J Evid Based Dent Prac*. 2014;14:127–132.
35. Hotamisligil GS. Molecular mechanisms of insulin resistance and the role of the adipocyte. *Int J Obes Relat Metab Disord*. 2000;24(suppl 4):S23–S27.
36. Hotamisligil GS. Inflammation and metabolic disorders. *Nature*. 2006;444:860–867.
37. Rotter V, Nagaev I, Smith U. Interleukin-6 (IL-6) induces insulin resistance in 3T3-L1 adipocytes and is, like IL-8 and tumor necrosis factor-α, overexpressed in human fat cells from insulin-resistant subjects. *J Biol Chem*. 2003;278:45777–45784.
38. Loos BG. Systemic markers of inflammation in periodontitis. *J Periodontol*. 2005;76:2106–2115.
39. Tomas I, Diz P, Tobias A, et al. Periodontal health status and bacteraemia from daily oral activities: systematic review/meta-analysis. *J Clin Periodontol*. 2012;39:213–228.
40. Reyes L, Herrera D, Kozarov E, et al. Periodontal bacterial invasion and infection: contribution to atherosclerotic pathology. *J Clin Periodontol*. 2013;40(suppl 14):S30–S50.
41. Tonetti MS, Van Dyke TE. Periodontitis and atherosclerotic cardiovascular disease: consensus report of the Joint EFP/AAP Workshop on Periodontitis and Systemic Diseases. *J Clin Periodontol*. 2013;40(suppl 14):S24–S29.
42. Dietrich T, Sharma P, Walter C, et al. The epidemiological evidence behind the association between periodontitis and incident atherosclerotic cardiovascular disease. *J Clin Periodontol*. 2013;40(suppl 14):S70–S84.
43. Schenkein HA, Loos BG. Inflammatory mechanisms linking periodontal diseases to cardiovascular diseases. *J Clin Periodontol*. 2013;40(suppl 14):S51–S69.
44. Choi HM, Han K, Park YG, et al. Associations among oral hygiene behavior and hypertension prevalence and control: the 2008 to 2010 Korea National Health and Nutrition Examination Survey. *J Periodontol*. 2015;86:866–873.
45. Tonetti MS, D'Aiuto F, Nibali L, et al. Treatment of periodontitis and endothelial function. *N Engl J Med*. 2007;356:911–920.
46. D'Aiuto F, Orlandi M, Gunsolley JC. Evidence that periodontal treatment improves biomarkers and CVD outcomes. *J Clin Periodontol*. 2013;40(suppl 14):S85–S105.
47. Sanz M, Kornman K. Periodontitis and adverse pregnancy outcomes: consensus report of the Joint EFP/AAP Workshop on Periodontitis and Systemic Diseases. *J Clin Periodontol*. 2013;40(suppl 14):S164–S169.
48. Ide M, Papapanou PN. Epidemiology of association between maternal periodontal disease and adverse pregnancy outcomes systematic review. *J Clin Periodontol*. 2013;40(suppl 14):S181–S194.
49. Madianos PN, Bobetsis YA, Offenbacher S. Adverse pregnancy outcomes (APOs) and periodontal disease: pathogenic mechanisms. *J Clin Periodontol*. 2013;40(suppl 14):S170–S180.
50. Michalowicz BS, Gustafsson A, Thumbigere-Math V, et al. The effects of periodontal treatment on pregnancy outcomes. *J Clin Periodontol*. 2013;40(suppl 14):S195–S208.
51. Oral health: prevention is key. *Lancet*. 2009;373:1.
52. Sjogren P, Nilsson E, Forsell M, et al. A systematic review of the preventive effect of oral hygiene on pneumonia and respiratory tract infection in elderly people in hospitals and nursing homes: effect estimates and methodological quality of randomized controlled trials. *J Am Geriatr Soc*. 2008;56:2124–2130.
53. Labeau SO, Van de Vyver K, Brusselaers N, et al. Prevention of ventilator-associated pneumonia with oral antiseptics: a systematic review and meta-analysis. *Lancet Infect Dis*. 2011;11:845–854.
54. Davies MJ, Heller S, Khunti K, et al. The DESMOND educational intervention. *Chronic Illn*. 2008;4:38–40.

55. Gillett M, Dallosso HM, Dixon S, et al. Delivering the diabetes education and self management for ongoing and newly diagnosed (DESMOND) programme for people with newly diagnosed type 2 diabetes: cost effectiveness analysis. *BMJ.* 2010;341:c4093.
56. Jonsson B, Ohrn K, Oscarson N, et al. The effectiveness of an individually tailored oral health educational programme on oral hygiene behaviour in patients with periodontal disease: a blinded randomized-controlled clinical trial (one-year follow-up). *J Clin Periodontol.* 2009;36:1025–1034.
57. Jonsson B, Ohrn K, Oscarson N, et al. An individually tailored treatment programme for improved oral hygiene: introduction of a new course of action in health education for patients with periodontitis. *Int J Dent Hyg.* 2009;7:166–175.
58. Lalla E, Cheng B, Kunzel C, et al. Six-month outcomes in dental patients identified with hyperglycaemia: a randomized clinical trial. *J Clin Periodontol.* 2015;42:228–235.
59. Wright D, Muirhead V, Weston-Price S, et al. Type 2 diabetes risk screening in dental practice settings: a pilot study. *Br Dent J.* 2014;216:E15.
60. Strauss SM, Rosedale MT, Pesce MA, et al. The potential for glycemic control monitoring and screening for diabetes at dental visits using oral blood. *Am J Public Health.* 2015;105:796–801.
61. Chapple IL, Genco R. Diabetes and periodontal diseases: consensus report of the Joint EFP/AAP Workshop on Periodontitis and Systemic Diseases. *J Clin Periodontol.* 2013;40(suppl 14):S106–S112.
62. Genco RJ, Williams RC, eds. *Periodontal Disease and Oral Health: A Clinician's Guide*. 2nd ed. Yardley, PA: Professional Audience Communications, Inc.; 2014.
63. Linden GJ, Lyons A, Scannapieco FA. Periodontal systemic associations: review of the evidence. *J Clin Periodontol.* 2013;40(suppl 14):S8–S19.
64. Tonetti MS, Eickholz P, Loos BG, et al. Principles in prevention of periodontal diseases: Consensus report of group 1 of the 11th European Workshop on Periodontology on effective prevention of periodontal and peri-implant diseases. *J Clin Periodontol.* 2015;42(suppl 16):S5–S11.

Chapter 13

Preventive Considerations in Special Care Dentistry

Roseann Mulligan, Phuu Pwint Han, and Piedad Suarez-Durall

SPECIAL NEEDS PATIENTS AND DENTAL HEALTH

The increase in the number of individuals with disabilities is a worldwide phenomenon, in part due to growth in the number of people who are living into chronologically older ages and in part due to premature aging and the resulting susceptibility to aging diseases experienced by many people with disabilities, especially those of the developmental type.[1] Individuals with disabilities are likely to have poorer health as a result of barriers to care that can include physical impediments, prohibitive costs, and limited availability.[1] In dentistry, the care of people with disabilities is that branch of dentistry that provides oral care services for people with physical, medical, developmental, or cognitive conditions that limit their ability to receive routine dental care.[2]

ORAL DISEASE BURDEN AND BARRIERS TO CARE IN SPECIAL NEEDS PATIENTS

As noted in the US Surgeon General's report on oral health, people with special needs have disproportionately high levels of oral disease due to the nature and limitations of access to care.[3] Frequently, patients with special care needs, especially those with developmental disabilities, are cared for by pediatric dentists with whom they continue their treatment even after entering adulthood. Yet these patients often have comorbidities, secondary health conditions, and age-related ailments that are not within the purview of the pediatric dentist. For them, an adult-centered dental home would be much more appropriate.[4] Because of the all-inclusive definition of special care needs, the increasing population of the United States, and the disproportionately high level of oral disease in patients with special healthcare needs, all dental care providers need to be willing and competent to treat patients in the primary care setting.[5,6] This situation is true for all countries, even those where special care dentistry is considered a dental specialty.[7]

In the best of situations and even when a patient with special needs has access to care, his or her ability to cooperate in receiving dental care may be a huge barrier to receiving preventive or curative treatments for dental diseases.[8] The most effective and efficient way to reduce the dental disease burden is by prevention, which in the past has been provided to the general population mainly by water fluoridation, the widespread use of fluoride-containing toothpastes and mouthrinses,[9] and regular dental care according to the patient's risk for dental disease.[10] However, patients with special healthcare needs have extra barriers to receiving routine care. This is especially true of those patients presenting with a variety of cognitive and physical disabilities that may impede their ability to understand the importance of preventive care or how to access it and to safely tolerate dental care delivery without the use of a sedative.[6,11] With new and better diagnostic and interventional medical procedures, people are living longer, even those diagnosed with multiple medical conditions, thus necessitating a manageable lifelong preventive care approach to reach and maintain a positive level of oral health.

IMPORTANCE OF PREVENTIVE CARE OF ORAL HEALTH

When discussing preventive dentistry it is impossible to describe the one best approach, as every patient is different. Announcements of new dental materials and technologies occur almost daily.[12] However evidence-based articles on the best techniques to be used for people with certain disabilities are not readily available. The alternative is to review the basic principles of preventive dentistry and extrapolate those concepts to the preventive care of individuals with special needs. DePaola and Cheney described two basic preventive principles that should serve as the foundation of preventive programs: (1) an accurate diagnosis that allows development of a detailed treatment plan reflective of the patient's needs; and (2) reinforcement of the prevention program at various steps, with the understanding that the patient or caregiver, or both, would be able to accomplish each of those steps.[13] In order to accomplish this outcome, knowledge of behavioral guidance methods is vital for the entire prevention team.

BEHAVIOR AND PSYCHOLOGICAL INTERVENTIONS

Behavior guidance techniques have been widely used in pediatric dental care because they model appropriate coping behavior during dental treatment.[6,14] Such techniques can be used to reduce the patient's anxiety, and to promote positive dental care experiences and attitudes, thus allowing the dental healthcare provider to perform safe and efficient oral healthcare services.[14] These same behavioral guidance techniques can be useful for all patients, including those with limited cooperative ability (e.g., patients with high fear and dental anxiety) and some older adult patients with cognitive impairment.[15,16]

The American Academy of Pediatric Dentistry (AADP) identifies 11 different approaches to nonpharmacological behavioral guidance: communication and communicative guidance, positive previsit imagery, direct observation, tell-show-do, ask-tell-ask, voice control, nonverbal communication, positive reinforcement and descriptive praise, distraction, memory restructuring, and parental presence or absence.[14] Different strategies described by other resources include modeling, shaping, flexibility, visualization, relaxation, consistency, desensitization and repetitive tasking, contingent and noncontingent escape, hypnosis, and escape extinction.[6] These behavioral strategies have overlapping principles and as one becomes more comfortable using the techniques and appreciating the principles that drive them, multiple techniques can be combined. For example, hypnosis is a formalized process of suggestion, visualization, and distraction, whereas tell-show-do utilizes similar components of suggestion and visualization.[16] If treatment failure occurs using one type of therapeutic approach, an alternative approach may lead to success. When used consistently over time, these approaches can assist the patient in developing behavioral responses that are conducive to receiving preventive and curative dental care without the need for sedation modalities.

Systematic Desensitization

Kemp defined desensitization as the gradual exposure of the patient to the feared object or situation, with the concurrent training of and reinforcement of relaxation as a response that was incompatible with anxiety or fear.[17] Desensitization can be conducted systematically in one's imagination, by video or computer program, or by clinical simulation.[17,18] The goal is to increase compliance or to reduce the amount of behavioral support, restraint, or sedation needed by the patient in order to receive dental care.[6] The desensitization process for patients with special needs often involves repeating more steps to reach the end goal of actual treatment more gradually.[17] This strategy can become costly as it often requires more visits to the dental office, and predicting when the end point will be achieved may be difficult due to individual variability. Creative approaches to dental visits that involve a few minutes' visit with a staff member rather than the clinician to assess how home care is going and provide feedback help keep costs down and take advantage of the engagement of the entire clinical staff in a preventive focus.

For many people with special needs, the foundation of desensitization is heavily dependent on caregivers—in partnership with the oral healthcare team—teaching tolerance of daily toothbrushing or flossing in incremental steps. Repetitive tasks that involve prompting or shaping of cooperative behavior consistent with actions necessary to achieve the target goal behavior are a component of the desensitization.[6] Positive reinforcement through use of small tangible rewards and verbal praise for achieving each step of desensitization will facilitate success. This technique is especially helpful for patients whose behavior is influenced by fear and anxiety.

Shaping Through Successive Approximation
The tell-show-do method is the most widely used behavioral management method of successive approximation.[19] For individuals who have receptive language capabilities, the provider first explains the procedure verbally, in language appropriate to the developmental level of the patient. Descriptions are given of what is about to happen, what instruments will be used, and the reason (the "tell" component), followed by demonstrations of the sensory cues of the procedures in a carefully defined, nonthreatening setting (the "show"); then, the actual procedure is completed (the "do").[6,14,18,19] "Foreshadowing" and visualization are similar concepts to tell-show-do.[6,18] Successive approximation can be used to gain patient acceptance of operative or other, more invasive, procedures as well.[19]

If the patient has an intellectual disability or cognitive impairment, oral hygiene techniques must be broken down into simple, multiple, discrete steps. Steps should be addressed one at a time, making sure the patient understands and masters each step before advancing to the next. Instructions should be short and simple. Written or recorded reminders can be given to the patient or the caregiver, or both. The technique should be monitored and reinforced, with encouragement (and perhaps some brightly colored new toothbrushes or other attractive oral hygiene aids) serving as positive reinforcement until the patient or caregiver can adequately incorporate the new behaviors into the patient's daily routine.

Contingent and Noncontingent Escape
It is not a surprise that individuals with special needs would be eager to escape from a dental appointment that can prove difficult to tolerate even for patients without special needs.[20,21] Neurobiological changes in certain brain regions of special needs patients can trigger the "flight or fight" reaction that manifests as fighting or attempts to escape from what is perceived as threatening or uncomfortable behaviors.

Contingent escape offers the opportunity to stop the immediate activity after a period of acceptable behavior is achieved. An example might be a rest period after a treatment interval in which the patient did not engage in any mouth closing or struggling activity. This is positive reinforcement of the targeted behavior.[6] On the other hand, noncontingent escape provides breaks from demands in relation to a prescribed period of time and is not related to the individual's compliance. For example, the provider could include a rest period after a quadrant of sealants is placed before moving on to another quadrant, whether or not the patient's behavior was conducive to the treatment. These temporary escape periods can give the patient some degree of control over the situation and the ability to communicate with the provider when rest is needed.[16] In fearful and anxious patients, pausing the procedure can allow patients to calm down, and the provider should initiate the rest breaks.[18] It is important that these rest breaks be initiated before the tolerance level of the patient has been exceeded and the break being called due to lack of cooperation.

When seen in demented patients, such care-resistant behavior (CRB) is likely to progress over time as the severity of the dementia increases, due to causative neurological deterioration.[22] Methods to overcome CRB in individuals with dementia impact the effectiveness of caregivers in providing adequate caregiving interventions[23] and will be discussed in a later section.

Consistency and Role Modeling
When a message or situation is regularly and repeatedly presented, patients with special healthcare needs can adapt, learn, and function more predictably. This sensitization can help make what was previously an intolerable situation, tolerable. The necessity for familiarity may translate to the same operatory, same dentist and dental assistant, same check-in protocol at the front desk, and so on. To encourage the impression of "sameness," it can help immeasurably to allow the attendant from the facility or a family caregiver to accompany the patient into the operatory and possibly stay there during care provision.

Role modeling involves having patients observe

the positive behavior of someone being treated, either in a video or in vivo. It could be watching the care delivery of a relative or of another patient from the same setting or facility. The important component of this strategy is being certain that the model will demonstrate positive behavior when engaged in the same or a similar task that is planned for the patient with special needs. While role modeling has been shown to be effective for children and many patients who have special needs, with increasing severity of the patient's disabilities, the likelihood of success lessens.[6]

Escape Extinction
When patients become physically resistant and thus require the cessation of dental treatment, the success of their disruptive behavior at escaping the threat (dental care) reinforces the resistive behavior and sets the stage for future episodes of disruption. It is important to prevent or address escape; however, escape extinction utilizes medical immobilization or physical guidance, or both, in order to proceed with dental care. Providers should be very careful in using these techniques and ideally need to have a plan that shows how these initial strategies will be used less often in the future. These techniques are mainly used for patients for whom other behavioral guidance techniques cannot be employed and when sedative techniques are not available. National guidelines[16] and the laws of individual jurisdictions should be consulted relative to the interpretation of these types of interventions within the political and geographical boundaries of the dental delivery site where they are to be utilized.

CLASSIFICATIONS OF PREVENTIVE DENTISTRY FOR THE GERIATRIC PATIENT

When discussing preventive dentistry, it is impossible to describe the one best approach since every patient is different and announcements of new dental materials and technologies occur almost daily.[12] Historically few evidence-based articles have been published on the best preventive techniques to be used for people with certain disabilities. There are also few national guidelines. One that we were able to locate, authored by Johnson and Chalmers (2011), focused on the care of older adults who are functionally dependent; have cognitive impairments; have intraoral conditions that negatively impact the oral milieu, resulting in dry mouth; or have lesions associated with diabetes, anticancer therapy, and so on.[24] This guideline identifies risk factors, provides an instrument for assessing baseline and ongoing oral health status, helps to lay out an oral health plan, and discusses specific approaches to mitigating individual findings, including disruptive behavior, cognitive impairment, and medication use.

In order to develop a preventive program for each individual patient, the dental office needs to be aware of the latest scientific findings related to the prevention of oral disease in general and map out the roles of each member on the prevention team: the patient or patient helper, the dental staff member, and the dentist or dental hygienist. When no resources relative to a specific condition are discoverable, the alternative is to review the two basic principles of preventive dentistry recommended by DePaola and Cheney, as mentioned earlier, and extrapolate those concepts into the preventive care of individuals with special needs.[13]

For the most part, few dental problems are linked to only one specific condition. Therefore, it is critically important to determine the nature of the patient's medical conditions, including whether they are progressive, and whether they involve the central nervous system, sensory organs, cognition, or frailty—for all of these factors will influence the ultimate preventive strategy chosen for each patient. However, determining the individual's ability to accomplish or tolerate oral hygiene procedures relates far more to his or her functional capabilities than to the number or type of medical diagnoses.

A dental office team can provide information about prevention with an enthusiastic commitment from the entire staff to be an active part of the patient's preventive oral health team. One size or style does not fit all offices; each clinic needs to develop a strategy that works in that setting and for the personnel who will attempt to motivate the patient member of the preventive team.[25] Providing training and an understanding of behavioral techniques, motivational methods, and prevention strategies for the entire dental team is critical to achieving success.

In developing a treatment plan, the preventive aspect of care cannot be an afterthought, the last item in the list of "things to do," or relegated only to actions that are described by a procedural code. Prevention should be an important part of every patient interaction. DePaola and Cheney describe five types of prevention that should occur in the dental office, with the first occurring at the initial encounter.[26]

Predictive Prevention[26]

In predictive prevention, the patient is observed as he or she comes into the dental office. Aspects such as how the patient ambulates and transfers or sits in the dental chair (with or without assistance) can provide clues to his or her functionality. For example, a patient's gait could suggest the amount of motor ability remaining for a patient with Parkinson's disease. This could then translate into a more informed assessment and discussion about the patient's ability to manage dentures now and in the future. Or, if a patient has consistent repetitive movements of the mandible, this could be a possible indicator of dystonia or bruxism and the need for a night guard. The flexed arm and circumduction of the leg seen in the hemiplegic gait of a patient following a stroke alerts to possible problems not only with prostheses but overall oral hygiene skills. Some patients may present with multiple bruises of the legs and arms that could be indicative of anticoagulant medication use or possible elder abuse; swollen ankles may be a sign of heart disease; and a patient who is short of breath and unable to lie back in the dental chair may have chronic obstructive pulmonary disease. The observation of these conditions or signs and a good review of the medical history in this first appointment are important first steps in developing not only successful treatment but also a successful prevention plan.

Clinical Prevention[26]

It is important to delay or arrest problems with interceptive or corrective actions at chairside. Consulting with the patient's physician is highly appropriate in certain circumstances, such as when intraoral manifestations occur as a result of medication side effects or due to chronic disease comorbidities that affect the oral cavity. The dentist has the responsibility to understand and differentiate changes in the oral cavity due to aging from pathology in older adults. Gaining a better understanding of chronic diseases will assist dental professionals in providing appropriate preventive care to all patients to help promote and preserve a healthy mouth for their lifetimes. When treating older adults, adherence to the *three R's* in dentistry serves as a guide: **R**epair, **R**emove, and **R**eplace, utilizing chemotherapeutic preventive agents to minimize further damage. In patients who are chronically ill and debilitated or terminally ill, these three R's are modified to RRI—**R**epair, **R**eline, and **I**gnore—as in some complex cases, the best treatment could be not to perform any procedure and just observe or maintain the status quo.

Empirical Prevention[26]

The empirical method of trial and error is often necessary when dealing with patients who have complex intraoral and disability issues, present with rare conditions, or may not be able to tolerate a complex dental treatment protocol, or because of uncertainty about the etiology of the disease. At this time, instituting a practical, palliative treatment strategy could be of value.

Conservative Prevention[26]

When the goal is limited to preserving healthy tissue and removing the foci of infection, conservative prevention principles are invoked. Such action might be confined to eliminating calculus or overt periodontal disease, active decay, or teeth with a poor prognosis. Conservative prevention is likely to be considered for the older adult who is unable to tolerate dental care due to significant medical issues, has poor oral tissue tolerance, has a very limited life expectancy, could cooperate with care but is unwilling to do so, or has no way to fund his or her care. Taking this approach will, at a minimum, allow the patient to regain comfort and many times restore nutritional support.

Aggressive Prevention

Good oral health is an important component of quality of life for the older adult. Being aggressive in applying a preventive strategy before disease and destruction occur will help maintain the health of the dentition and periodontium. Such health will have a significant effect on a variety of components that make up the psychological and emotional well-being of the individual, as reflected in his or her oral health-related quality of life profile.[27] Beyond the impact that oral health can play on nutrition, mastication, digestion, and esthetic appearance, enjoyment of food and the socialization that occurs at mealtimes are also important.[28] Self-esteem is significantly linked to quality of life and is a contributor to socialization. An older adult with a lot of calculus, missing teeth, or bad breath is not socially acceptable. Communication and social interaction decline, leaving the individual feeling lonely and depressed. Once teeth are lost, there may be many impediments that preclude getting proper treatment, ranging from an inability to tolerate care to lack of financial resources to pay for it.[29] If aggressive prevention were introduced early into the care regimen, these highly negative outcomes could be forestalled. Examples of aggressive prevention include regular recare appointments for prophylaxis and examination scheduled at short intervals, and application of chlorhexidine varnish or fluoride varnish every 3 months, depending upon a patient's needs.

PREVENTIVE DENTAL CARE CONSIDERATIONS

First Visit and Annual Visits

One of the main goals of prevention is to have zero or minimal oral problems, especially those related to dental plaque, caries, and periodontal disease. Therefore, to be optimally effective, any prevention program must focus on intervening at incipient stages of these developing conditions. This approach will allow the dental professional to move from what has typically been a traditional emphasis on secondary and tertiary preventive dentistry to primary preventive care.[30] Critical to this process is determining the follow-up visit interval, consideration of which actually starts at the first visit in the reception area as the patient is completing the medical history questionnaire. Before the clinical examination, the dental professional should review in detail the patient's medical history information for both evidence of transmissible disease and systemic conditions with potential for oral manifestations. For example, patients with depression and hypertension who are taking medications may experience dry mouth, putting them at risk for a higher incidence of caries. The initial and subsequent annual exams should include not only the detailed intraoral examination findings, but also the disabilities of the patient. This information will help determine the level of prevention needed by the patient. Dental professionals should have the knowledge and experience to develop an appropriate preventive treatment plan, including use of behavior modification and related strategies.[31]

Periodic Preventive Maintenance

The timing of preventive maintenance appointments should be individualized and should reflect the patient's or caregiver's ability to successfully perform oral hygiene procedures at home. While development of the preventive plan should occur at the initial visit, during each follow-up or recare appointment, that plan should be reviewed to see if it has been successful at preventing oral disease. If not, both the frequency of the recare interval and the components of the preventive plan should be reconsidered. Often, medically compromised patients are on fixed or limited incomes and have difficulty financing their oral health care, including their preventive visits. While some are eligible for government insurance plans, they may have little access to clinics accepting such plans. Many patients with disabilities rely on family members who can, once educated about the importance of preventive care, assist the patient with performing self-care at home.[31]

Adjuvant Interventions

Older adults are retaining their natural teeth longer. However, the prevalence of gingival recession and the exposure of root surfaces increases susceptibility to root caries. Since root caries develops more rapidly in dentin than in enamel due to the presence and the pH of the surrounding dental biofilm, preventive interventions are critical for reducing risk of this disease.[32,33] In 2015, Wierichs and Meyer-Lueckel performed a systematic review of noninvasive treatment of root caries lesions, summarizing the results of clinical studies investigating professional or home use of chemical agents.[34] Many studies included in their review reported that regular dental prophylaxis and motivation of patients improves and intensifies patient oral hygiene care. Findings also supported regular control of plaque as the first choice among interventions to manage root caries lesions.[34] This systematic review also identified different agents that can be used to keep root caries from forming or to inactivate them if they do, such as daily use of dentifrices containing 5,000 ppm fluoride, professionally applied chlorhexidine varnish (1% or 10%), or silver diamine fluoride varnish (38%). However, Wierichs and Meyer-Lueckel recommended interpreting these results with caution because the clinical trials were few and had both high potential for bias and lower levels of evidence.

Impact of Systemic or Psychological Declines
Recently, chronic periodontitis (CP), a prevalent inflammatory disease, has become a focus of increasing interest in relation to other chronic inflammatory conditions in the body.[35] CP is highly prevalent in adults and is associated with life-threatening systemic disorders, such as atherosclerosis, autoimmune diseases, neurodegenerative and neuroprogressive conditions, and aspiration pneumonia. CP is characterized by chronic immune activation, oxidative and nitrosative stress, and systemic inflammation.[36] However, there is a lack of consensus among experts about the nature of these associations and confusion among healthcare providers and the public on how to interpret this rapidly growing body of science.[37]

The geriatric literature includes little written about the concept of psychological frailty encompassing cognitive, mood, and motivational components. The concept considers brain changes that are beyond normal aging, but not necessarily inclusive of disease. Most studies exploring the interface among cognition, mood, and physical frailty have demonstrated a bidirectional association between the domains. Psychological symptoms or deficits have been described as either worsening the degree of physical frailty, or physical frailty has been viewed as a risk to worsening cognition or depression.[38]

Anxiety associated with a potential or actual diagnosis of dementia is common among older adults. Patients with Alzheimer's disease tend to express fear of further cognitive decline.[39-42] Mental and physical well-being are intrinsic components in the dialogue of the concerned older adults. Well-being studies support that some individuals are motivated to maintain mental and physical health by implementation of compensatory or preventative strategies to impede further cognitive decline. Evidence supports the need for physical exercise, healthy diet, and maintenance of social interactions as early preventive strategies for a range of diseases, including cognitive decline.[43-45] All of these topics are very important to consider when formulating the best prevention plan for our patients, especially the involvement of family members or caregivers. As cognitive impairment increases, an individual may experience an increase in tooth loss, dental decay, gum disease, and denture-related problems, all of which negatively affect nutrition.[28,46,47]

Dietary Considerations[31,48]
For some patients with special needs, foods high in sugar are distributed throughout the day as rewards for having been compliant. In a study done by Fure in 2004, it was found that the frequency of daily carbohydrate intake increased with age, from around five times per day in the 55-year-old to seven times per day in the 85-year-old.[49] No difference was found between men and women. A significantly higher caries incidence was found in those who had a carbohydrate intake of six times or more per day. With patients who have

decreased neuromuscular coordination, decreased salivary flow, or both, it may be difficult to adequately clean the mouth of food debris. Food may remain in the buccal vestibule and interproximally until the next brushing. To decrease the risk of caries, we often tell patients that it is necessary to restrict between-meal snacking and limit the use of highly cariogenic food. Yet, some are encouraged to eat multiple small meals a day for a variety of medical reasons and encouraged to eat high-carbohydrate foods to keep their weight up.[31] We know that if sweets are to be consumed, they should be consumed at mealtime, when salivary flow is best. If bedtime snacking cannot be avoided, the patient should be encouraged to brush immediately after eating.

Home Care Need for Parent and Family Involvement

It is extremely important for dental clinicians to collaborate with other healthcare professionals as well as with family members or caregivers who are responsible for the care of the patient. A high and consistent quality of care can only be provided with the cooperation of primary caregivers and the full knowledge of the personal and social life of the patient and environment. Often the future health of the older adult with physical or mental disability is uncertain. Caregivers and patients are sometimes so overwhelmed in dealing with medical or social challenges that oral health concerns are given lesser priority, which can lead to neglect of dental problems. An additional challenge occurs when dental treatment is sought: patients and their caregivers may be unable to find dentists who are trained in the unique issues of older adults.[50]

CARE DELIVERY PROBLEMS SPECIFIC TO PATIENTS WITH SPECIAL NEEDS

Patients with Neurodegenerative Diseases

Patients with neurodegenerative diseases should have preventive care and aggressive treatment in preparation for the classic progressive nature of these conditions that result in functional decline. These disorders—including stroke, multiple sclerosis, amyotrophic lateral sclerosis (ALS), Alzheimer's disease, Parkinson's disease, and Huntington's disease—are among the most challenging and devastating illnesses. Dental professionals who are treating patients affected by any of these disorders are confronted with major challenges of cognitive decline, mobility losses, and behavioral changes, as well as the physical limitations that preclude being able to manage regular dental homecare and professional dental visits.[51] The dental problems associated with these conditions mainly include poor oral hygiene; difficulty in wearing, cleaning, and retaining dentures; and root caries and recurrent decay as a result of medication-induced hyposalivation.[51]

Daily oral hygiene care with toothbrushing and flossing requires fine motor skills and dexterity of the small muscles of the fingers and hands as well as the gross motor skills of the larger muscle groups in the upper extremities.[52] Either hypoactive or hyperactive muscles and nerves of the head, neck, and upper extremities affected by neurodegenerative conditions will influence dexterity, motor skills, and range of motion of the bones and joints.

It is important to assess the functional capacity of the patient and his or her ability to perform oral hygiene. A modified device, power device, or caregiver assistance may be needed to compensate for the patient's limitations. The gross motor skills needed to grasp a toothbrush handle and move the brush to the mouth can be improved with the use of orthotic devices such as splints and braces to support a deformed, constricted, or weakened limb (arm or shoulder). However, the skill and dexterity needed to apply fine vibratory brushing motions and properly utilize dental floss typically cannot be enhanced with orthotics or physical medicine modalities.[31] In such cases, modified power toothbrushes or flossing devices may be beneficial.

Patients with Sensory Disorders

Patients with sensory disorders that impair hearing, vision, or speech will have communication barriers. Those with significant visual impairment may need to be escorted to the operatory. Such individuals may be carrying a cane, arrive with an escort (human or animal), or have no obvious outward signs of visual impairment except the inability to read a treatment consent form. If a patient requests that a companion be allowed in the treatment area, such a request should be accommodated. While a human escort may be involved in learning about oral hygiene instructions and participating in demonstrations, animal companions may be equally as important to keep the patient calm so that he or she can pay attention to instructions. Dental professionals must ensure that their patients are able to fully participate in their care. They can do so by using appropriate communication strategies so that patients understand their dental treatment needs, are able to provide informed consent, and commit to proposed preventive homecare recommendations. Custom-tailored instruction sheets with large black letters of at least 12-point font size, typed onto white paper,[53] and use of oversized dental models and oversized toothbrushes for demonstrations can be helpful. Colored floss and magnifying mirrors can be used to help patients observe the effectiveness of their oral hygiene skills. Other recommendations include checking to be sure that all demonstrations are performed within the patient's visual field and preventing possible discomfort from the glare of the dental light by carefully focusing and positioning the operatory light. If a patient is blind, he or she can be taught to feel how to perform self-care using an individualized training technique in the patient's mouth, and sensitizing the patient to the "feeling" and "smell" of a clean mouth to ensure the success of oral hygiene measures.[54]

Patients with hearing impairments can be negatively impacted by the sound of dental equipment, background noises from music and televisions, and street noises. Ideally these noises should be silenced; if that is not possible, noise should be minimized so that it does not interfere with the communication going on in the dental operatory. The individual who is communicating with the patient with a hearing impairment needs to lower or remove his or her face mask and stay directly in front of the patient at the same eye level to allow the patient to lip read and take cues from the speaker's facial expression and body posture.[55] Speaking distinctly and slightly slower in a well-modulated voice can facilitate communication.[56] Shouting at the person is not recommended. Patients who have hearing aids may prefer to remove them or turn them off prior to dental treatment to avoid the electronic feedback that frequently results in noxious sounds. Ensuring that the hearing aids are in place and turned back on for postoperative instructions is critical. If the patient with a hearing impairment communicates through sign language, the dentist must retain and pay for a sign language interpreter's services if, in fact, an interpreter is needed to achieve the same "effective communication" for the patient as would occur for a patient without hearing impairment.[57]

Patients with Speech and Language Impairment
Several motor or cognitive impairment disorders can affect a patient's speech or language ability. The patient with cerebral palsy may have a speech impairment due to central nervous system involvement affecting the muscle movements needed for speech. Patients with neuromuscular diseases such as Parkinson's or ALS may have severe weakness of the muscles, resulting in an inability to articulate sounds (dysarthria). A patient may experience a language disorder such as aphasia (an inability to express or understand speech) following a stroke. In these circumstances, it is helpful for the patient's caregiver or family member, who is attuned to "reading" the patient's needs, to be readily available to help interpret the patient's nonverbal actions. Aphasia may present differently in affected individuals, with retention of some speech, although the actual words used may not be appropriate. Listening to the emphasis the patient places on the words spoken frequently helps to clarify his or her intent.

Patients with Autism Spectrum Disorders
The number of patients who present with autism spectrum disorders (ASD) continues to grow. An increased prevalence of ASD over the past decade

requires familiarity with this diagnosis and its potential impact on oral health.[58] Patients with ASD have an overly sensitive nervous system[59] and, as a result, exhibit extreme and peculiar responses to visual, auditory, tactile, olfactory, and gustatory signals, all of which invariably occur as part of a dental appointment.[60] Thus, sensory overload during a dental appointment can quickly lead to overstimulation and subsequent challenging behaviors, including noncompliance, hyperactivity, sensory hypersensitivity, and self-injurious behavior.[59,60]

Communicating with patients who have ASD can be difficult due to language deficits, poor comprehension of speech, or difficulties reading social cues. Moreover, many patients with ASD insist on sameness, adhere to strict routines, demonstrate rigid thinking patterns, and may react adversely to even minor changes in their daily routine.[61] These impediments to care can be overcome in some patients with ASD using traditional approaches or basic behavioral guidance strategies. Unique strategies have been developed for approaching the dental care of the individual with ASD. Nontraditional approaches of behavior guidance, such as visual pedagogy (a strategy that takes advantage of the ability of patients with autism to respond better to pictures than words), social stories, and video modeling have been used in conjunction with traditional behavior guidance approaches.[59,62] More recent successes in the dental office have been found when a sensory-adapted dental environment (SADE) is provided for the patient with ASD.[63]

Patients with ASD may present with hypersensitivity to the oral region, and in fact, oral defensiveness has been reported to be evident in 50% of children with this condition.[64] Experimental introduction of relaxing light conditions, rhythmic music, and deep pressure applications in the dental setting,[65] together with using the shortest possible duration of the dental visit and minimum sensory stimulation, can reduce the patient's anxiety and enhance positive participation in the dental care visit. Parental input regarding the behaviors and preferences of the patient can be of tremendous value to the success of the oral healthcare appointment. Parents can bring the child's favorite music, video, movie, or toy to help encourage the patient to relax. Treating the patient in the same operatory with the same dentist and dental assistant, and designating a separate waiting area for patients with ASD, are recommended.[59]

Preventive Dental Care for Geriatric Patients

Older adults are the fastest growing segment of the population in the United States; population projections indicate that by 2030, more than 20% of US residents will be aged 65 years and older.[66] Dentists are challenged with treating community dwelling older adults who have chronic stable systemic diseases as well as with caring for the dental needs of frail homebound or institutionalized older adults. Preventive dental care for geriatric patients is complicated by the presence of systemic diseases, medications taken for these comorbid conditions, and disease- and drug-induced adverse effects on the oral tissues.[67] Oral problems in dentate or partially edentulous geriatric patients include dental caries, periodontal disease, chronic facial pain or temporomandibular dysfunction, and benign or malignant lesions of the oral mucosa or the jaws. Medications taken for medical conditions may result in decreased salivary flow that impairs the patient's ability to chew, swallow, or clean the oral cavity. Some medications and systemic conditions, such as orthostatic hypotension[68] and medication-related osteonecrosis of the jaw,[69] can have significant effects on the well-being of older adults.

In vulnerable older adults, oral infections can cause significant morbidity and mortality. Aspiration pneumonia is the most common infection in nursing home residents, who are particularly at risk for dysphagia secondary to neurological disease.[70] Aspiration pneumonia is the most common reason for hospitalization and is the leading cause of death from infection in these frail older patients.[71]

Residents of nursing homes are prone to poor oral health and present with increased periodontal and dental disease burden due to lack of oral hygiene care. Although the complex nature of periodontal disease and aspiration pneumonia make direct cause-and-effect connections challenging, many studies suggest an association between poor oral hygiene and respiratory pathogens. In one National Institutes of Health study, poor oral hygiene was implicated as a common risk factor for aspiration, accounting for 21% of such cases.[72] A decrease in the incidence of respiratory complications was noted when patients were provided with chemical or mechanical interventions to improve oral conditions.[70] Clearly, regular oral hygiene care for this population is of prime importance. However as previously discussed, brain-related changes often cause CRB in these patients, so much so that 80% of the certified nursing assistants (CNAs) report experiencing CRB from elderly patients with whom they have worked.[73]

CNAs may benefit from instructional programs about behavioral management strategies that can be used with patients while providing oral hygiene care. Such strategies include approaching the patient at eye level and within the patient's visual field to avoid startling the patient, smiling, providing positive reinforcements such as compliments, engaging in simple positive conversations, and accompanying interactions with gentle touches. These strategies work best when performed in a relaxing, quiet environment with minimal disruptions.[22]

For those who are not bedbound, engaging in oral healthcare behavior in the patient's bathroom in front of a sink can serve as cue to similar behavior from past memories. Having the CNA stand behind the patient and having both in front of the bathroom mirror can prompt mouth opening when oral hygiene aids are placed in sight. Handing the toothbrush to the patient and cueing him or her to begin brushing is especially helpful to those who have lost language ability. Hand-over-hand prompting can serve as gentle reminders of the task to be accomplished.

Respectful communication and delivery of simple, one-step commands, as well as the elimination of disrespectful "baby talk," have been shown to be helpful in promoting self-care and eliminating CRB.[23] Distraction techniques such as singing or talking can be uniquely helpful or cause negative reactions, depending on the individual patient with whom they are used. When various techniques are not successful and CRBs begin to occur, a rescue strategy should be invoked, wherein one caregiver is replaced with another in an attempt to rescue the oral healthcare effort.[74] Such a tradeoff is often successful in salvaging the experience.

PROVIDERS' READINESS TO CONSIDER UNIQUE NEEDS OF SPECIAL PATIENTS

It should not be presumed that it is only the patient or caregiver who may or may not have the capability and motivation to improve the oral health of the patient with special needs. The practitioner must also be willing and able to develop his or her skills with communication, motivation, planning, and patient management. Watching a patient with a disability progress from being virtually unapproachable in the dental office to being able to maintain his or her home care at an acceptable level, and smiling with self-satisfaction when complimented on these efforts, brings a sense of satisfaction and accomplishment to the clinician as well.

Individuals with special healthcare needs have disproportionate amounts of oral disease and are more likely to have barriers when attempting to receive oral healthcare services. Studies show that dentists who feel that they were adequately educated in how to manage patients with special needs are more likely to treat these patients after graduation. The dental educational system has an important role to play in ensuring that future healthcare professionals are well-educated to meet the complex needs and overcome the healthcare disparities experienced by these patients.[75]

Dental education must address developing the appropriate attitudes and skill required to provide care as a part of an interprofessional team in a variety of settings.[5] Adequate educational preparation is essential to support the delivery of effective and efficient preventive care to meet the unique needs of special patient populations.

REFERENCES

1. World Health Organization. Disability and health. Fact sheet No. 352. Available at: http://www.who.int/mediacentre/factsheets/fs352/en/.
2. Special Care Dentistry Association. SCDA definition. Available at: http://www.scdaonline.org/?SCDA Definitions
3. *Oral Health in America: A Report of the Surgeon General.* Rockville, MD: U.S. Department of Health and Human Services, National Institutes of Health, National Institute of Dental and Craniofacial Research; 2000.
4. Council of Clinical Affairs, American Academy of Pediatric Dentistry. Policy on transitioning from a pediatric-centered to an adult-centered dental home for individuals with special health care needs. In: *American Acadamy of Pediatric Dentistry Reference Manual.* Vol 37. Chicago, IL: American Academy of Pediatric Dentistry; 2011:108–110.
5. Albino JE, Ingelhart MR, Tedesco LA. Dental education and changing oral health care needs: dispartities and demands. *J Dent Educ.* 2012;76:75–88.
6. Lyons RA. Understanding basic behavioral support techniques as an alterative to sedation and anesthesia. *Spec Care Dentist.* 2009;29:39–50.
7. Greig V, Sweeney P. Special care dentistry for general dental practice. *Dental Update.* 2012;40:452–454.
8. Gordon SM, Dionne RA, Snyder J. Dental fear and anxiety as a barrier to accessing oral health care among patients with special health care needs. *Spec Care Dentist.* 1998;18:88–92.
9. Bansal A, Ingle NA, Kaur N, Ingle E. Recent advancements in fluoride: a systematic review. *J Int Soc Prev Community Dent.* 2015;5:341–346.
10. Giannobile WV, Braun TM, Caplis AK, Doucette-Stamm L, Duff GW, Kornman KS. Patient stratification for preventive care in dentistry. *J Dent Res.* 2013;92:694–701.
11. Horner-Johnson W, Dobbertin K, Beilstein-Wedel E. Disparities in dental care associated with disability and race and ethnicity. *J Am Dent Assoc.* 2015;146:366–374.
12. Scheller-Sheridan C. *Basic Guide to Dental Materials.* Chichester, UK: Wiley-Blackwell; 2010:2.
13. DePaola DP, Cheney HG. Commentary on preventive dentistry for the individual. In: *Preventive Dentistry.* Littleton, CO: PSG Publishing Company; 1979:37.
14. American Academy of Pediatric Dentistry Clinical Affairs Committee–Subcommittee on Behavior Management. Guideline on behavior guidance for the pediatric dental patient. In: *Clinical Practice Guidelines Reference Manual.* Vol 37. Chicago, IL: American Academy of Pediatric Dentistry; 2015:180–192.
15. Newton T., et al. The management of dental anxiety: time for a sense of proportion? *Br Dent J.* 2012;213(6) 271–274.
16. Oliver K, Manton DJ. Contemporary behavior management techniques in clinical pediatric dentistry: out with the old and in with the new? *J Dent Child.* 2015;82:22–28.
17. Kemp F. Alternatives: a review of non-pharmacologic approaches to increasing the cooperation of patients with special needs to inherently unpleasant dental procedures. *Behavior Analyst Today.* 2005;6:88–108.
18. Armfield JM, Heaton LJ. Management of fear and anxiety in the dental clinic. *Aust Dent J.* 2013;58:390–407.
19. Law CS, Blain S. Approaching the pediatric dental patient: a review of nonpharmacologic behavior management strategies. *CDA J.* 2003;31:703–713.
20. Do C. Applying the social learning theory to children with dental anxiety. *J Contemp Dent Pract.* 2004;5:1–8.
21. Allen KD, Wallace DP. Effectiveness of using noncontingent escape for general behavior managment in a pediatric dental clinic. *J Appl Behav Anal.* 2013;46:723–737.
22. Jablonski RA, Therrien B, Kolanowski A. No more fighting and biting during mouth care: applying the theroretical contructs of threat perception to clinical practice. *Res Theory Nurs Pract.* 2011;25:163–175.
23. Jablonski RA, Therrien B, Mahoney EK, Kolanowski A, Gabello M, Brock A. An intervention to reduce care-resistant behavior in persons with dementia during oral hygiene: a pilot study. *Spec Care Dentist.* 2011;31:77–87.
24. Johnson VB, Chalmers J. *Oral Hygiene Care for Functionally Dependent and Cognitively Impaired Older Adults.* Iowa City, IA: University of Iowa College of Nursing, John A. Hartford Foundation Center of Geriatric Excellence; 2011. Available from the National Guideline Clearinghouse (NGC), Agency for Healthcare Research and Quality at: http://www.guideline.gov/content.aspx?id=34447&search=oral+health.
25. Mobley CC, Rugh J, Karotkin JW, Bhatt AA. Enhancing patient adherence to preventive programs. In: Mobley CC, Cappelli DP, eds. *Prevention in Clinical Oral Health Care.* St. Louis, MO: Mosby; 2008:chap 11, p. 140.
26. Freedman KA. Geriatric oral health care. In: DePaola DP, Cheney HG, eds. *Preventive Dentistry.* Littleton, CO: PSG Publishing Company; 1979:chap 11, pp. 199–200.
27. Jensen PM, Saunders RL, Thierer T, Friedman B. Factors associated with oral health-related quality of life in community-dwelling elderly persons with disabilities. *J Am Geriatr Soc.* 2008;56:711–717.
28. Daly B, Smith K. Promoting good dental health in older adults: role of community nurse. *Br J Community Nurs.* 2015;20:431–436.
29. Freedman KA. Geriatric oral health care. In: DePaola DP, Cheney HG, eds. *Preventive Dentistry.* Littleton, CO: PSG Publishing Group; 1979:chap 11, p. 208.
30. Freedman KA. Geriatric oral health care. In: DePaola DP, Cheney HG, eds. *Preventive Dentistry.* Littleton, CO: PSG Publishing Company; 1979:chap 11, p. 196.

31. Mulligan R, Sobel S. Preventive oral health care for compromised individuals. In: Garcia-Godoy F, Harris NO, eds. *Primary Preventive Dentistry*. 6th ed. Englewood Cliffs, NJ: Prentice-Hall; 2003:559–588.
32. Peters MC. Strategies for noninvasive demineralized tissue repair. *Dent Clin North Am*. 2010;54:507–525.
33. Schiffner U, Hoffmann T, Kerschbaum T, Micheelis W. Oral health in German children, adolescents, adults and senior citizens in 2005. *Community Dent Health*. 2009;26:18–22.
34. Wierichs RJ, Meyer-Lueckel H. Systematic review on noninvasive treatment of root caries lesions. *J Dent Res*. 2015;94:261–271.
35. Thornton-Evans G, Eke P, Wei L, et al. Centers for Disease Control and Prevention (CDC). Periodontitis among adults aged ≥ 30 years—United States, 2009–2010. *MMWR Suppl*. 2013;62(3):129–135.
36. Hajishengallis G. Periodontitis from microbial immune subversion to systemic inflammation. *Nat Rev Immunol*. 2015;15:30–44.
37. Otomo-Corgel J, Pucher JJ, Rethman MP, Reynolds MA. State of the science: chronic periodontitis and systemic health. *J Evid Based Dent Pract*. 2012;12(suppl 3):20–28.
38. Fitten LJ. Psychological frailty in the aging patient. *Nestle Nutr Inst Workshop Ser*. 2015;83:45–53.
39. Begum A, Whitley R, Banerjee S, Matthews D, Stewart R, Morgan C. Help-seeking response to subjective memory complaints in older adults: toward a conceptual model. *Gerontologist*. 2013;53:462–473.
40. Lingler JH, Nightingale MC, Erlen JA, et al. Making sense of mild cognitive impairment: a qualitative exploration of the patient's experience. *Gerontologist*. 2006;46:791–800.
41. Lawrence V, Samsi K, Banerjee S, Morgan C, Murray J. Threat to valued elements of life: the experience of dementia across three ethnic groups. *Gerontologist*. 2011;51:39–50.
42. Sabat SR. Voices of Alzheimer's disease sufferers: a call for treatment based on personhood. *J Clin Ethics*. 1998;9:35–48.
43. Stathi A, Fox KR, McKenna J. Physical activity and dimensions of subjective well-being in older adults. *J Aging Phys Act*. 2002;10:76–92.
44. Corner L, Bond J. Being at risk of dementia: fears and anxieties of older adults. *J Aging Studies*. 2004;18:143–155.
45. Friedman DB, Laditka JN, Hunter R, et al. Getting the message out about cognitive health: a cross-cultural comparison of older adults' media awareness and communication needs on how to maintain a healthy brain. *Gerontologist*. 2009;49(suppl 1):S50–60.
46. Chalmers JM, Hodge C, Fuss JM, Spencer AJ, Carter KD. The prevalance and experience of oral diseases in Adelaide nursing home residents. *Aust Dent J*. 2002;47:123–130.
47. Zimmerman S, Solane PD, Cohen LW, Barrick AL. Changing the culture of mouth care: mouth care without a battle. *Gerontologist*. 2014;54(suppl 1):S25–34.
48. Hayes M, Allen E, da Mata C, McKenna G, Burke F. Minimal intervention dentistry and older patients. Part 1: Risk assessment and caries prevention. *Dent Update*. 2014 Jun;41(5):406-8, 411-2.
49. Fure S. Ten-year cross-sectional and incidence study of coronal and root caries and some related factors in elderly Swedish individuals. *Gerodontology*. 2004;21(3):130–140.
50. Freedman KA. Geriatric oral health care. In: DePaola DP, Cheney HG, eds. *Preventive Dentistry*. Littleton, CO: PSG Publishing Company; 1979:chap 11, pp. 212–214, 223.
51. Kieser J, Jones G, Borlase G, MacFadyen E. Dental treatment of patients with neurodegenerative disease. *N Z Dent J*. 1999;95:130–134.
52. Mulligan R, Wilson S. Design characteristics of floss holding devices for persons with upper extremity disabilities. *Spec Care Dent*. 1984;4:168–172.
53. American Dental Association. Patients with physical and mental disabilities. In: *Oral Health Care Guidelines*. Chicago, IL: American Dental Association; 1991:19.
54. Morsey S. Communicating with and treating the blind child. *Dent Hygiene*. 1980;54:288–290.
55. Cherney LR. The effects of aging on communication. In: Lewis BC, ed. *Aging: The Health Care Challenge*. Philadelphia, PA: FA Davis; 1996:103.
56. Lange BM, Entwistle BM, Lipson LF. *Dental Management of the Handicapped: Approaches for Dental Auxiliaries*. Philadelphia, PA: Lee & Febiger; 1983.
57. Sfikas PM. Treating hearing-impaired people. *J Am Dent Assoc*. 2000;131:108–110.
58. Perou R, Bitsko RH, Blumberg SJ, et al. Centers for Disease Control and Prevention (CDC). Mental health surveillance among children—United States, 2005–2011. *MMWR Suppl*. 2013;62(2):1–35.
59. Gandhi RP, Klein U. Autism spectrum disorders: An update on oral health managment. *J Evid Base Dent Pract*. 2014;14S:115–126.
60. Delli K, Reichart PA, Bornstein MM, Livas C. Management of children with autism spectrum disorder in the dental setting: concerns, behavioural approaches and recommendations. *Med Oral Patol Oral Cir Bucal*. 2013;18:e862–868.
61. American Psychiatric Association. *Diagnostic and Statistical Manual of Mental Disorders*. 5th ed. Arlington, VA: American Psychiatric Association; 2013.
62. Pilebro C, Backman B. Visual pedagogy in dentistry for children with autism. *ASDC J Dent Child*. 1999;66:325–331.
63. Cermak SA, Stein Duker LI, Williams ME, et al. Feasibility of a sensory-adapted dental environment for children with autism. *Am J Occup Ther*. 2014;69:6903220020p1–10.
64. DeMattei R, Cuvo A, Maurizio S. Oral assessment of

children with an autism spectrum disorder. *J Dent Hyg.* 2007;81:65.
65. Shapiro M, Sgan-Cohen HD, Parush S, Melmed RN. Influence of adapted environment on the anxiety of medically treated children with developmental disability. *J Pediatr.* 2009;154:546–550.
66. Ortman JM, Velkoff VA, Hogan H. *An Aging Nation: The Older Population in the United States. Population Estimates and Projections.* Washington, DC: US Census Bureau; 2014:25–1140.
67. Schreiber A, Glickman R. Geriatric dentistry: maintaining oral health in the geriatric population. In: Fillit HM, Rockwood K, Woodhouse K, eds. *Brocklehurst's Textbook of Geriatric Medicine and Gerontology.* Philadelphia, PA: Elsevier Health Sciences; 2010:chap 75, pp. 599–607.
68. Figueroa JJ, Basford JR, Low PA. Preventing and treating orthostatic hypotension: as easy as A, B, C. *Cleve Clin J Med.* 2010;77:298–306.
69. McClung M, Harris ST, Miller PD, et al. Bisphosphonate therapy for osteoporosis: benefits, risks, and drug holiday. *Am J Med.* 2013;126:13–20.
70. Pace CC, McCullogh GC. The association between oral micororganisms and aspiration penumonia in the institutionalized elderly: review and recommendations. *Dysphagia.* 2010;25:307–322.
71. Oh E, Weintraub N, Dhanani S. Can we prevent aspiration pneumonia in the nursing home? *J Am Med Dir Assoc.* 2004;5:174–179.
72. Quagliarello V, Ginter S, Han L, Van Ness P, Allore H, Tinetti M. Modifiable risk factors for nursing home-acquired pneumonia. *Clin Infect Dis.* 2005;40:1–6.
73. Frenkel HF. Behind the screens: care staff observations on delivery of oral health care in nursing homes. *Gerodontology.* 1999;16:75–80.
74. Chalmers JM. Behavior management and communication strategies for dental professionals when caring for patients with dementia. *Spec Care Dent.* 2000;20:147–154.
75. Dao LP, Zwetchkenbaum S, Inglehart MR. General dentists and special needs patients: does dental education matter? *J Dent Educ.* 2005;69:1107–1115.

Chapter 14
Fluorides

I. A. Pretty

Fluoride has been employed in dentistry for over 100 years for the prevention and treatment of dental caries.[1] Despite this long history there has been considerable debate over its mode of action, the optimal way of delivering fluoride to different patient groups, and risks associated with its use.[2] This chapter examines the background, history, and current application of fluorides for individual patients, considering the life course and risk as a context for determining optimal fluoride therapies for individual patients as well as populations.

HISTORY OF FLUORIDES

Since the late nineteenth century, fluoride has been employed by those concerned with the prevention and treatment of dental caries. The first use of fluorides was as powders, often calcium or potassium fluoride, and it was Denninger whose early clinical trials suggested that children and expectant mothers would benefit from their use.[3]

It is paradoxical that the benefit of fluoride was first established from studies that assessed its detrimental effects. A Colorado dentist, Dr. Frederick McKay, had observed that many of his patients had a unique appearance to their teeth—an appearance that became known as "Colorado brown stain," now referred to as *enamel fluorosis*. (See Figure 1.) The presence of the stain was associated with patients who had had exposure to naturally fluoridated water.[3] Norman Ainsworth, an English dentist, subsequently found that patients who presented with enamel fluorosis had fewer caries—approximately half the decay of patients without enamel mottling.

These initial findings, of a relationship between mottled enamel and reduced caries, were further investigated in a series of landmark epidemiological studies by H. Trendley Dean. Dean found that children between the ages of 12 and 14 years who were living in communities with water fluoridation had roughly half the caries experience of children living in areas where the water supply had low levels of fluoride.[4] Encouraged by these findings, the "21 Cities" study was undertaken that aimed to determine the optimal level of fluoride needed to reduce caries while reducing the risk of enamel fluorosis.[4] This study established 1.0 to 1.2 mg of fluoride (F)/L as the optimal level, which has remained largely unchanged until recently by, among others, the Irish and US regulators to 0.7 mg F/L.

What Is Fluoride?

Fluoride is the ionic form of the trace element fluorine and is commonly found in the natural environment. Most individuals acquire fluoride from dietary sources such as foodstuffs and beverages; however, this can vary from individual to individual. The accidental swallowing of dental products containing fluoride (such as toothpaste in young children) can exceed that consumed through dietary intake.

Benefits of Fluoride?

Fluoride is used for the prevention and treatment (arrest) of both enamel and dentin (root) caries. In the early part of the twentieth century, fluoridation of public water supplies was the main focus of fluoride applications. Use of fluoridated toothpaste is now the most common means of delivering fluoride and has been largely credited

Figure 1. Enamel Mottling (now known as dental fluorosis)

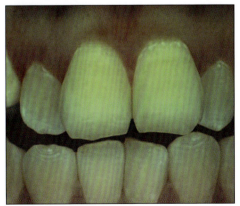

with the significant decrease in caries prevalence seen across Western populations.[5]

How Does Fluoride Work?

Fluoride was long considered to exert its beneficial effect as a result of systemic ingestion and subsequent incorporation into developing enamel. However, since the 1980s this view has changed; the majority of the benefit is now thought to be secured by topical application of fluoride to tooth surfaces.[3] There are three main means by which this topical effect is secured:

1. When fluoride is present, hard tissue remineralization is encouraged.
2. The mineral that is formed in the presence of fluoride has an increased resistance to acid attack.
3. Fluoride may inhibit bacterial metabolism (and hence reduce acid production).

Caries is now understood to be a dynamic process of de- and remineralization that occurs throughout the day.[6] (See Figure 2.) Caries progresses when protective factors are overwhelmed by those favoring mineral loss. If not corrected, the continual mineral loss from the tooth surface progresses, leading to an initial lesion and ultimately to cavitation and involvement of the dentin and pulp, and potential tooth loss.[6] When fluoride is present in the oral environment surrounding the tooth surface during remineralization, it adsorbs onto the developing mineral surface where it attracts calcium and phosphate ions. The newly formed mineral excludes carbonate and hence has an increased resistance to acid dissolution.[7]

It has been suggested that the fluoride incorporated into teeth during development is insufficient to play a key role in caries protection. The primary effect of fluoride is posteruptive.

How Can We Deliver Fluoride?

By the late twentieth century, waterborne sources of fluoride were replaced by fluoridated dentifrice. Crest®, the first clinically proven toothpaste, was marketed in 1955. Early toothpastes used stannous fluoride as their active ingredient; this was not only astringent but caused staining of teeth

Figure 2. The Dynamic Process of Demineralization and Remineralization

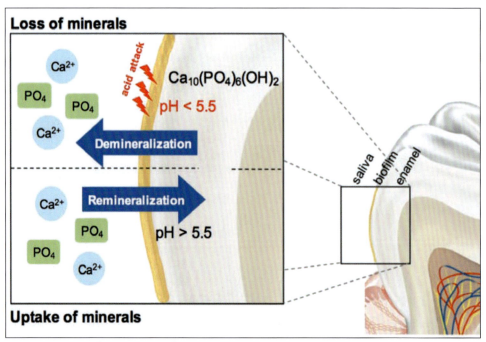

Source: Image courtesy of the Colgate-Palmolive Company.

and silicone-based restorative materials. Modern fluorides, sodium fluoride and sodium monofluorophosphate, were introduced in the 1970s and 1980s.

While dentifrices remain the main source of fluoride, there are supplemental or adjunct sources that include rinses, tablets, drops, varnishes, gels, and foodstuffs such as salt, milk, and juices. Restorative filling materials were developed that claimed to release fluorides with the potential to reduce the incidence of secondary caries. These include glass ionomer, compomers, and resin-modified glass-ionomer cements.[8]

Risks of Fluoride Use

Early water fluoridation studies demonstrated that very high levels of fluoride can be detrimental. The main risk of fluoride ingestion, for levels seen in populations with optimally fluoridated water, is enamel fluorosis. This results from the ingestion of sufficiently high levels of fluoride over a prolonged period during tooth development.[9] Those who have all of their adult teeth developed are not at risk of fluorosis. Fluorosis at the levels seen within the normal therapeutic use of fluorides is typically mild and generally not of aesthetic concern.[10]

Optimal Delivery

Given the risk of fluorosis for children (generally those younger than 6 years old) and the mechanism of fluoride action, topical fluoride systems that are easily ingested or are designed to be swallowed are generally discouraged. For example, fluoride tablets are rapidly ingested and hence have little benefit, but they increase the risk of fluorosis. Therefore, it is not surprising that the main contemporary delivery methods of fluoride are toothpaste, mouthrinses, gels, and varnishes.

The rest of this chapter describes the evidence base for use of these products within the context of the life course.

A LIFE COURSE APPROACH

Caries is a lifelong disease experienced by individuals of all ages that is characterized by periods of higher and lower risk at both an individual patient level and a population level. For example, young children are regarded as being at high risk for caries due to difficulties with toothbrushing, dietary challenges, and erupting teeth. Older adults, who have a similar level of caries incidence as children, face other challenges such as loss of manual dexterity, cognitive impairment, and polypharmacy that can lead to a dry mouth and hence loss of the protective effect of saliva.

Individual patients present with their own risk profiles. These include
- Previous caries experience
- Diet and, in particular, sugar consumption and grazing behaviors
- Presence of restorations and plaque-retentive areas
- Level of oral health literacy
- Medical conditions and special care needs
- Prescribed medicines
- Dental-attending behavior
- Oral hygiene behavior and individual fluoride use
- Bacterial composition of plaque biofilm
- Socioeconomic status
- Education level

There are many tools available to assess caries risk, and it is beyond the scope of this chapter to examine these in detail. The reader is referred to Chapter 3, "Risk Assessment."

When considering either populations or individual patients, it is useful to consider the life course,[11] as shown in Figure 3. A "typical" life course provides a framework to understand opportunities for caries prevention among patients as they age. Periods of vulnerability have a higher risk for caries that are associated with events in the life course. These include birth and early childhood, a recognized period of risk, and later life, where increased general vulnerability, often referred to as frailty, increases caries risk.

The consideration of life course encourages clinicians to assess their patients' risk factors, not only at the time of presentation, but for the future. In particular, clinicians can introduce preventive strategies in a timely manner and improve the likelihood of effectiveness. Considering risk, age, and level of vul-

Figure 3. The Life Course and Vulnerability

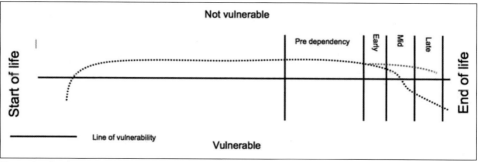

Source: Gerodontology. 2014;31(suppl 1):1–8,[11] with permission.

nerability (at any age) enables a tailored, personalized preventive strategy for oral health to be developed. This strategy should include both professional preventive therapies and a comprehensive, deliverable self-care plan. For many patients, an effective self-care plan will be the main means of preventing caries.

Caries Detection and Diagnosis

While the broader topic of caries detection and diagnosis is beyond the scope of this chapter, it is important to consider diagnostic thresholding. Typically, detection has occurred when the caries encroached into the dentin threshold. While reliable and simple, this level of detection precludes effective prevention and arrest. There have been extensive developments to help facilitate early caries detection in primary care dental practice. Detection at an early stage, when the lesion is restricted to enamel or the outer layer of dentin, is the most effective point at which to arrest caries and achieve maximum benefit from fluoride therapies.

Systems such as International Caries Detection and Assessment System (ICDAS) advocate for careful, methodical examination of teeth that have been subjected to a thorough preexamination prophylaxis. The addition of appropriate clinical illumination and a ball-ended probe, to note differences in texture of hard surfaces rather than to probe softness, ensures that the clinical examination will detect these early lesions and inform diagnosis, risk assessment, and treatment planning.

Using Fluorides to Prevent and Treat Caries

The following sections consider the evidence-based interventions that are available to prevent and treat caries in various age groups across the life course. Each is predicated on a careful assessment of the individual patient that considers risk factors and presentation. The interventions include those that are professionally delivered and those suitable for home care.

Every patient should be provided with simple, consistent, and evidence-based messages regarding caries prevention:

- Use a commercially available fluoride toothpaste for 2 minutes twice daily.
- Reduce sugary snacks, and avoid eating or drinking anything in the hour before bed.
- Visit a dental professional regularly.

CHILDREN AND ADOLESCENTS
Evidence

Fluoride products for children include toothpaste, mouthrinses, gels, foams, fluoride varnish, and dietary supplements.[12] (See Table 1.)

Toothpaste for Self-Care

Consumer toothpaste for children is available in a range of fluoride concentrations dependent upon the geographical market. Irrespective of this, all children should use a commercially available fluoride toothpaste—one with 1,000 parts per million (ppm) F or higher. This recommendation is based on evidence from the Cochrane systematic review that found that a significant anticaries benefit was not seen in concentrations below 1,000 ppm, and that,

Table 1. Summary of Fluoride Modalities for Children and Adolescents

Fluoride Modality	Lower Caries Risk	Higher Caries Risk
Toothpaste	Commence at emergence of first tooth using a smear of toothpaste until age 3 and then a pea-sized amount until 6 years; toothpaste should be 1,000 ppm F or higher	Commence at emergence of first tooth using a smear of toothpaste until age 3 and then a pea-sized amount until 6 years; consider prescription of higher fluoride dentifrice but never less than 1,000 ppm
Mouthrinses, gels, and foams		Starting at age 6, and consider use of daily versus weekly rinses dependent on risk
Fluoride varnish <AU: I've resequenced entries for mouthrinse and varnish to match the order of text discussion; OK?>	At discretion of dentist, but consider every 3–6 months following emergence of teeth	Every 3–6 months following emergence of teeth
Dietary supplements		See text

Source: Modified from *Pediatrics.* 2014;134:626–633.[12]

as the concentration of fluoride increases, greater benefit is seen.[5] Indeed, there is good evidence of a dose–response relationship between fluoride concentration and caries prevention up to 2,800 ppm.[5]

Clinical trial evidence over the past 50 years supports the use of toothpaste for children, with those using fluoride having fewer decayed, missing, or filled permanent teeth irrespective of the presence of fluoridated water. There is also strong evidence to support that twice-daily use increases this benefit.[13] The effectiveness of toothpaste use can also be increased by advising the patient to spit, rather than rinse, after toothbrushing to maintain fluoride levels.[14] The use of a cup to rinse the mouth out after brushing should be positively discouraged.[14]

Initiating a good toothbrushing regimen from an early age is essential, and the recommendation is to commence brushing as soon as the first tooth emerges. Reviews suggest that there is only weak, unreliable evidence of an increased risk of fluorosis in children younger than 12 months of age, and this should be set against the clear evidence of benefit.[13] Flavored toothpastes, such as those with fruit flavors, should be discouraged as these promote swallowing of dentifrice in younger children.

Frequency of brushing is important and should feature as a key message in self-care plans. Clinical trials have shown that children who brushed once a day or less had 20% to 30% more caries than those who brushed twice a day or more.[14] (See Figure 4.)

The timing of brushing is a matter of some debate and many would argue irrelevant against the more important driver that teeth are brushed at all. Mealtimes are when the cariogenic challenge is greatest and hence offer an ideal opportunity for brushing. Some authorities argue for brushing before meals, thus reducing the plaque bulk and maximizing the fluoride levels when food is con-

Figure 4. Caries Experience in Children Who Brush Once or Less, or Twice or More

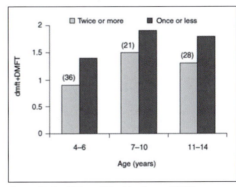

Source: National Diet and Nutrition Survey; 2000.[15]

sumed. However, others advocate for brushing after meals, thus ensuring that the fluoride is not washed away by the stimulated saliva and that food debris is removed. In reality, the logistics of toothbrushing will probably be determined by morning and evening routines within the family setting, although the low saliva rate during sleeping lends some credibility to the recommendation that the last activity before sleep should be toothbrushing.

The amount of toothpaste to be used is less important than the frequency of exposure and fluoride content. Clinical trials have found no association with amount of toothpaste used and anticaries efficacy, but the amount of paste on the brush is important in relation to fluorosis risk and recommendations for smear and pea-sized amounts for younger children. Using appropriate concentrations, twice daily, with spitting and no rising will maximize the anticaries benefit and minimize the fluorosis risk.[14]

In summary, good toothbrushing advice for patients, parents, and caregivers would be the use of fluoride toothpaste with no less than 1,000 ppm F, twice daily, once after or before a meal and once before bed with no rinsing.

Fluoride Mouthrinses

Mouthrinses are most commonly available as daily (227 ppm F) and weekly (909 ppm F) products, and typical use consists of rinsing with 10 mL of solution for approximately 1 minute. Mouthrinses offer an excellent risk–benefit profile when used appropriately as they maximize topical exposure and minimize the risk of fluorosis. Clinical trials demonstrate caries reductions of around 30%,[16] although the differences in those areas served by water fluoridation are lower. A Cochrane review of evidence for the use of mouthrinses found that at either strength (daily or weekly), their use was associated with a clear reduction (23% to 30%) in caries.[17]

Patients and parents should be advised to use mouthrinses and toothpaste at different times of the day to maximize efficacy.[18] Use of mouthrinses for children younger than age 6 years is not recommended due to risk of swallowing and ingestion.

Fluoride Gels and Foams

In many parts of the world, fluoride gels and foams are available as either self-care or professionally applied products. They typically have fluoride concentrations similar to those found in mouthrinses, although some may have up to 5,000 ppm. They are generally highly viscous and are placed in either custom or preformed trays. A Cochrane review found moderate-quality evidence to support a large caries-inhibiting effect (approximately 28%) from clinical studies that were largely school based, making gels and foams similar in efficacy to mouthrinsing.[19] It is interesting to note that the use of chlorhexidine in gels (or indeed varnishes) was not shown to have any effect.[20]

Fluoride Dietary Supplements

Fluoride tablets were introduced in the 1940s to act as an alternative to water fluoridation, and dosage was based on delivering the equivalent of 1 ppm based on average water consumption. This calculation is fundamentally flawed as it should have been based on the dose per kilogram weight of the child—as for any other drug. As previously described, the action of fluoride is now understood to be topical and posteruptive; therefore, any ingestion of fluoride will have little impact on caries but will significantly increase the risk of fluorosis. Despite this risk, many professional dental organizations recommend the use of supplements in areas without water fluoridation. Use of lozenges that are chewed or sucked (and provide a topical effect) is preferable to tablets or drops that are swallowed. Evidence from clinical trials supports the use of lozenges and suggests a 20% to 28% reduction in caries.[21,22] However, one should consider the continuing risk from fluoride ingestion versus the use of professional products such as fluoride varnish prior to advising patients to use supplements of this kind.

Professional Fluoride Interventions for Children and Adolescents

In addition to a custom-tailored self-care plan, patients can also benefit from professional prevention, which should be considered as active treatment within the treatment planning process. The need for a professionally applied fluoride treatment should also be informed by the clinical examination and risk assessment process and should be reassessed on a regular basis. Recall intervals for such patients should reflect their higher risk.

Fluoride Varnish

The popularity of fluoride varnish for the treatment and prevention of caries has increased over the past decade with increasing use and a wider professional team involved in its application. Across healthcare systems, physicians, nurses, and the dental team have all been involved in the delivery of fluoride varnish, both in the private setting and in community-based health programs.

Fluoride varnish is used in a targeted fashion on specific risk sites, or applied on a whole mouth basis for those at greatest risk. Varnishes are applied usually every 3 to 6 months and contain high levels of sodium fluoride (22,600 ppm F). These fluoride products are designed to be highly retentive in the oral environment by hardening on the tooth surface after application following contact with saliva. (See Figure 5.) It is thought that the local delivery of high levels of fluoride produces local areas of calcium fluoride that acts as a reservoir for subsequent slow release of fluoride.[23] There is strong evidence for the use of fluoride varnish in children and adolescents, with a Cochrane systematic review concluding that there is a substantial caries-inhibiting effect of fluoride varnish in both permanent (43% reduction) and primary teeth (37%).[24] Fluoride varnish represents an important, cost-effective, and easily applied mechanism for the management and prevention of caries in children and adolescents.

Fluoride varnish application is simple, non–operator sensitive, and well-tolerated by patients. Early carious lesions, especially those restricted to enamel, are especially suitable for varnish application, but it appears that whole mouth treatments are an effective means of prevention.[24] A systematic review examining the evidence base for professionally applied fluoride treatments, including silicon tetrafluoride, fluoride gel, and traditional sodium fluoride varnishes, found that only sodium fluoride gel and silver diamine fluoride (not widely used in Western populations) have significant benefit.[25]

Toothpaste: Professional Prescriptions

Children and adolescents at higher risk of caries will benefit from toothpastes with higher concentrations of fluoride. The available levels of higher fluoride pastes vary between markets. For example, in Europe products with 2,800 ppm and 5,000 ppm are available, whereas in North America, only a 5,000 ppm product is available. There is a well-recognized dose–response relationship between the concentration of fluoride and caries prevention, and the evidence to support the use of fluoridated toothpastes is described by Cochrane as unequivocal.[13] A recent Cochrane review examined the use of fluoride toothpastes containing up to 2,800 ppm and described a dose–response effect up to this level, but stated that this was not always statistically significant. The review found that the highest probability of caries preventive benefits was found in those toothpastes containing greater fluoride concentrations.[5] In comparisons to placebos, low-concentration pastes (400 to 550 ppm) demonstrated no significant benefit, those with "standard" levels of fluoride having a median prevented fraction of 25%, and those with the highest levels of fluoride one of 45%. These findings were mirrored in an earlier review by Ammari and colleagues that considered differences between pastes ranging from a low of 250 ppm up to 1,055 ppm.[26]

Toothpastes with higher concentrations of fluoride should therefore be considered for those at higher risk of caries and may be prescribed for those with transitory increased risk—for example, adolescents wearing fixed orthodontic appliances as well as patients with special needs. The decision

Figure 5. Application of Fluoride Varnish to a Tooth Surface

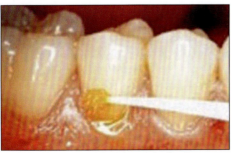

Source: Image courtesy of the Colgate-Palmolive Company.

to prescribe these toothpastes should be revisited on a regular basis and should reflect the current risk assessment of the patient.

ADULTS AND OLDER ADULTS
Evidence

Evidence for the use of fluoride products in adults is relatively scarce. This is largely due to the fact that the caries studies are traditionally undertaken in school settings where large numbers of study participants are easily reached and assessed. Studies undertaken using long-term care and nursing home residents have largely examined the use of professional fluoride applications to prevent and arrest root caries.[27] However, large-scale trials of fluorides in adults are not available; thus, professionals must also rely on their judgment to make the best decisions for their patients.

For nonfrail, nonvulnerable adults, self-care and professional interventions are broadly similar to those for children and adolescents. This reflects the fact that caries is a lifelong disease and that the etiology of the disease is constant across the life course. Treatment planning should reflect changes in risk and risk factors of the adult population.[27] Sugar consumption, for example, can change with a reduced intake of candies but an increased consumption of carbonated drinks, contributing not only to caries but also erosion risk. The presence of restorations, both extra- and intracoronal, needs to be considered with respect to secondary caries and diagnosis of early lesions, and the assessment of their activity can be complicated by the presence of dietary and other habitual stains.[27]

The responsibility of the dental professional is to assess when the patient is at a life stage where, owing to a range of internal and external factors, that risk may increase.[28] (See Figure 3, earlier.) This increased vulnerability is often, but not exclusively, associated with older adults, can occur at any time, and may be manifested by physical or cognitive impairment, or both.[28] Although the research base for older adults largely comprises long-term care and nursing home residents, it should be recognized that this is a function of clinical trial efficiency rather than population-specific interventions. The nursing home setting largely mirrors that of the school—an accessible population for interventions. It is crucial that the predependency stage be identified and that care plans that reflect the increasing risk of caries in this group be put in place for both professional care and self-care.[28]

Older adults with predependency and early dependency have a range of risk factors that differ from those of children or nondependent adults. These include

- *Cognitive impairment:* This can manifest as simply forgetting to brush the teeth or can lead to combative behavior, preventing caregivers from undertaking oral hygiene procedures.[29]
- *Manual dexterity:* Toothbrushing requires a high degree of manual dexterity, which is slowly lost with aging and may be adversely affected by conditions such as rheumatoid arthritis or Parkinson's disease.[30]
- *Polypharmacy:* The number of medications prescribed increases with age. Either as individual agents or as a function of their collective physiological effects, medications can cause decreased salivary flow, reducing the protective effect of saliva and also encouraging behaviors to stimulate saliva that further increase caries risk.[31]
- *Finances and access to care:* Older adults served by insurance-based dental care may find financial barriers to continuing access to services, and there is evidence to suggest that dental professionals in primary care settings are reluctant to treat patients with extensive, complex medical histories or conditions.

Published in 2014, "The Seattle Care Pathway for Securing Oral Health in Older Patients" describes an evidence-based approach to managing older adults with increased dependency. Provided as an open access document, it is recommended for all practitioners who serve older patients.[28]

Therapies available for older adults are the same as those for children and adolescents. The provision of a detailed and achievable self-care plan (which may include the prescription of a high-fluoride dentifrice) and professional application of fluoride (typically in the form of varnish) are recommended.[7] Both sodium fluoride and silver diamine fluoride varnishes have significant levels of trial evidence to support efficacy.[32] Dental professionals should also consider how they can help to mediate the risk factors associated with increased vulnerability by undertaking a personalized assessment of the patient's needs. This may involve recommendations for toothbrush modifications (e.g., power brushes) or consultation with the patient's physician to alter an existing medication to one that causes less xerostomia.[28]

Using Skill Mix to Deliver Fluoride-Based Prevention

There is a growing trend to extend the application of fluoride beyond the traditional dental practice model to expand the reach of this effective preventive intervention.[32] The use of midlevel providers, while not without its detractors, presents an opportunity for both dental practice–based and population-based fluoride interventions to be delivered in an effective and efficient manner. By using the principle of "every contact counts," pediatricians and nurse practitioners are now applying fluoride varnish to patients seen in their practice settings, as are other healthcare professionals in school-based programs. The simple, safe and effective technique of fluoride varnish means that it can be adopted across populations rather than just individuals, and for those areas where water fluoridation is either logistically or politically impossible, it offers an alternative strategy.[33]

Population-Based Fluoride Interventions

Community (or population) prescriptions for high-fluoride toothpastes are being considered, whereby a lead dentist will undertake to prescribe not to an individual, but to a defined population. This could enable, for example, all long-term care or nursing home residents to be provided with 5,000 ppm toothpaste. While such population interventions should not be seen as negating the need for dental attendance and personalized care, this approach may help in areas where access to care is restricted.

Community-based water fluoridation remains the population fluoride intervention of choice, but it is not always physically possible (e.g., due to the water provision infrastructure) or may be problematic due to regulatory or legislative issues.[34] Dietary fluorides, such as those in salt or milk, are considered as alternatives,[35,36] although their evidence base is weaker.

The integration of fluoride into public health systems and population interventions is best achieved in a holistic manner. By working within wider public health concerns, such as childhood obesity, the integration of dental prevention is aligned to other work streams and program efficiency is increased. Dental professionals have an important advocacy role to ensure that oral health is featured in community health plans and that emphasis that is placed, quite correctly, on young children, is not at the expense of older adults who have similar needs for oral health improvement.

FUTURE DIRECTIONS AND BEST PRACTICE

Fluoride remains the mainstay of caries prevention and, in the case of early lesions, treatment. Although other technologies show promise (e.g., arginine and casein phosphopetides-amorphous calcium phosphate [CP-ACP]), the use of fluoride in toothpaste, gels, and varnishes will continue to be the therapy of choice for consumers, professionals, and populations.[37,38]

Technologies for delivering fluoride remain largely unchanged since the introduction of varnishes to supplement dentifrices. The incorporation of fluoride into restorative materials continues and new-generation materials may offer the potential for slower fluoride release and improved recharge properties.[8] There has been considerable interest in the development of further slow-release materials, possibly using degradable glass beads bonded to a tooth surface that then release fluoride over a long period. Despite initial promise, concerns about the beads being swallowed (and risk for toxicity or fluorosis in appropriately aged children) and a lack of evidence of efficacy persist.[39] It is likely that the best means of improving the efficacy of fluoride will be ensuring that compliance is optimized; concentration levels are appropriate to risk; and simple, consistent messages regarding rinsing, timing, and amount are provided.

SUMMARY

Caries is a lifelong condition that is characterized by periods of increased risk, but it should be remembered that some individuals will be considered at high risk throughout life.[11] Caries risk is associated with a number of physical and psychosocial factors, and risk assessment is the cornerstone of any preventive treatment program, which should include consideration for self-care and professional interventions.[40] Caries is a dynamic process in which alternate periods of demineralization and remineralization occur, and caries lesions can be prevented and, if detected in early stages, reversed.[41]

Fluoride is the main therapeutic agent for the prevention and arrest of dental caries and can be delivered through population, professional, or individual routes using a range of delivery systems.[42] Evidence is clear that fluoride exerts its caries-preventive effects topically, and there is little justification for the use of fluoride delivery systems based on systemic use. For population prevention, water fluoridation remains the intervention of choice, whereas the vast majority of fluoride is delivered by means of fluoridated dentifrices.[43,44] The efficacy of such pastes, which remain the mainstay of preventive self-care plans for adults and children, can be increased by simple messages on utilization, including avoidance of rinsing, using twice daily for 2 minutes, and appropriate dosage and concentration based on age, risk of fluorosis, and caries risk.[44] The risk of fluorosis in younger children should always be balanced against the risk of dental caries.[45]

Professional application of fluorides, using varnishes, gels, or foams has a strong and sound evidence base established by systematic reviews.[25] Their use is to be encouraged within a wider preventive plan that considers physical barriers such as pit and fissure sealants. The effectiveness of both the self-care plan and any professional application of fluorides is predicated on the detection of early caries lesions (those limited to enamel or the very outer aspects of dentin). Dental professionals should recognize members of the wider healthcare team for fluoride delivery and advocate for population-based programs within integrated public health programs.

REFERENCES

1. Rugg-Gunn A. Dental caries: strategies to control this preventable disease. *Acta Med Acad.* 2013;42:117–130.
2. Buzalaf MA, Pessan JP, Honório HM, ten Cate JM. Mechanisms of action of fluoride for caries control. *Monogr Oral Sci.* 2011;22:97–114.
3. McGrady MG, Ellwood RP, Pretty IA. Why fluoride? *Dent Update.* 2010;37:595–598, 601–602.
4. Dean H. Nutrition classics. Public Health Reports, Volume 56, 1941, pages 761–792. In: Dean HT, Jay P, Arnold FA Jr, Elvove E, eds. Domestic water and dental caries. II. A study of 2,832 white children, aged 12–14 years, of 8 suburban Chicago communities, including Lactobacillus acidophilus studies of 1,761 children. *Nutr Rev.* 1976;34:116–118.
5. Walsh T, Worthington HV, Glenny AM, Appelbe P, Marinho VC, Shi X. Fluoride toothpastes of different concentrations for preventing dental caries in children and adolescents. *Cochrane Database Syst Rev.* 2010(1):CD007868.
6. Featherstone JD. The continuum of dental caries—evidence for a dynamic disease process. *J Dent Res.* 2004;83(special no. C):C39–42.
7. Wierichs RJ, Meyer-Lueckel H. Systematic review on noninvasive treatment of root caries lesions. *J Dent Res.* 2015;94:261–271.
8. Raggio DP, Tedesco TK, Calvo AF, Braga MM. Do glass ionomer cements prevent caries lesions in margins of restorations in primary teeth?: A systematic review and meta-analysis. *J Am Dent Assoc.* 2016;147:177–185.
9. Iheozor-Ejiofor Z, Worthington HV, Walsh T, et al. Water fluoridation for the prevention of dental caries. *Cochrane Database Syst Rev.* 2015;(6):CD010856.
10. Whelton HP, Ketley CE, McSweeney F, O'Mullane DM. A review of fluorosis in the European Union: prevalence, risk factors and aesthetic issues. *Community Dent Oral Epidemiol.* 2004;32(suppl 1):9–18.
11. Pretty IA. The life course, care pathways and elements of vulnerability. A picture of health needs in a vulnerable population. *Gerodontology.* 2014;31(suppl 1):1–8.
12. Clark MB, Slayton RL, Section on Oral Health. Fluoride use in caries prevention in the primary care setting. *Pediatrics.* 2014;134:626–633.
13. Wong MC, Clarkson J, Glenny AM, et al. Cochrane reviews on the benefits/risks of fluoride toothpastes. *J Dent Res.* 2011;90:573–579.
14. Chesters RK, Huntington E, Burchell CK, Stephen

KW. Effect of oral care habits on caries in adolescents. *Caries Res.* 1992;26:299–304.
15. Walker A. *National Diet and Nutrition Survey: Young People Aged 4–18 Years. Volume 2. Report of the Oral Health Survey.* London, England: Stationery Office; 2000.
16. Ripa LW. A critique of topical fluoride methods (dentifrices, mouthrinses, operator-, and self-applied gels) in an era of decreased caries and increased fluorosis prevalence. *J Public Health Dent.* 1991;51:23–41.
17. Marinho VC, Higgins JP, Logan S, Sheiham A. Fluoride mouthrinses for preventing dental caries in children and adolescents. *Cochrane Database Syst Rev.* 2003;(3):CD002284.
18. Blinkhorn AS, Holloway PJ, Davies TG. Combined effects of a fluoride dentifrice and mouthrinse on the incidence of dental caries. *Community Dent Oral Epidemiol.* 1983;11:7–11.
19. Marinho VC, Worthington HV, Walsh T, Chong LY. Fluoride gels for preventing dental caries in children and adolescents. *Cochrane Database Syst Rev.* 2015;(6):CD002280.
20. Walsh T, Oliveira-Neto JM, Moore D. Chlorhexidine treatment for the prevention of dental caries in children and adolescents. *Cochrane Database Syst Rev.* 2015;(4):CD008457.
21. Driscoll WS, Heifetz SB, Korts DC, Meyers RJ, Horowitz HS. Effect of acidulated phosphate-fluoride chewable tablets in schoolchildren: results after 55 months. *J Am Dent Assoc.* 1977;94:537–543.
22. DePaola PF, Lax M. The caries-inhibiting effect of acidulated phosphate-fluoride chewable tablets: a two-year double-blind study. *J Am Dent Assoc.* 1968;76:554–557.
23. Ripa LW. An evaluation of the use of professional (operator-applied) topical fluorides. *J Dent Res.* 1990;69(special no.):786–796; discussion 820–823.
24. Marinho VC, Worthington HV, Walsh T, Clarkson JE. Fluoride varnishes for preventing dental caries in children and adolescents. *Cochrane Database Syst Rev.* 2013;(7):CD002279.
25. Gao SS, Zhang S, Mei ML, Lo EC, Chu CH. Caries remineralisation and arresting effect in children by professionally applied fluoride treatment—a systematic review. *BMC Oral Health.* 2016;16:12.
26. Ammari AB, Bloch-Zupan A, Ashley PF. Systematic review of studies comparing the anti-caries efficacy of children's toothpaste containing 600 ppm of fluoride or less with high fluoride toothpastes of 1,000 ppm or above. *Caries Res.* 2003;37:85–92.
27. Pretty I. The Seattle Care Pathway: defining dental care for older adults. *J Calif Dent Assoc.* 2015;43:429–437.
28. Pretty IA, Ellwood RP, Lo EC, et al. The Seattle Care Pathway for securing oral health in older patients. *Gerodontology.* 2014;31(suppl 1):77–87.
29. Chen X, Clark JJ, Naorungroj S. Oral health in older adults with dementia living in different environments: a propensity analysis. *Spec Care Dentist.* 2013;33:239–247.
30. Marchini L, Vieira PC, Bossan TP, Montenegro FL, Cunha VP. Self-reported oral hygiene habits among institutionalised elderly and their relationship to the condition of oral tissues in Taubate, Brazil. *Gerodontology.* 2006;23:33–37.
31. Närhi TO, Vehkalahti MM, Siukosaari P, Ainamo A. Salivary findings, daily medication and root caries in the old elderly. *Caries Res.* 1998;32:5–9.
32. Gluzman R, Katz RV, Frey BJ, McGowan R. Prevention of root caries: a literature review of primary and secondary preventive agents. *Spec Care Dentist.* 2013;33:133–140.
33. Brocklehurst P, Macey R. Skill-mix in preventive dental practice—will it help address need in the future? *BMC Oral Health.* 2015;15(suppl 1):S10.
34. Melbye ML, Armfield JM. The dentist's role in promoting community water fluoridation: a call to action for dentists and educators. *J Am Dent Assoc.* 2013;144:65–75.
35. Marthaler TM. Salt fluoridation and oral health. *Acta Med Acad.* 2013;42:140–155.
36. Yeung CA, Chong LY, Glenny AM. Fluoridated milk for preventing dental caries. *Cochrane Database Syst Rev.* 2015;(9):CD003876.
37. Cummins D. Dental caries: a disease which remains a public health concern in the 21st century—the exploration of a breakthrough technology for caries prevention. *J Clin Dent.* 2013;24(special no. A):A1–14.
38. Reema SD, Lahiri PK, Roy SS. Review of casein phosphopeptides-amorphous calcium phosphate. *Chin J Dent Res.* 2014;17:7–14.
39. Chong LY, Clarkson JE, Dobbyn-Ross L, Bhakta S. Slow-release fluoride devices for the control of dental decay. *Cochrane Database Syst Rev.* 2014;(11):CD005101.
40. Senneby A, Mejàre I, Sahlin NE, Svensäter, Rohlin M. Diagnostic accuracy of different caries risk assessment methods. A systematic review. *J Dent.* 2015;43:1385–1393.
41. Fejerskov O. Changing paradigms in concepts on dental caries: consequences for oral health care. *Caries Res.* 2004;38:182–191.
42. Lenzi TL, Montagner AF, Soares FZ, de Oliveira Rocha R. Are topical fluorides effective for treating incipient carious lesions?: A systematic review and meta-analysis. *J Am Dent Assoc.* 2016;147:84–91 e1.
43. McGrady MG, Ellwood RP, Maguire A, Goodwin M, Boothman N, Pretty IA. The association between social deprivation and the prevalence and severity of dental caries and fluorosis in populations with and without water fluoridation. *BMC Public Health.* 2012;12:1122.
44. McGrady MG, Ellwood RP, Pretty IA. Water fluoridation as a public health measure. *Dent Update.* 2010;37:658–660, 662–664.
45. Goodwin M, Sanders C, Davies G, Walsh T, Pretty IA. Issues arising following a referral and subsequent wait for extraction under general anaesthetic: impact on children. *BMC Oral Health.* 2015;15:3.

Chapter 15
Non-Fluoride Remineralization Therapies

Mark S. Wolff and Michael P. Rethman

The utilization of low concentrations of the fluoride ion as a caries prevention tactic is well established and has been in wide use for nearly 60 years. Contemporary approaches include a number of fluoride delivery regimens that are well supported by research. Fluoride-containing dentifrices, high-concentration fluoride compounds, and low-concentration fluoride in community water supplies have all had significant beneficial effects on the public's oral health. Nevertheless, all dental clinicians are aware that the use of fluoride-containing products alone does not prevent or arrest all tooth decay.[1-3] Indeed, caries remains a problem for many patients despite widespread utilization of fluoride-containing products.[4] This chapter examines the notion that patients with high caries risk, such as those with xerostomia or poor diets, may fare better if fluoride-based therapeutics are supplemented with other non-fluoride-based regimens aimed at countering the etiology of caries or by making the teeth more resistant to cavitation.

Utilizing an individualized caries risk assessment facilitates a customized approach to oral health based on an individual's specific needs (see Chapter 3, Risk Assessment). As noted, the use of non-fluoride preventive interventions and remineralization agents may help prevent or better mitigate caries in some patients. However, the cost-effectiveness of these agents has been questioned, particularly for patients with low caries risk. This is because such individuals are unlikely to develop caries with or without these interventions. It is for this reason that non-fluoride caries preventive and remineralization agents are not appropriate for every patient. On the other hand, higher risk individuals may benefit from these agents. The bottom line is that a customized anticaries regimen for every patient (that may be adjusted as risks change over time) is considered optimal.[5]

As clinicians consider using or recommending non-fluoride preventive interventions or remineralization agents, they should keep in mind that fluoridated community water supplies (or supplemental systemic fluoride if community water supplies are fluoride-free), good home oral hygiene, limited dietary intake of fermentable carbohydrates, local application of high-concentration fluoride compounds (when or where indicated), and the consistent use of fluoride-containing dentifrices are the pillars of any well-reasoned anticaries program.[5] Thus, non-fluoride preventive and remineralization agents should be considered adjunctive.

BEYOND FLUORIDES: FINDING OTHER METHODS TO REDUCE CARIES

Dental biofilm, also known as dental plaque, has long been implicated in the etiology of caries. In 1973, Miller proposed a two-step process of caries development. The first step involves tooth-adherent oral bacteria that produce acids when exposed to fermentable carbohydrates. In the second step, the acids act on tooth structure to dissolve mineral components of teeth (hydroxyapatite), eventually causing cavitation.[6] The production of bacterial acids within plaque in response to fermentable carbohydrates and the subsequent slow recovery toward a neutral plaque pH was demonstrated by Stephan.[7,8] The consumption of dietary carbohydrates (especially sugars), even if only thin layers of dental biofilm are present, results in significant bacterial acid production. Such acid acts immediately to begin dissolving the mineral components of the teeth. The amount and duration of the pH drop are related to the amount of dissolution and are to some degree mitigated by the natural acid–base buffering capabilities of saliva and nearby dental plaque.[9,10] Dental plaque is a highly diverse, temporally dynamic, three-dimensional community embedded in a polymeric matrix of bacterial and salivary origins.[11] Marsh demonstrated that the nature of this bacterial community is dependent, in part, on the ongoing "feeding" of the biofilm.[12] For example, frequent consumption of sugars (highly fermentable carbohydrates) favors the vitality of acidogenic bacteria, thereby tailoring an environment that quickly becomes less attractive to other bacterial species that produce high-pH metabolites. Thus, tooth-adherent supragingival dental plaque is where acid-producing bacteria can proliferate (under certain conditions), where acid–base chemistry occurs, and also serves as a temporary reservoir for inorganic ions such as calcium that are continuously exchanged between tooth surfaces and the saliva[13] (see Figure 1).

Saliva, when present in adequate quantities, is a potent protector against caries.[7] A significant loss of salivary secretions is termed *xerostomia*. Xerostomia may be caused by systemic diseases (e.g., Sjögren's syndrome), therapeutic antitumor irradiation, or any of nearly a thousand drugs that have hyposalivation as a side effect.[14] Adequate amounts of normal saliva supply the necessary ingredients for successful remineralization of early carious lesions once the acidic environment is countered either naturally or through therapeutic intervention. Saliva is also critical in terms of protecting teeth against the acidic changes that occur in dental plaque when plaque bacteria digest fermentable carbohydrates. Salivary bicarbonate, phosphate, urea, amino acids, and peptides collectively work to buffer or raise plaque pH.[15] In some circumstances, salivary peptides containing arginine are utilized to raise the pH of dental plaque by favoring the growth of base-forming bacteria.[16] The natural flow of salivary fluids through tooth-adherent dental plaque helps raise plaque pH by diluting bacterial acids. Saliva also acts to cleanse the mouth of particulate food, dissolved cariogenic compounds such as sucrose, as well as some microbes. Indeed, in patients in good health, the rapid clearance of carbohydrates by appropriate quantities of saliva helps protect against caries. Furthermore, the calcium and phosphate ions in saliva help protect the teeth from acid dissolution while also coming into play with regard to remineralization of the tooth when the local environment is favorable[17] (see Figure 2). Saliva also contains calcium-phosphate-carbohydrate-protein complexes named *salivary precipitin*.[18] These calcium and phosphate complexes help prevent the dissolution of enamel in mildly acidic environments.

Figure 1. Progression of Caries Formation

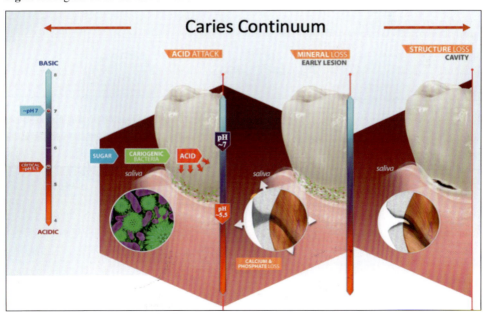

Source: Image courtesy of the Colgate-Palmolive Company.

Indeed, in neutral to slightly basic environments, these complexes appear to assist the deposition of calcium onto tooth surfaces at risk for or already affected by caries, or precipitate on intact tooth surfaces in the form of calculus.

At the enamel surface, small-chain acids produced by cariogenic bacteria (e.g., formic, lactic, acetic, and propionic acids) enter the slightly porous enamel through small diffusion channels that allow these tiny molecules to demineralize tooth surfaces and subsurfaces.[19] In turn, freed calcium and phosphate ions diffuse to the tooth surface through the biofilm and beyond along concentration gradients. So long as the tooth surface is in an acidic environment and is undersaturated with respect to the calcium and phosphate, the mineral components of the tooth will continue to dissolve. However, demineralization at the tooth surface may be slowed, at least somewhat, because of the resulting and often transitory accumulations of calcium and phosphate ions at the tooth surface and in overlying plaque, as well as that which is diffusing from dissolving tooth minerals immediately below. This same proximity of saturated solutions of calcium and phosphate ions facilitates remineralization of the tooth as acid–base chemistry of the local environment is buffered or otherwise altered toward a neutral pH. In conditions such as ongoing exposure to fermentable carbohydrates, acid production is continuous. As an early lesion progresses, bacterial acids diffuse into an increasingly accessible enamel subsurface, resulting in the ever-greater demineralization of enamel crystals as mineral ions diffuse into the biofilm and eventually into the saliva. If not countered, the result is a net loss of mineral from the tooth and cavitation.

The acidic pH generated by cariogenic microbes can be neutralized by saliva in several ways. In the simplest mechanism, saliva dilutes and washes the acids away (although this may act to also remove inorganic minerals such as calcium and phosphate ions).[13] Saliva also contains bicarbonate ions that buffer bacteria-produced acids. Another mechanism of neutralizing acids is also present. Saliva passively transports (along concentration gradients) other bacterial nutrients such as arginine and urea. Because dental plaque is a mixed bacterial culture containing numerous bacterial species, arginine, urea, and other like molecules supply energy

Figure 2. The Demineralization/Remineralization Process

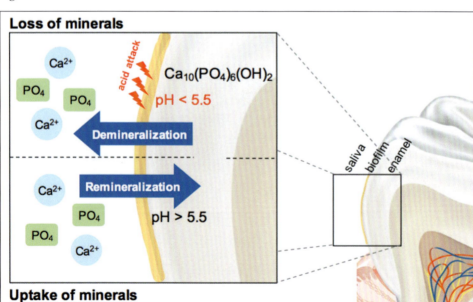

Source: Image courtesy of the Colgate-Palmolive Company.

to arginolytic bacteria that, in turn, produce high-pH metabolites that serve to neutralize the plaque acids produced by cariogenic bacteria.[16]

It is noteworthy that if the enamel surface remains intact, bacteria have no way of invading the dentin because enamel diffusion channels are too small to permit bacterial invasion. This is true even though radiography may reveal significant decreases in enamel radiodensity. This observation of an early enamel-only lesion provides the rationale for therapies aimed at chemical remineralization of partially demineralized enamel. This is in lieu of traditional surgical interventions (i.e., preparing the site for a dental restoration) for early carious lesions. Indeed, a remineralization approach is usually indicated when bacterial acids have penetrated but not completely destroyed the enamel.[20] However, clinicians would do well to remember that remineralization is a microscopic phenomenon and will not macroscopically replace tooth structure. Once frank cavitation occurs, surgical restoration is often indicated.[13]

NON-FLUORIDE STRATEGIES FOR MANAGING CARIOGENIC BIOFILMS
Traditional Approaches
Three strategies have dominated the history of modern dentistry, namely (1) brush one's teeth with fluoride toothpaste, (2) use dental floss every day, and (3) decrease the consumption of fermentable carbohydrates ("cut down on sweets"). Combinations of these strategies have been responsible for substantial reductions in the rates of dental caries.

Oral hygiene education has been shown to reduce bacterial counts but not reduce the bacterial burden by clinically significant amounts.[21] Plaque elimination by toothbrushing has been well documented. A review of the literature related to flossing revealed that self-flossing failed to produce effective reductions in caries.[22] However, it must be remembered that comparative studies report average responses in what are thought to be sufficiently large groups of patients selected to reflect the population as a whole. No one is average. This means that while flossing (or perhaps brushing using a non-fluoride dentifrice) may not produce dramatic population effects in terms of reducing caries, toothbrushing and daily flossing still make sense for individuals. Furthermore, when reviewing studies related to toothbrushing effectiveness and caries, it is difficult to separate out the beneficial effects of frequent toothbrushing using fluoride-containing dentifrices—an intervention that has been repeatedly demonstrated to reduce caries rates. Incremental reduction in caries increases with the concentration of fluoride in the dentifrice and the frequency of its use. Not surprising, such benefits are more noticeable in those patients most prone to caries.[23]

Attempts to decrease the rate of dental caries by lowering the consumption of sugars have met with less success. The Vipeholm studies of the mid-20th century demonstrated that the nature of sugar exposures affects the risk of caries, with sticky foods and frequent consumption increasing caries rates.[24-26] Despite this information, caries management by dietary control of sugar has remained difficult. Draconian decreases in sugar consumption, such as that which occurred in post-World War II Japan and later in trade-embargoed Iraq, demonstrated that dramatic reductions in the consumption of sugars could decrease caries incidence.[27,28] However, voluntary dietary restrictions that largely eliminate the consumption of dietary sugars necessitate lifelong changes in habits that are seldom sustainable.[29]

Targeted Antimicrobial Therapies
Modifying the dental plaque to be less cariogenic is a more recent and logical strategy. Multiple methodologies have been suggested to manage the bacterial constituents of dental biofilms. Stannous fluoride and amine fluoride (as well as numerous metallic ions) have demonstrated antimicrobial effectiveness.[30,31] Naturally high levels of tin, zinc, copper, and other ions dissolved in community water supplies have demonstrated antimicrobial effects, but none of these ions have demonstrated anticaries effectiveness. Taste, safety, and lack of clinical trials make any recommendation difficult.[32,33] Essential oils (a mixture of thymol, eucalyptol, methyl salicylate, and

menthol) have been demonstrated to be effective in limiting accumulations of supragingival plaque, acid-producing *Streptococcus mutans*, and gingivitis,[34-37] but have failed to demonstrate effectiveness against caries. Triclosan/copolymer has demonstrated clinical effectiveness in reducing plaque and gingivitis. Research conducted by several groups has demonstrated that the addition of triclosan/copolymer enhances the caries-preventative effect of fluoride.[38-40] A recent Cochrane Collaboration review of the body of evidence for the clinical benefit of triclosan/copolymer toothpaste confirmed a 5% reduction in caries above what was seen in toothpastes that contain fluoride alone.[41] Certain silver compounds, especially diamine fluoride, have demonstrated effectiveness in arresting active caries, although they are not considered non-fluoride remineralizing agents.[42,43]

Chlorhexidine, a bisguanide, is a broad-spectrum antimicrobial that functions by disturbing the cell membrane of bacteria. It is available in combination with thymol in a varnish, a 0.12% or 0.2% mouthrinse, and a 10% to 40% varnish in many parts of the world. Studies have demonstrated that chlorhexidine, administered frequently enough and in high enough doses, can reduce *Streptococcal* bioburden in the mouth.[44] Unfortunately, clinical studies assessing caries reduction have been equivocal, especially in high-risk cases where beneficial effects would be most likely detected.[45,46] One use for which there is positive evidence is for adults and elderly people prone to root caries. In this population, a 1:1 chlorhexidine:thymol varnish produced significant reductions in caries and should be considered as adjunctive therapy.[47-49]

Polyol-sweetened chewing gums, candies, and pastes have been suggested as methods of preferentially altering the bacterial contents of the biofilm. Xylitol is a low-calorie polyol that is a five-carbon sugar alcohol. Xylitol is widely available in lozenges, gum, and other foods. Polyols are metabolized by plaque bacteria slowly and do not result in a decrease in plaque pH.[50] Multiple studies have also demonstrated that xylitol reduces the growth of *S. mutans*.[51] It has been suggested that the consumption of 6 to 10 grams of xylitol per day may reduce dental caries.[52] However, in studies, reductions in caries incidence have been confounded by the effects of supplemental fluorides, the effects of fluoride dentifrices, or the positive effects of chewing gums on saliva production.[53] Nevertheless, many low-evidence quality studies have reported positive effects on caries rates with substantial daily amounts of xylitol delivered in syrups, gums, and confections.[45,54-57] Unfortunately, low doses of xylitol have failed to demonstrate similar positive effects.[58,59] Data on other polyols are equivocal.[44]

Multiple modifiers to the activity and viability of specific biofilm bacteria have been suggested. Koo (2009) suggested the utilization of naturally occurring molecules, such as apigenin, a potent inhibitor of insoluble-glucan synthesis, and tt-farnesol, a disrupter of *S. mutans* cell membranes, aimed at reducing counts of this cariogenic species in dental biofilms.[60,61] These methods have yet to yield commercial products. Others have recommended the introduction of antimicrobial peptides that can kill target organisms by attaching to and altering electrostatic charges on bacterial cell walls. Combined peptide–cetylpyridinium chloride combinations have shown promise in regulating *S. mutans* in the biofilm but to date have not achieved clinical utility.[62] Another antimicrobial peptide, termed *specifically targeted antimicrobial peptide* (STAMP), targets a pheromone produced by *S. mutans*.[63] STAMP is now being investigated in vivo for its effectiveness in the reduction of *S. mutans* within the mixed ecology of dental plaque. Results are promising, but STAMP has thus far not been evaluated with regard to its effects on caries.[64]

The microenvironment of supragingival plaque has a tendency to become increasingly acidic, thereby favoring overpopulation of the biofilm with acidogenic bacteria such as *S. mutans* and *Lactobacillus* species.[9,11,12] Other commensal bacterial species in the plaque, such as *Streptococcus sanguinis*, are suppressed in an acidic biofilm.[65] However, *S. sanguinis* metabolizes the amino acid arginine that is naturally found in saliva, producing ammonia and carbon dioxide.[16,66] Supplemental arginine, when provided to the mixed ecology of plaque, promotes the reproduction of arginolytic bacteria, such as *S. sanguinis*. Ammonia production is thereby enhanced. Ammonia in aqueous solution is basic. It neutralizes the acids produced by cariogenic bacteria and alters the acid–base balance of plaque toward a more neutral pH.[66,67] A new acid-neutralizing toothpaste containing arginine is now available in much of the world (Colgate Maximum Cavity Protection plus Sugar Acid Neutralizer™). This dentifrice also contains typical concentrations of fluoride ion. The new dentifrice has demonstrated greater caries prevention capabilities than a control dentifrice that contains fluoride ion alone.[67–70] However, the new dentifrice also contains insoluble calcium that might also have a beneficial effect on caries rates. The observed improvement over fluoride-containing dentifrice is likely due, at least in part, to the ability of ammonia to neutralize acids produced by cariogenic bacteria.[71]

Stimulating Salivary Flow

The concept of stimulating salivary flow as a means to reduce caries seems notionally sound. Saliva has many properties that are beneficial in terms of reducing caries. Saliva contains bicarbonate, a potent buffer to acidic challenges, and also contains calcium and phosphate ions, both of which are useful in terms of remineralizing early carious lesions. Saliva also has a slightly basic pH of 7.4. Saliva washes away sugar-containing foods, serves to dilute and neutralize cariogenic acids, and stocks the dental biofilm with calcium and phosphate ions that help prevent tooth demineralization while encouraging remineralization.

Chewing gum can produce and sustain up to a 10- to 12-fold increase in salivary flow compared with unstimulated salivary flow.[72–74] Stimulated salivary flow has been demonstrated to neutralize acids, clear debris, and return the plaque pH to neutrality.[75–77] Both experimental evidence and expert opinions recommend that sugarless chewing gums, particularly those containing polyols, be utilized multiple times per day in patients at high risk of caries.[45,78,79]

Calcium-Based Remineralization

Remineralization of the tooth utilizing calcium is not a new concept. A classic chemistry equation (see Figure 3) describes the relationship between bacterial acids and the eventual release of calcium and phosphate ions into the plaque and eventually the saliva. Increasing calcium and phosphate ion concentrations proximate to the tooth helps prevent demineralization and may force remineralization by the law of mass action.[80] Calcium-containing products have been recommended for decades in the wake of in vitro data that demonstrated the filling of exposed dentinal tubules treated with calcium hydroxide.[81] A key problem associated with local application of calcium hydroxide is its high solubility in water and saliva.

In more recent decades, numerous calcium-based desensitizing products have appeared. In the early 1990s, an amorphous calcium phosphate (ACP)–based dentifrice became commercially available. It contained sodium fluoride, calcium salts, and phosphate salts. Calcium hydroxide was separated from the phosphate and fluoride by a plastic divider inside the tube to prevent chemical interactions while stored. In an 8-week clinical trial, the product was shown to reduce sensitivity

Figure 3. Relationship of Bacterial Acids to Calcium and Phosphate Ions

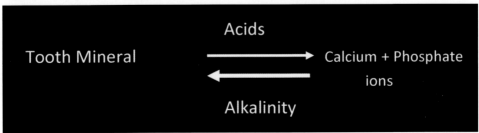

Source: Image courtesy of the Colgate-Palmolive Company.

about as well as nondentifrice products available at the time.[82] ACP has recently been incorporated into a commercially available dentifrice that also contains bicarbonate. ACP is also included in a number of prophylactic polishing pastes and dental varnishes.

In the late 1990s, a calcium-based remineralizing product was introduced that demonstrated desensitization capabilities as both a toothpaste and a prophylaxis paste. This product is an arginine bicarbonate/calcium carbonate compound (formally known as Cavistat™, Ortek Therapeutics, Garden City, NY, USA) that can be incorporated into multiple delivery platforms to assist in mineralization. It is currently available on the market in many countries in dentifrice form (Colgate Maximum Cavity Protection Plus Sugar Acid Neutralizer™, Colgate-Palmolive Company, New York, NY, USA). The mechanism of action is described as follows:

The highly soluble arginine bicarbonate component surrounds, or is surrounded by, particles of less soluble calcium carbonate, and because of the adhesive qualities of this composition, forms a paste-like plug that not only fills but also adheres to the dentinal tubule walls. Because of its alkalinity, the arginine bicarbonate/calcium carbonate also reacts with the calcium and phosphate ions of the dentinal fluid to make the plug chemically contiguous with the dentinal walls.[83]

Twice-daily self-application of the dentifrice containing arginine bicarbonate/calcium carbonate achieved similar results in clinical trials. Two studies, including one double-blind, placebo-controlled study utilizing a chewable mint and a cohort-controlled study of a Cavistat™-containing dentifrice, demonstrated reductions in new decayed, missing, filled surfaces (DMFS), as well as reversals of early carious lesions.[84,85] Subsequently, a similar 1.5% arginine carbonate/insoluble calcium carbonate compound has been incorporated into a commercial dentifrice and has demonstrated both remineralization of early lesions and caries-preventive capabilities.[69,70]

Also in late 1990s, another calcium-based remineralizing technology became available. This technology addressed the problem of stabilizing amorphous calcium phosphate under neutral or alkaline conditions in an effort to increase the plaque content of calcium and phosphate. This goal was achieved by the development of a casein phosphopeptide linked to amorphous calcium phosphate (CPP-ACP; Recaldent™, Cadbury Enterprises Pte Ltd, Parsippany, NJ, USA).[86] This product, in a series of in situ studies, has demonstrated the ability to remineralize enamel that was previously demineralized.[87] The effectiveness of the CPP-ACP product in reducing dentin hypersensitivity was demonstrated utilizing a dentifrice delivery system. In a small study of patients with Sjögren's syndrome, a casein derivative coupled with calcium phosphate was used to slightly reduce the caries incidence without a statistically significant difference being noted.[88] A 2,720-patient, 2-year, double-blind clinical study used digital bitewing radiographs to assess the progression or regression of interproximal caries in adolescent subjects chewing a sugar-free gum containing CPP-ACP. Caries progression or regression was analyzed and, for subjects chewing the CPP-ACP gum, the odds of a surface experiencing caries progression were 18% less than for those chewing a control gum.[89] In 2010, a study using light-induced fluorescence analyzed the effects of CPP-ACP on demineralized white spots after orthodontic treatment. No apparent differences in remineralization were observed when compared with controls.[90] Another study found that patients with xerostomia who used a supersaturated $Ca^{2+}/PO_4^{(3-)}$ and fluoride-containing rinse demonstrated significantly fewer caries than those who did not use a fluoride-containing rinse. Unfortunately fluoride usage was a confounding variable in this study.[91]

CONCLUSION

Decisions related to reducing caries risk must be simple, cost-effective, and individualized. All recommendations start with an understanding of what causes the disease. The consistent use of a fluoride-containing dentifrice, professionally applied high-concentration fluoride applications (e.g., fluoride varnishes), and at-home supplemental fluorides (e.g., 5,000 ppm sodium fluoride) are the cornerstones of most evidence-based oral health recommendations. This includes proper toothbrushing technique and regular brushing habits. Dietary issues must also be considered by encouraging patients to tightly limit the frequency of highly fermentable carbohydrate intake. This may require major and lifelong changes to familial habits.

Patients at high risk for developing caries should substitute polyols, particularly xylitol (at a minimum of 6 grams per day), for sugar where possible so as to gain the benefits of decreased bacterial acids as well as the inhibitory effects of xylitol on cariogenic bacteria. Antimicrobial rinses, such as those that contain chlorhexidine, should be approached with caution because evidence for anticaries effectiveness is weak and because chlorhexidine rinses are expensive and can cause side effects such as tooth staining and taste alteration. However, for patients who have developed or are at risk for root caries, the use of chlorhexidine-containing varnishes should be considered. The use of calcium-containing pastes should only be considered in patients who are at the highest risk and *never* as a substitute for a fluoride-containing dentifrice. Unfortunately, the incorporation of calcium into fluoride dentifrices may alter the anticaries capabilities of the fluoride ions. These dentifrices should undergo additional clinical studies to support the hypothesis that calcium compounds do not reduce the effectiveness the fluorides.

In closing, clinicians need to fully appreciate that non-fluoride anticaries preventive interventions or remineralization agents should almost always be considered as adjunctive to therapies aimed at patients for whom quality self-care and the full use of a wide range of fluoride-containing products does not seem to be enough to eliminate or otherwise control dental caries.

Dr. Mark Wolff is a paid consultant, lecturer, and researcher for the Colgate-Palmolive Company and C3-Jian, Inc.
Dr. Michael Rethman is a paid consultant for the Colgate-Palmolive Company and Interleukin Genetics Inc.

REFERENCES

1. Marinho VC, Higgins JP, Sheiham A, Logan S. Combinations of topical fluoride (toothpastes, mouthrinses, gels, varnishes) versus single topical fluoride for preventing dental caries in children and adolescents. *Cochrane Database Syst Rev.* 2004;(1):CD002781.
2. Marinho VC, Worthington HV, Walsh T, Clarkson JE. Fluoride varnishes for preventing dental caries in children and adolescents. *Cochrane Database Syst Rev.* 2013;(7):CD002279.
3. Featherstone JD. Delivery challenges for fluoride, chlorhexidine and xylitol. *BMC Oral Health.* 2006;6(suppl 1):S8.
4. Beltran-Aguilar ED, Barker LK, Canto MT, et al. Surveillance for dental caries, dental sealants, tooth retention, edentulism, and enamel fluorosis—United States, 1988–1994 and 1999–2002. *MMWR Surveill Summ.* 2005;54(3):1–43.
5. Twetman S. Treatment protocols: nonfluoride management of the caries disease process and available diagnostics. *Dent Clin North Am.* 2010;54:527–540.
6. Miller WD. *The Micro-Organisms of the Human Mouth; the Local and General Diseases Which Are Caused by Them.* Basel, Switzerland: S. Karger; 1973.
7. Stephan RM. Changes in hydrogen ion concentration or tooth surfaces and in carious lesions. *J Am Dent Assoc.* 1940;27:718–723.
8. Stephan RM. Intra oral hydrogen ion concentrations associated with dental caries activity. *J Dent Res.* 1944;23:257–266.
9. Kleinberg I. Formation and accumulation of acid on the tooth surface. *J Dent Res.* 1970;49:1300–1317.
10. Kleinberg I, Jenkins GN, Chatterjee R, Wijeyeweera L. The antimony pH electrode and its role in the assessment and interpretation of dental plaque pH. *J Dent Res.* 1982;61:1139–1147.
11. Marsh P, Martin M. *Oral Microbiology.* 3rd ed. London, England: Chapman & Hall; 1992.
12. Marsh PD, Bradshaw DJ. Dental plaque as a biofilm. *J Ind Microbiol.* 1995;15:169–175.
13. Wolff MS, Larson C. The cariogenic dental biofilm: good, bad or just something to control? *Braz Oral Res.* 2009;23(suppl 1):31–38.
14. Sreebny LM, Schwartz SS. A reference guide to drugs and dry mouth—2nd edition. *Gerodontology.* 1997;14:33–47.
15. Mandel ID. The functions of saliva. *J Dent Res.* 1987;66(special no.):623–627.
16. Kleinberg I, Kanapka J, Chatterjee R, et al. Metabolism of nitrogen by mixed bacteria. In: Kleinberg I, Ellison SA, Mandel ID, eds. *Proceedings: Saliva and Caries.* Special Supplement, *Microbiology Abstracts.* New York, NY: Information Retrieval; 1979:357–377.
17. Kleinberg I, Chatterjee R, Denepetya L. Effects of saliva and dietary eating habits on the pH and demineralisation-remineralisation potential of dental plaque. In:

Demineralisation-Remineralisation of the Teeth. Oxford, England: IRL Press; 1983:25–50.
18. Kleinberg I, Kaufman HW, Wolff M. Measurement of tooth hypersensitivity and oral factors involved in its development. *Arch Oral Biol.* 1994;39(suppl):63S–71S.
19. Featherstone JD, Holmen L, Thylstrup A, Fredebo L, Shariati M. Chemical and histological changes during development of artificial caries. *Caries Res.* 1985;19:1–10.
20. Featherstone JD, Cutress TW, Rodgers BE, Dennison PJ. Remineralization of artificial caries-like lesions in vivo by a self-administered mouthrinse or paste. *Caries Res.* 1982;16:235–242.
21. Smiech-Slomkowska G, Jablonska-Zrobek J. The effect of oral health education on dental plaque development and the level of caries-related *Streptococcus mutans* and *Lactobacillus* spp. *Eur J Orthod.* 2007;29:157–160.
22. Hujoel PP, Cunha-Cruz J, Banting DW, Loesche WJ. Dental flossing and interproximal caries: a systematic review. *J Dent Res.* 2006;85:298–305.
23. Marinho VC, Higgins JP, Sheiham A, Logan S. Fluoride toothpastes for preventing dental caries in children and adolescents. *Cochrane Database Syst Rev.* 2003;(1):CD002278.
24. Gustafsson BE, Quensel CE, Lanke LS, et al. The Vipeholm dental caries study; the effect of different levels of carbohydrate intake on caries activity in 436 individuals observed for five years. *Acta Odontol Scand.* 1954;11:232–264.
25. Krasse B. The Vipeholm Dental Caries Study: recollections and reflections 50 years later. *J Dent Res.* 2001;80:1785–1788.
26. Newbrun E. Frequent sugar intake—then and now: interpretation of the main results. *Scand J Dent Res.* 1989;97:103–109.
27. Moynihan PJ, Kelly SA. Effect on caries of restricting sugars intake: systematic review to inform WHO guidelines. *J Dent Res.* 2014;93:8–18.
28. Sheiham A, James WP. A new understanding of the relationship between sugars, dental caries and fluoride use: implications for limits on sugars consumption. *Public Health Nutr.* 2014;17:2176–2184.
29. Sheiham A, James WP. Diet and dental caries: The pivotal role of free sugars reemphasized. *J Dent Res.* 2015;94:1341–1347.
30. Gaffar A, Afflitto J, Nabi N. Chemical agents for the control of plaque and plaque microflora: an overview. *Eur J Oral Sci.* 1997;105(5 pt 2):502–507.
31. Scheie AA, Fejerskov O, Assev S, Rolla G. Ultrastructural changes in *Streptococcus sobrinus* induced by xylitol, NaF and ZnCl2. *Caries Res.* 1989;23:320–327.
32. Glass RL, Rothman KJ, Espinal F, Velez H, Smith NJ. The prevalence of human dental caries and water-borne trace metals. *Arch Oral Biol.* 1973;18:1099–1104.
33. Navia JM. Evaluation of nutritional and dietary factors that modify animal caries. *J Dent Res.* 1970;49:1213–1228.
34. Walker CB. Microbiological effects of mouthrinses containing antimicrobials. *J Clin Periodontol.* 1988;15:499–505.
35. Charles CH, Vincent JW, Borycheski L, et al. Effect of an essential oil-containing dentifrice on dental plaque microbial composition. *Am J Dent.* 2000;13(special no.):26C–30C.
36. Fine DH, Furgang D, Barnett ML, et al. Effect of an essential oil-containing antiseptic mouthrinse on plaque and salivary *Streptococcus mutans* levels. *J Clin Periodontol.* 2000;27:157–161.
37. Lobo PL, Fonteles CS, Marques LA, et al. The efficacy of three formulations of *Lippia sidoides Cham.* essential oil in the reduction of salivary *Streptococcus mutans* in children with caries: a randomized, double-blind, controlled study. *Phytomedicine.* 2014;21:1043–1047.
38. Gjermo P, Saxton CA. Antibacterial dentifrices. Clinical data and relevance with emphasis on zinc/triclosan. *J Clin Periodontol.* 1991;18:468–473.
39. Mann J, Vered Y, Babayof I, et al. The comparative anticaries efficacy of a dentifrice containing 0.3% triclosan and 2.0% copolymer in a 0.243% sodium fluoride/silica base and a dentifrice containing 0.243% sodium fluoride/silica base: a two-year coronal caries clinical trial on adults in Israel. *J Clin Dent.* 2001;12:71–76.
40. Vered Y, Zini A, Mann J, et al. Comparison of a dentifrice containing 0.243% sodium fluoride, 0.3% triclosan, and 2.0% copolymer in a silica base, and a dentifrice containing 0.243% sodium fluoride in a silica base: a three-year clinical trial of root caries and dental crowns among adults. *J Clin Dent.* 2009;20:62–65.
41. Riley P, Lamont T. Triclosan/copolymer containing toothpastes for oral health. *Cochrane Database Syst Rev.* 2013;(12):CD010514.
42. Rosenblatt A, Stamford TC, Niederman R. Silver diamine fluoride: a caries "silver-fluoride bullet". *J Dent Res.* 2009;88:116–125.
43. Zhang W, McGrath C, Lo EC, Li JY. Silver diamine fluoride and education to prevent and arrest root caries among community-dwelling elders. *Caries Res.* 2013;47:284–290.
44. Ribeiro LG, Hashizume LN, Maltz M. The effect of different formulations of chlorhexidine in reducing levels of mutans streptococci in the oral cavity: A systematic review of the literature. *J Dent.* 2007;35:359–370.
45. Rethman MP, Beltran-Aguilar ED, Billings RJ, et al. Nonfluoride caries-preventive agents: executive summary of evidence-based clinical recommendations. *J Am Dent Assoc.* 2011;142:1065–1071.
46. Petti S, Hausen H. Caries-preventive effect of chlorhexidine gel applications among high-risk children. *Caries Res.* 2006;40:514–521.
47. Baca P, Clavero J, Baca AP, Gonzalez-Rodriguez MP, Bravo M, Valderrama MJ. Effect of chlorhexidine-thymol varnish on root caries in a geriatric population: a randomized double-blind clinical trial. *J Dent.* 2009;37:679–685.
48. Brailsford SR, Fiske J, Gilbert S, Clark D, Beighton D. The effects of the combination of chlorhexidine/thymol- and fluoride-containing varnishes on the severity of root

caries lesions in frail institutionalised elderly people. *J Dent.* 2002;30:319–324.
49. Tan HP, Lo EC, Dyson JE, Luo Y, Corbet EF. A randomized trial on root caries prevention in elders. *J Dent Res.* 2010;89:1086–1090.
50. Dodds MW. The oral health benefits of chewing gum. *J Irish Dent Assoc.* 2012;58:253–261.
51. Van Loveren C. Sugar alcohols: what is the evidence for caries-preventive and caries-therapeutic effects? *Caries Res.* 2004;38:286–293.
52. Milgrom P, Ly KA, Roberts MC, Rothen M, Mueller G, Yamaguchi DK. Mutans streptococci dose response to xylitol chewing gum. *J Dent Res.* 2006;85:177–181.
53. Maguire A, Rugg-Gunn AJ. Xylitol and caries prevention—is it a magic bullet? *Br Dent J.* 2003;194:429–436.
54. Alanen P, Isokangas P, Gutmann K. Xylitol candies in caries prevention: results of a field study in Estonian children. *Community Dent Oral Epidemiol.* 2000;28:218–224.
55. Honkala E, Honkala S, Shyama M, Al-Mutawa SA. Field trial on caries prevention with xylitol candies among disabled school students. *Caries Res.* 2006;40:508–513.
56. Isokangas P, Soderling E, Pienihakkinen K, Alanen P. Occurrence of dental decay in children after maternal consumption of xylitol chewing gum, a follow-up from 0 to 5 years of age. *J Dent Res.* 2000;79:1885–1889.
57. Riley P, Moore D, Ahmed F, Sharif MO, Worthington HV. Xylitol-containing products for preventing dental caries in children and adults. *Cochrane Database Syst Rev.* 2015;(3):CD010743.
58. Kovari H, Pienihakkinen K, Alanen P. Use of xylitol chewing gum in daycare centers: a follow-up study in Savonlinna, Finland. *Acta Odontol Scand.* 2003;61:367–370.
59. Oscarson P, Lif Holgerson P, Sjostrom I, Twetman S, Stecksen-Blicks C. Influence of a low xylitol-dose on mutans streptococci colonisation and caries development in preschool children. *Eur Arch Paediatr Dent.* 2006;7:142–147.
60. Jeon JG, Klein MI, Xiao J, Gregoire S, Rosalen PL, Koo H. Influences of naturally occurring agents in combination with fluoride on gene expression and structural organization of *Streptococcus mutans* in biofilms. *BMC Microbiol.* 2009;9:228.
61. Koo H, Jeon JG. Naturally occurring molecules as alternative therapeutic agents against cariogenic biofilms. *Adv Dent Res.* 2009;21:63–68.
62. Leung KP, Abercrombie JJ, Campbell TM, et al. Antimicrobial peptides for plaque control. *Adv Dent Res.* 2009;21:57–62.
63. Eckert R, He J, Yarbrough DK, Qi F, Anderson MH, Shi W. Targeted killing of *Streptococcus mutans* by a pheromone-guided "smart" antimicrobial peptide. *Antimicrob Agents Chemother.* 2006;50:3651–3657.
64. Guo L, McLean JS, Yang Y, et al. Precision-guided antimicrobial peptide as a targeted modulator of human microbial ecology. *Proc Natl Acad Sci U S A.* 2015;112:7569–7574.
65. Caufield PW, Dasanayake AP, Li Y, Pan Y, Hsu J, Hardin JM. Natural history of *Streptococcus sanguinis* in the oral cavity of infants: evidence for a discrete window of infectivity. *Infect Immun.* 2000;68:4018–4023.
66. Cummins D. Dental caries: a disease which remains a public health concern in the 21st century—the exploration of a breakthrough technology for caries prevention. *J Clin Dent.* 2013;24(special no. A):A1–14.
67. Wolff M, Corby P, Klaczany G, et al. In vivo effects of a new dentifrice containing 1.5% arginine and 1450 ppm fluoride on plaque metabolism. *J Clin Dent.* 2013;24(special no. A):A45–54.
68. Kleinberg I. A new saliva-based anticaries composition. *Dent Today.* 1999;18:98–103.
69. Yin W, Hu DY, Fan X, et al. A clinical investigation using quantitative light-induced fluorescence (QLF) of the anticaries efficacy of a dentifrice containing 1.5% arginine and 1450 ppm fluoride as sodium monofluorophosphate. *J Clin Dent.* 2013;24(special no. A):A15–22.
70. Hu DY, Yin W, Li X, et al. A clinical investigation of the efficacy of a dentifrice containing 1.5% arginine and 1450 ppm fluoride, as sodium monofluorophosphate in a calcium base, on primary root caries. *J Clin Dent.* 2013;24(special no. A):A23–31.
71. ten Cate JM, Cummins D. Fluoride toothpaste containing 1.5% arginine and insoluble calcium as a new standard of care in caries prevention. *J Clin Dent.* 2013;24:79–87.
72. Dawes C. The unstimulated salivary flow rate after prolonged gum chewing. *Arch Oral Biol.* 2005;50:561–563.
73. Dawes C, Kubieniec K. The effects of prolonged gum chewing on salivary flow rate and composition. *Arch Oral Biol.* 2004;49:665–669.
74. Dawes C, Macpherson LM. Effects of nine different chewing-gums and lozenges on salivary flow rate and pH. *Caries Res.* 1992;26:176–182.
75. Dodds MW, Hsieh SC, Johnson DA. The effect of increased mastication by daily gum-chewing on salivary gland output and dental plaque acidogenicity. *J Dent Res.* 1991;70:1474–1478.
76. Fu Y, Li X, Ma H, et al. Assessment of chewing sugar-free gums for oral debris reduction: a randomized controlled crossover clinical trial. *Am J Dent.* 2012;25: 118–122.
77. Jenkins GN, Edgar WM. The effect of daily gum-chewing on salivary flow rates in man. *J Dent Res.* 1989;68:786–790.
78. Deshpande A, Jadad AR. The impact of polyol-containing chewing gums on dental caries: a systematic review of original randomized controlled trials and observational studies. *J Am Dent Assoc.* 2008;139:1602–1614.
79. Mickenautsch S, Leal SC, Yengopal V, Bezerra AC, Cruvinel V. Sugar-free chewing gum and dental caries: a systematic review. *J Appl Oral Sci.* 2007;15:83–88.
80. Voit EO, Martens HA, Omholt SW. 150 years of the

mass action law. *PLoS Comput Biol.* 2015;11:e1004012.
81. Brannstrom M, Isacsson G, Johnson G. The effect of calcium hydroxide and fluorides on human dentine. *Acta Odontol Scand.* 1976;34:59–67.
82. Kaufman HW, Wolff MS, Winston AE, Triol CW. Clinical evaluation of the effect of a remineralizing toothpaste on dentinal sensitivity. *J Clin Dent.* 1999;10(1 special no.):50–54.
83. Kleinberg I. SensiStat. A new saliva-based composition for simple and effective treatment of dentinal sensitivity pain. *Dent Today.* 2002;21:42–47.
84. Acevedo AM, Machado C, Rivera LE, Wolff M, Kleinberg I. The inhibitory effect of an arginine bicarbonate/calcium carbonate CaviStat-containing dentifrice on the development of dental caries in Venezuelan school children. *J Clin Dent.* 2005;16:63–70.
85. Acevedo AM, Montero M, Rojas-Sanchez F, et al. Clinical evaluation of the ability of CaviStat in a mint confection to inhibit the development of dental caries in children. *J Clin Dent.* 2008;19:1–8.
86. Reynolds EC. Anticariogenic complexes of amorphous calcium phosphate stabilized by casein phosphopeptides: a review. *Spec Care Dentist* 1998;18:8–16.
87. Cai F, Shen P, Morgan MV, Reynolds EC. Remineralization of enamel subsurface lesions in situ by sugar-free lozenges containing casein phosphopeptide-amorphous calcium phosphate. *Aust Dent J.* 2003;48:240–243.
88. Hay KD, Thomson WM. A clinical trial of the anticaries efficacy of casein derivatives complexed with calcium phosphate in patients with salivary gland dysfunction. *Oral Surg Oral Med Oral Pathol Oral Radiol Endod.* 2002;93:271–275.
89. Morgan MV, Adams GG, Bailey DL, Tsao CE, Fischman SL, Reynolds EC. The anticariogenic effect of sugar-free gum containing CPP-ACP nanocomplexes on approximal caries determined using digital bitewing radiography. *Caries Res.* 2008;42:171–184.
90. Beerens MW, van der Veen MH, van Beek H, ten Cate JM. Effects of casein phosphopeptide amorphous calcium fluoride phosphate paste on white spot lesions and dental plaque after orthodontic treatment: a 3-month follow-up. *Eur J Oral Sci.* 2010;118:610–617.
91. Singh ML, Papas AS. Long-term clinical observation of dental caries in salivary hypofunction patients using a supersaturated calcium-phosphate remineralizing rinse. *J Clin Dent.* 2009;20:87–92.

Chapter 16
Chemotherapeutic Agents

Harlan J. Shiau and Louis G. DePaola

At the patient level, prevention of the major oral maladies, caries and periodontitis, requires clinician-inspired health literacy and instruction in essential home care. The prevention of dental caries seeks to stem the development of incipient lesions. Primary prevention of periodontal diseases, including gingivitis, focuses on thwarting their clinical onset. Secondary prevention, especially in the context of chronic periodontitis, aims to avoid progression or exacerbation of the conditions. At the individual level, oral hygiene is the single most effective means for prevention of periodontal disease, and it also has a crucial role in dental caries prevention.

Chemotherapeutics is a general term often used to designate the application of an active compound or agent with intended beneficial clinical effects. For example, in the treatment of periodontal diseases, such as aggressive or chronic periodontitis, this entails adjunctive use of antimicrobials or antibiotics.[1] Chemotherapeutics, in the context of prevention, refers to a strategy of employing active compounds to counter disease onset or recurrence. The term *chemotherapeutics* is also used to contrast mechanical approaches to oral disease prevention. Specifically, plaque biofilm is an etiologic agent of both caries and periodontal diseases; mechanical removal or reduction of supragingival and subgingival plaque, whether professionally or by the individual, is the intervention target. With that same end goal in mind, chemical plaque-control agents are commonly used in the management of caries and periodontal disease—whether for prevention or treatment. As discussed later in this chapter, targeting the etiology is but one of the available approaches in preventive chemotherapeutics.

KEY CONSIDERATIONS
Clinical Evaluation of Preventive Chemotherapeutics

Published studies in the 1960s bolstered the view that routine removal of plaque was essential to establish and maintain oral health. Mechanical toothbrushing and flossing was universally accepted by the profession to this end; when properly and precisely performed, mechanical practices proved sufficient.[2] However, most patients do not adequately brush and floss effectively and do not remove dental plaque on a daily basis. An amount of manual dexterity is needed to achieve qualitatively acceptable results for mechanical therapy, as well as a patient commitment to the necessary time to achieve acceptable results. Furthermore, physical removal of plaque biofilm is often challenging in difficult-to-access regions of the mouth, and in the presence of anatomical contributing factors (furcations, malpositioned teeth, developmental grooves, cervical enamel projections, etc.) or iatrogenic factors (poorly contoured restorations, overhanging crown margins, etc.). A final consideration is that beyond the hard surfaces of teeth—the customary target of mechanical home care—there exist additional sites of bacterial colonization in the mouth, such as the dorsum of the tongue and oral mucosal sites.[3]

In the early 1980s, chemotherapeutic agents were introduced as adjuncts to brushing and flossing. It should be noted, however, that these agents, often dispensed in the vehicle of an oral rinse, had historically been in use for centuries; only in modern history have attempts been made to adjudicate clinical claims in a systematic manner. In fact, the historic formulations in many instances were perhaps reasonable in their concept but questionable in their intended biological activity. In the early twentieth century, some advocated use of compounds, such as sulfuric acid, mercuric chloride, and formaldehyde, which had the potential to induce local damage or systemic toxicity.[4]

Thus, guidelines for evaluating the safety and efficacy of putative chemotherapeutic agents became necessary. In 1985 the American Dental Association (ADA) recognized the need and potential benefits of some chemotherapeutic formulations, giving rise to the development and publication of guidelines for the evaluation of antiplaque and antigingivitis chemotherapeutic agents. Even today, these parameters serve a crucial role to protect the public by ensuring safety and utility of clinical agents and their claims; guidelines have been established to provide appropriate preclinical and clinical support[5] (see Figure 1).

This comprehensive set of criteria requires that a study population of typical product users be evaluated in a randomized, parallel group that is active or placebo-controlled. Two 6-month studies, conducted at independent sites, are required, with qualitative and quantitative sampling performed at baseline, an intermediate point (usually 3 months), and 6 months. Documentation of a significant reduction of plaque and gingivitis is required to demonstrate product efficacy as compared

Figure 1. Recognition and Regulatory Process of Antigingivitis Chemotherapeutic Properties in the United States

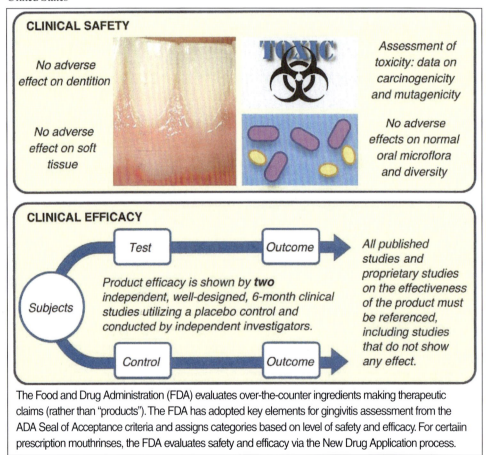

Sources: American Dental Association, Council on Scientific Affairs Acceptance Program;[5] and *Periodontol 2000.* 2002;28:91–105.[6]

with a control. In addition to efficacy, each agent has to establish safety of the formulation, which mandates microbiological profiles to evaluate possible adverse shifts in microbial populations and resistance, as well as toxicological testing. Notably in the United States, the Food and Drug Administration has accepted the ADA guidelines for determination of over-the-counter products that reduce or prevent dental plaque and gingivitis.[6]

Overview of Active Agents of Chemotherapeutics

Conceptually, active agents target the etiologic agent—plaque bacteria—or confer a defensive advantage to the host. The former approach describes the majority of prevalently used or prescribed preventive chemotherapeutics. As has been described earlier in the chapter, this is not surprising given the established pathogenesis paradigms of caries, gingivitis, and destructive periodontal disease. Table 1 presents the major strategies employed by chemotherapeutic agents. Note that some groups, such as antibiotics or the host-modulation approach, are not used in *preventive* applications.[7] Other strategic approaches, such as antiadhesive agents, lack any relevant examples with robust clinical support for efficacy. The majority of commercially available preventive chemotherapeutic products, to date, follow an *antiseptic* approach. Some preclinical data exist indicating that these chemotherapeutics exhibit additional properties—such as anti-inflammatory properties or the ability to interfere with plaque colonization—that might contribute to overall efficacy.[8]

By definition, antimicrobials that are antiseptic in nature aim to kill or prevent proliferation of bacteria within the plaque biofilm. There are, of course, many antiseptic agents or specific formulations of agents in existence not appropriated for intraoral use. The literature is replete with applications such as surgical wound management, patient perioperative skin preparation, standard hand washing, and general hard-surface asepsis. Antiseptics are an indispensable part of infection control practices and help in the prevention of nosocomial infections.[9] In spite of their usage, less is known about antiseptics relative to antibiotics. In the United States, a recent Food and Drug Administration advisory committee cautiously seeks more scientific data on safety and effectiveness of active ingredients of antiseptics present in hand soaps in response to concerns. Because of the inherent biological activity of these chemotherapeutics, the conventional wisdom is that evidence-based safety in the context of oral application must be established.

Safety of Active Agents in Preventive Chemotherapeutics

In the context of *intraoral* chemotherapeutics, investigations have addressed the safety and compatibility of long-term use. Pragmatic safety concerns include effect on existing biomaterials in the mouth, whether aesthetic or functional, and generation of xerostomia-like

Table 1. Major Strategies for Effective Chemotherapeutic Agents

Antimicrobials: Target the Biofilm					Host Modulation: Attenuates Disease Pathogenesis
Antiseptic	**Antibiotic**	**Enzyme or Dispersal Agent**		**Antiadhesive**	**Antiproteinase, anti-inflammatory or bone sparing strategies**
Broad-spectrum chemical agents that slow or stop the growth of microorganisms	Agents capable of killing and inhibiting growth of specific microorganisms, such as infectious bacteria and fungi	Alters the structure or the metabolic activity of plaque biofilm		Interferes with bacteria attachment to aquired pellicle or bacterial coaggregation	Agent provides interference to key components of disease pathogenesis

conditions. But perhaps the concerns with the most potential for patient harm and morbidity are the following: (1) Do active agents in preventive chemotherapeutics have an adverse effect on the balance of commensal oral microflora? (2) Do active agents damage the soft tissues or increase risk for oral or oropharyngeal cancer? (see Figure 2).[10,11]

Effect of Preventive Chemotherapeutic Use on Microbial Diversity

Do preventive chemotherapeutics have an adverse impact on the normal microbial diversity and dynamics of the oral cavity? The selective killing or inhibition of flora followed by repopulation with opportunistic organisms, including those that are more pathogenic and resistant, is not desirable. There are concerns that opportunistic organisms such as *Candida* might thrive in long-term routine use of antiseptic-type chemotherapeutics. Studies document no adverse effects on supragingival dental plaque microflora after 6 months of continued use with either a mixture of combination essential oil mouthrinse (CEOM) or 0.12% chlorhexidine gluconate (CHX).[12–14] In a long-term study over more than 6 months, dental plaque was harvested at baseline, at midpoint, and at the end of the trial. The microbial organisms and quantitative data were collected and the minimum inhibitory concentration (MIC) for isolates was determined. The routine use of CEOM and CHX on a long-term basis (6 months) was not associated with adverse shifts in plaque ecology, the emergence of opportunistic pathogens, the

Figure 2. Summary of Safety Concerns for Major Preventive Use of Chemotherapeutic Agents

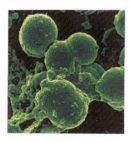

Does the use of preventive chemotherapeutic agents cause adverse outcomes to the diversity and dynamics of the oral microflora?
- Studies indicate that active agents EO, CHX, and triclosan do not cause undue harm to the oral microbiota diversity.
- To date there is little to no evidence that bacterial resistance develops with long–term use of active agents, for example, such as triclosan.

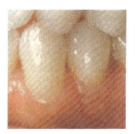

Does the use of alcohol-containing preventive chemotherapeutic agents cause adverse effects to the oral mucosa, such as cancer?
- The association between alcohol and cancer fuels speculation into putative relationships between alcohol-containing rinses and carcinoma.
- An appraisal of evidence finds that the routine use of alcohol-containing mouthrinse (ACM) **does not** cause oral cancer.

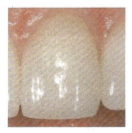

Does the use of preventive chemotherapeutic agents cause structural damage to restorative materials?
- In vitro studies have evaluated exposure of various biomaterials to common actiive agents, such as EO-containing mouthrinses.
- Outcome measures of resin hardness, resin bond strength, and porosity were evaluated in these experiments; no significant adverse effects were noted.
- Extrinsic staining is a known side effect of active agents such as CHX and CPC.

Sources: J Dent Hygiene. 2007;81(5) and *Ann Agric Environ Med.* 2012;19:173–180.[10,11]

emergence of resistance strains, or changes in microbial susceptibility.[14]

Triclosan is an antimicrobial agent used in consumer preventive products to reduce dental plaque, gingivitis, and oral malodor. This broad-spectrum chemotherapeutic has utility against gram-positive and gram-negative bacteria, fungi, and yeasts. Triclosan has been used in oral preventive applications since the 1980s in Europe and subsequently beginning in the 1990s in the United States. Notably, the body of science evaluating triclosan safety is substantial because of applications in nonoral consumer products for skincare, cosmetics, deodorants/antiperspirants, and even products such as clothing, utensils, trash bags, and toys.[15] With its prolific use, one area of concern raised is the development of bacterial resistance; there have been studies related to this concern in oral preventive applications. Multiple clinical trials 6 months in duration[16-18] and a long-term community assessment, with plaque samples collected over 19 years,[19] have found no evidence of unfavorable shifts in bacteria and no evidence of development of bacterial resistance to the active agent, triclosan. Plaque samples collected from participants in a 5-year clinical, randomized control trial have also yielded similar conclusions.[20] The use of the triclosan dentifrice does not increase triclosan MICs for oral bacteria and does not result in triclosan-resistant oral bacteria.

Potential toxicity of triclosan is a secondary safety concern raised, as the mechanism of triclosan is to disrupt cell cytoplasmic membranes. Reviewed human safety studies on the use of triclosan-containing dentifrice or rinses, measuring hematological and clinical chemistry, reveal no difference compared with controls.[21] Rodricks and colleagues confirm safety of triclosan, and present a comprehensive review detailing acute and chronic toxicity studies, issues of pharmacokinetics, and effects on carcinogenesis.[21] Furthermore, triclosan has not been found to be a dermal or oral mucosal irritant.[22]

Available research does not support the notion that the CEOM group of antiseptic agents can induce significant bacterial resistance.[23] The potential for a selective increase of *Streptococcus mutans*, with a possible negative impact on caries rate, was addressed by Fine and colleagues.[24] In this randomized crossover study, 29 adults with recoverable salivary *S. mutans* levels were evaluated after rinsing with CEOM-containing mouthrinse versus placebo. Recoverable *S. mutans* counts from interproximal spaces were reduced by 75.4% with the essential oil compared with the control. Total streptococci in interproximal plaque were reduced by 69.9%, and activity of the essential oil was 37.1% greater against *S. mutans* than against other streptococci.[24] The data clearly document a reduction rather than an increase of *S. mutans*. While there is no intentional claim of anticariogenicity of CEOM rinses, there certainly appears to be no increase in caries risk with routine use. Interestingly, recent clinical research has proposed the alternative use of CEOM-type antiseptics *in response* to trends of increasing drug-resistant bacteria. The combination of phytochemicals, such as essential oils, with traditional systemic antibiotics has been proposed; in vitro studies have shown synergism or additive effects when these combinations are used together.[23] Further research is needed to build on the possibility of essential oils being used in an adjunctive manner.

Opportunistic infections, such as fungal overgrowth during long-term antiseptic use, would seem to be a possibility given analogous trends with traditional antibiotic use. Yet, studies seem to indicate the contrary. Antiseptic mouthrinses appear to decrease the levels of viable *Candida* species, for example. In an in vitro investigation, five species of *Candida* (*albicans, dubliniensis, krusei, glabrata,* and *tropicalis*) were grown and treated with CEOM and 0.12% CHX. Antifungal activity was measured, and both agents were found to be effective at commercially available concentrations with comparable inhibition between CEOM and CHX.[25] A series of investigations in patients presenting with denture stomatitis caused by an overgrowth of *C. albicans* and other fungal species in maxillary prostheses documented that rinsing with CEOM twice daily was as effective as nystatin oral suspension in reducing clinical palatal inflammation and candidiasis.[26,27] Thus, rather than promoting fungal growth, antiseptic mouthrinses have substantial antifungal properties, providing a potential benefit. The evidence confirms that daily, long-term use ($\geq$ 6 months) of antiseptic chemotherapeutic CEOM and CHX does not adversely affect the oral microbial flora; there was no microbial overgrowth, opportunistic infection, or development of microbial resistance.

Effects on Oral Mucosal Tissues

A second concern with routine use of preventive chemotherapeutics is adverse effects on oral mucosa. Perhaps the single most cited issue is the potential association of oral pharyngeal cancer and alcohol-containing oral rinses. In many preventive chemotherapeutic rinses, alcohol is a component necessary to solubilize essential oils and other active ingredients. Alcohol is also used in products to dissolve flavoring agents. The range of alcohol in commercially available and over-the-counter products is generally 10% to 27%. Whether the concerns are founded or unfounded, development of low-percentage alcohol-containing products has occurred recently in response to unease about a possible association between alcohol-containing oral rinses and oropharyngeal cancer (see Table 2).[28]

The aforementioned association rests on investigations that find both tobacco usage and beverage alcohol consumption as the traditional risk factors for oropharyngeal cancer.[29–31] Since the majority of preventive oral

Table 2. Composition of Preventive Chemotherapeutic Mouthrinses

Active Agent	Product Examples	OTC	Content	Alcohol (%)
Essential oil-containing mouthwash	Listerine®	Y	• Active ingredient: eucalyptol 0.092%, menthol 0.042%, methyl salicylate 0.06%, thymol 0.064% • Other: water, alcohol, sorbitol, flavoring, poloxamer 407, benzoic acid, sodium saccharin, sodium benzoate, green 3	21.6–26.9
Chlorhexidine (0.12%)*	Peridex®	N	• Active ingredient: chlorhexidine gluconate 0.12% • Other: water, alcohol, glycerin, PEG-40 sorbitan, diisostearate, flavoring, sodium saccharin, coloring	12.6
	Paroex®	N	• Active ingredient: chlorhexidine gluconate 0.12% • Other: water, propylene glycol, glycerin, polyoxyl 40 hydrogenated castor oil, mint flavor, potassium acesulfame, red 40, and red 33	0
Cetylpyridinium chloride (0.07%)	Colgate Total® Rinse	Y	• Active ingredient: cetylpyridinium chloride 0.07% • Other: water, glycerin, flavoring, poloxamer 407, sodium saccharin, methyl paraben, propyl paraben, propolyne glycol, blue 1, yellow 6, and green 3	0
	Crest Pro Health® Multi-Protection	Y	• Active ingredient: cetylpyridinium chloride 0.07% • Other: water, glycerin, flavoring, poloxamer 407, sodium saccharin, methyl paraben, propyl paraben, propolyne glycol, blue 1, yellow 6, and green 3	0
	Scope® (CPC 0.045%)	Y	• Active ingredient: cetylpyridinium chloride 0.045% • Other: water, alcohol, glycerin, flavoring, polysorbate 80, sodium saccharin, sodium benzoate, benzoic acid, blue 1, and yellow 5	15

OTC, over-the-counter product. *Also available in 0.2% formulation, in Europe.

rinses contain alcohol, the logical assumption would be that they potentially increase risk for oropharyngeal cancer as well. Gandini and colleagues identified epidemiological studies of mouthwash and oral cancer/oropharyngeal cancer, and conducted a quantitative meta-analysis.[11] They concluded from the 18 studies that routine mouthwash use and risk of oral cancer had no statistically significant association, or any trend in risk with increasing daily use.

Currie and colleagues reviewed 15 case-control studies evaluating the existence or lack of an association between the use of alcohol-containing mouthrinses and the development of oral squamous cell carcinoma (OSCC).[32] A solid consensus is lacking among these investigations, with six studies indicating positive and statistically significant associations, and nine reporting nonsignificant positive, none, or negative correlations between alcohol-containing mouthwash use and OSCC.

Other important considerations must also be weighed in building any substantial case for alcohol-containing rinses and associations with cancer.[33,34] Evidence-based appraisal of the literature should turn a critical eye to the following issues. First, available studies need to show a dose-response based on frequency or duration of mouthrinse use, or both. Second, studies need to offer a scientific or biological basis for inconsistent findings between men and women. Investigations may need to correct for combined alcoholic beverage ingestion *and* tobacco use. Finally, population data should exclude or at least separate the pharyngeal cancer and other head and neck carcinomas, lymphomas, and sarcomas that occur in regions with no regular oral rinse contact.

APPLICATION TO CLINICAL PRACTICE

This section focuses on the major commercially available or prescription preventive chemotherapeutics, reviewing their mechanism and claims to efficacy. Published systematic reviews are useful when taking steps to consider a particular active agent's effectiveness. Clinicians should be judicious in handling the "bottom line" results of these studies by considering magnitude of the effect, number of available studies, consistency of the results, and heterogeneity.

Chlorhexidine

Chlorhexidine (CHX 0.12%) is a cationic bisbiguanide antiseptic with a broad antimicrobial spectrum, demonstrating efficacy against a wide range of gram-positive and gram-negative organisms.[35] CHX 0.2% is also available as an over-the-counter product in Europe. The cationic property of CHX allows favorable interactions—that is, a strong binding—with anionic cell membrane and wall components. As such, CHX demonstrates inhibitory effects on a wide range of bacteria associated with periodontal disease and caries.[36] CHX also exhibits antiviral activity against herpes simplex viruses 1 and 2, HIV-1, cytomegalovirus, influenza A, human parainfluenza, and hepatitis B.[37,38] Finally, CHX has been shown to demonstrate antifungal properties, of note, against several *Candida* species and others.[39,40] In fact, CHX is often used either alone or in combination with other antifungal medications to reduce opportunistic infections in at-risk populations.[41] CHX binds to cell membranes and disrupts the bacterial cell membrane, catastrophically altering cell permeability.[42] In addition, CHX prevents colonization of plaque bacteria by binding to salivary mucins, which results in a reduced acquired pellicle formation.[43] CHX has high substantivity by binding tightly to tooth structure, dental plaque, and oral soft tissues; high substantivity greatly enhances its antibacterial properties.[44]

Long-term studies (≥ 6 months) have shown CHX is effective in reducing plaque and reducing gingivitis, as has been confirmed in systematic reviews.[45-47] In several controlled trials for periods of 6 months or longer, CHX demonstrated reduction in plaque ranging from 16% to 49%. In another systematic review on the efficacy of CHX in plaque reduction in gingivitis patients, the authors include studies as short as 4 weeks in duration, the rationale being that this duration represents the majority of CHX applications. In this investigation, when used as an adjunct to normal home care, an average of 33% plaque reduction was confirmed as compared with controls.[48] With respect to gingival health, as measured by gingival index, CHX use results in significant improvement.[47] A systematic review of randomized controlled clinical trials lasting 4 weeks or longer and comparing CHX to placebo or control found significant improvement in gingival health, as measured by gingival index scores.[48] The aforementioned trends in plaque and gingivitis reduction associated with CHX use have elevated the status of CHX, which is now considered the gold standard and is used as a positive control in many clinical investigations.

Cetylpyridinium Chloride

Cetylpyridinium chloride (CPC) is an antiseptic agent with evidence supporting effectiveness in preventing supragingival plaque accumulation and reducing signs of gingivitis. CPC is a quaternary ammonium compound that has broad-spectrum antimicrobial properties. In clinical studies, CPC has been primarily evaluated in an oral rinse format. CPC functions by disrupting the bacterial cell membrane, causing leakage of intracellular contents and ultimately cell death.

A 2006 review of long-term (≥ 6 months) studies on CPC efficacy produced equivocal conclusions.[45] A portion of the included studies, four of the seven, reported a statistically significant benefit over the control. A challenge in drawing strong conclusions was the heterogeneity in the type of CPC formulation used and the results.

A second systematic review, which included clinical trials as short as 4 weeks, found that CPC-containing mouthrinses provided a small but significant additional benefit—reducing plaque and gingival inflammation—when compared with toothbrushing only or toothbrushing followed by a placebo rinse.[49] A recent review on oral rinses notes that the limited number of controlled clinical trials investigating the same CPC formulations presents a challenge to issuing clinical recommendations.[50]

Combination Essential Oil

Antiseptics containing essential oils act by disrupting the microorganism cell wall and inhibiting enzymatic activity. Essential oils have been shown to prevent bacterial aggregation and slow bacterial multiplication. Commercially available CEOM is a mixture of thymol 0.063%, eucalyptol 0.091%, and menthol 0.042%, with other ingredients such as methyl salicylate 0.0660%.[51] Phenolic compounds exhibit anti-inflammatory properties by inhibiting prostaglandin synthetase, an enzyme involved in the formation of prostaglandins, which are primary inflammatory mediators. The anti-inflammatory effect occurs at concentrations lower that those needed for antibacterial activity.[52] Phenols, especially thymol, also reduce inflammation by altering neutrophil function, specifically by suppressing the formation of and scavenging existing free radicals generated in neutrophils, and by altering neutrophil chemotaxis.[53]

CEOM bactericidal activity has been demonstrated in situ to penetrate the bacterial biofilm.[51,54,55] CEOM kills a wide variety of aerobic and anaerobic bacteria associated with plaque and gingivitis, including *Actinobacillus actinomycetemcomitans*, *Actinomyces viscosus*, *Streptococcus sanguis*, *S. mutans*, and *Bacteroides* species.[56] Efficacy against gram-positive and gram-negative organisms occurs even at concentrations that are less than full strength.[56,57] A single 30-second rinse penetrates and exerts an antibacterial effect interproximally; this is an important consideration, given that periodontal disease and caries patterns initiate interproximally, and that patients usually demonstrate inadequate mechanical interproximal plaque control. The total recovered bacteria from proximal tooth surfaces was 43.8% lower following a single 30-second rinse of CEOM compared with a control ($P = 0.001$).[58] Rinsing twice daily with CEOM as an adjunct to brushing for 11 days reduced total recoverable streptococci in interproximal plaque by 69.9% ($P < 0.001$), with CEOM producing a 37.1% greater activity against *S. mutans* than other streptococci. A significant reduction of 75.4% in total recoverable *S. mutans* count was observed ($P < 0.001$).[24]

Essential oil antiseptic mouthrinses are able to reduce bacterial plaque and gingivitis, as evidenced in long-term studies. In a systematic review and meta-analysis, the majority of long-term studies investigating efficacy of CEOM-containing rinses found significant reduction in plaque.[45] There exists some heterogeneity in comparisons made within clinical trials. In these investigations, CEOM has been found superior in plaque reduction to negative control/placebo; also, studies find essential oil-containing mouthrinses to be as good or superior to positive controls (CHX).[46] Similarly, the antigingivitis effects of CEOM have been substantiated by systematic reviews. Again, the evidence supports, when used as an adjunct to at-home oral hygiene measures, that CEOM provide benefit in reduction of plaque and gingivitis compared with controls.[45,46]

The combined effectiveness of daily mechanical methods with CEOM was demonstrated in a study by Araujo and colleagues.[52] This meta-analysis demonstrated clinically significant, site-specific benefit of adjunctive essential oil mouthrinse application in subjects between routine 6-month dental visits.

Stannous Fluoride with Sodium Hexametaphosphate

Stannous fluoride is a broad-spectrum antimicrobial agent and had previously been identified for its plaque-control properties.[59] The mechanism of action of this active agent involves inhibition and reduction of bacterial plaque biomass, virulence, and metabolism. It is the formulation of stannous fluoride with sodium hexametaphosphate (SnF2) that has enabled the active agent to overcome undesirable properties of extrinsic staining and unpalatable taste.[60] SnF2 can be delivered in vehicles such as a dentifrice or gel, a mouthrinse, or even a regimen of combination dentifrice and mouthrinse.

The use of a stabilized 0.454% SnF2 dentifrice over a 6-month period provided statistically significant improvements in gingivitis, gingival bleeding, and plaque levels when compared with a negative control dentifrice.[61] Specifically, with 6 months of SnF2 usage, the experimental group had 21.7% less gingivitis ($P < 0.001$), 57.1% less bleeding ($P < 0.001$), and 6.9% less plaque ($P = 0.01$) on average compared with the negative control group. A similar 6-month controlled trial produced comparable improvements, with the experimental arm showing significant long-term reductions in gingival bleeding and gingival inflammation relative to a negative control.[62] In this analysis, the use of SnF2 dentifrice produced a 16.9% reduction in gingivitis ($P < 0.001$), a 40.8% reduction ($P < 0.001$) in gingival bleeding, and an 8.5% reduction in plaque levels compared with negative control.

Paraskevas and colleagues addressed the effects of SnF2-containing dentifrices or rinses on gingival health parameters in a systematic review/meta-analysis.[63] Randomized or controlled clinical trials having a minimum 6-month duration were considered. There were, overall, insufficient studies with regard to the effect of SnF2 mouthrinses as well as the combined (dentifrice/mouthrinse) regimen on gingivitis and plaque. SnF2 in dentifrice vehicles, however, yielded a significant albeit small improvement in plaque levels and gingivitis compared with control sodium fluoride dentifrices.

Triclosan and PVM/MA
As described previously, triclosan has been studied as an active agent for preventive chemotherapeutics owing to its antibacterial properties. First, at bacteriostatic concentrations, triclosan inhibits uptake of essential amino acids. At higher bactericidal levels, triclosan disrupts the bacterial cellular membrane causing fatal leakage of contents. In this scenario, the bacterial enzyme enoyl-acyl carrier protein reductase is the target of triclosan; this reductase is necessary for fatty acid synthesis, a process involved in bacterial cell membrane formation. Polyvinylmethyl ether/maleic acid copolymer (PVM/MA) is the carrier copolymer that enhances the delivery of triclosan.[64] Studies indicate that triclosan with PVM/MA (triclosan/PVM/MA) has enhanced binding to enamel surfaces and buccal epithelial cells compared with triclosan alone. Triclosan has demonstrated preclinical efficacy in altering levels of viable plaque, which is representative of both gram-positive bacteria and gram-negative periodontal pathogens.

Triclosan, in addition to actions on the bacterial plaque, may also exert clinical effects by modulation of host inflammatory response. There are preliminary in vitro and animal model data documenting the anti-inflammatory properties of triclosan. In vitro studies have shown triclosan provides inhibition of proinflammatory mediators and cytokines, including prostaglandin E_2, leukotriene, and interferon- pathways when challenged with lipopolysaccharide (LPS).[65–67] Finally, triclosan has been shown to be a potent inhibitor of oral epithelial cell LPS-induced proinflammatory responses by inducing mitochondrial RNA regulation of the toll-like receptor-signaling pathway.[68]

A substantial body of controlled long-term trials evaluated triclosan/PVM/MA–containing dentifrice in comparison to negative control or placebo. The effect of triclosan/PVM/MA on supragingival plaque accumulation and gingivitis development was measured.[8] With respect to plaque levels, on average these studies showed 25% (range, 12% to 59%) efficacies relative to the placebo control. Long-term clinical studies also support the efficacy of triclosan/PVM/MA in reducing gingivitis.[8] A Cochrane review found a 49% reduction in the proportion of sites with bleeding, when triclosan was compared with control fluoride dentifrice.[69] On average these studies showed 25% (range, 19% to 32%) efficacies relative to the placebo control. Triclosan use, as a preventive chemotherapeutic, may have considerable value in the maintained chronic periodontitis population of practices. Rosling and colleagues recruited maintenance patients showing signs of disease recurrence.[70] Specifically, the subjects were given either triclosan/PVM/MA or placebo dentifrice, and monitored up to 36 months. The triclosan arm exhibited quantitative and qualitative reduction in subgingival bacteria, and prevalence of recurrent periodontitis sites was reduced.

CONCLUSION

The supplemental use of chemotherapeutics, in concert with mechanical control, confers marked advantages in terms of aiding plaque biofilm control and the reduction of gingival inflammation. The current available evidence supports various applications, though to differing degrees (see Table 3).[71–78] The clinician should embrace a personalized medicine approach to disease prevention and treatment; this accounts for differences in people's genes, environments, and lifestyles—and from this assessment select an appropriate preventive chemotherapeutic approach. For example, although xerostomia is a concern when alcohol-containing mouthrinses are used, the clear preventive benefit of these agents would usually still not preclude their use in the majority of our patient population. Perhaps only in the most profoundly xerostomic patient cohort would alcohol not be a desired constituent of the preventive chemotherapeutic agent. The delivery format of the active agent might also be an important consideration. Selecting a

Table 3. Clinical Guide to Supported Benefits of Major Preventive Chemotherapeutic Rinses

Application	Strength of Evidence	Preventive Chemotherapeutic Agent	Comment
Prevention of oral candidosis in immuno-compromised population	🟠	CHX CHX-CPC combination	Some investigation has been made into use of chlorhexidine digluconate and CPC in prevention of mucositis in patients who have undergone chemotherapy or radiotherapy. Studies are of small sample size, and some find nonsignificant benefit with active agent rinses over placebo rinse. Traditional anti-fungal rinses such as fluconazole are still the accepted approach.[69,70]
Decontamination of dentures	🟡	CHX CHC-CPC combination EOMW	Limited studies support the efficacy of using agents to prevent stomatitis in denture wearers. Active agents would be used to disinfect denture appliances. The suggestion has been made that chlorhexidine is effective in disinfection of dentures contaminated with azole-resistant *Candida albicans*.[71]
Prevention of alveolar osteitis	🟡	CHX rinse or gel	A Cochrane review of 21 trials (2,570 participants) found some evidence that rinsing with chlorhexidine (0.12% and 0.2%) or placing chlorhexidine gel (0.2%) in the sockets of extracted teeth, provides a benefit in preventing alveolar osteitis (dry socket).[72]
Preprocedural rinsing	🟢	EOMW CHX	Preprocedural rinsing reduces the viable microbial count generated from aerosols during dental procedures. Together with standard use of personal protective equipment (PPE), preprocedural rinsing provides a safe measure to decrease the risk of contamination of dental healthcare providers. There is insufficient evidence to recommend use of preprocedural rinsing to decrease the chance of bacteremia, in the context of risk of the patient developing bacterial endocarditis.[73]
Halitosis	🟢	EOMW CHX CPC	Systematic reviews conclude that mouthrinses containing antimicrobials may help to reduce the levels of halitosis producing bacteria on the tongue.[74,75]
Prevention of ventilator-associated pneumonia	🟢	CHX rinse or gel	In critically ill adults, oral health care that includes either chlorhexidine mouthwash or gel is associated with a 40% reduction in the odds of developing ventilator-associated pneumonia. There is no evidence of a difference in the outcomes of mortality, duration of mechanical ventilation, or duration of ICU stay. This conclusion made from a review of 35 randomized controlled trials, representing 5,374 patients.[76]
Prevention of gingivitis	🟢	CPC 0.075% CHX EOMW	Studies from 4 weeks to 6 months in duration support efficacy of these active agents in reducing gingival inflammation. See chapter text for details.

CHX, chlorhexidine gluconate; CPC, cetylpyridinium chloride; EOMW, essential oil-containing mouth rinse; ICU, intensive care unit.

Strength of evidence:
🟢 High quality supporting data. Sound clinical application when weighed against alternative patient morbidity.
🟡 Fair quality supporting evidence presented.
🟠 Limited quality support, further studies warranted. Caution in recommendation of specific application.

dentifrice delivery vehicle for the active agent, as it is linked to "traditional" and "routine" mechanical toothbrushing, might be the appropriate route for our general patient cohort in maintaining reasonable compliance. The literature supports the efficacy of mouthrinses, and these products might be appropriate for at-risk or "downhill" periodontal maintenance patients, or in other similar clinical scenarios. All in all, achieving success at patient-level prevention requires clinicians to assess a patient's level of compliance and degree of motivation to attain his or her healthcare goals. In this regard, the use of preventive chemotherapeutics is a welcome addition to the complete armamentarium available to care for our patients.

With knowledge of preventive chemotherapeutics' established safety and efficacy, the oral healthcare team can suggest routine use—that is, applied in a truly *preventive* capacity. A large proportion of the general populace engages dentistry only on an urgent care basis, in response to oral disease and associated morbidity. This is diametrically opposed to the oral healthcare practitioner's value of preventive dentistry. The clinician and patient might do well to view appropriate chemotherapeutics as preventive, and not only for use after the appearance of disease. If we consider the overall disease mechanism of plaque-caused and inflammatory-driven diseases, this makes all the more sense. The clinical onset of disease (detection) lags behind the subclinical disease process that has already begun. Furthermore, preventive chemotherapeutics can serve as a buffer against poor patient compliance and the occasional below-standard mechanical oral hygiene measures. Preventive chemotherapeutics can augment existing oral hygiene measures, with an end goal of keeping the biofilm burden below a threshold for disease initiation.

REFERENCES

1. Feres M, Figueiredo LC, Soares GM, Faveri M. Systemic antibiotics in the treatment of periodontitis. *Periodontol 2000*. 2015;67:131–186.
2. Lang WP, Ronis DL, Farghaly MM. Preventive behaviors as correlates of periodontal health status. *J Public Health Dent*. 1995;55:10–17.
3. Paster BJ, Olsen I, Aas JA, Dewhirst FE. The breadth of bacterial diversity in the human periodontal pocket and other oral sites. *Periodontol 2000*. 2006;42:80–87.
4. Addy M, Moran JM. Evaluation of oral hygiene products: science is true; don't be misled by the facts. *Periodontol 2000*. 1997;15:40–51.
5. American Dental Association Council on Scientific Affairs, ed. *Acceptance Program Guidelines: Chemotherapeutic Products for Control of Gingivitis*. Chicago, IL: American Dental Association; 2011.
6. Wu CD, Savitt ED. Evaluation of the safety and efficacy of over-the-counter oral hygiene products for the reduction and control of plaque and gingivitis. *Periodontol 2000*. 2002;28:91–105.
7. Mandel ID. Chemotherapeutic agents for controlling plaque and gingivitis. *J Clin Periodontol*. 1988;15:488–498.
8. Panagakos FS, Volpe AR, Petrone ME, DeVizio W, Davies RM, Proskin HM. Advanced oral antibacterial/anti-inflammatory technology: a comprehensive review of the clinical benefits of a triclosan/copolymer/fluoride dentifrice. *J Clin Dent*. 2005;16(suppl):S1–19.
9. Siani H, Maillard JY. Best practice in healthcare environment decontamination. *Eur J Clin Microbiol Infect Dis*. 2015;34:1–11.
10. DePaola LG, Spolarich AE. Safety and efficacy of antimicrobial mouthrinses in clinical practice. *J Dental Hyg*. 2007;81(5).
11. Gandini S, Negri E, Boffetta P, La Vecchia C, Boyle P. Mouthwash and oral cancer risk quantitative meta-analysis of epidemiologic studies. *Ann Agric Environ Med*. 2012;19:173–180.
12. Emilson CG, Fornell J. Effect of toothbrushing with chlorhexidine gel on salivary microflora, oral hygiene, and caries. *Scand J Dent Res*. 1976;84:308–319.
13. Schiott CR, Briner WW, Loe H. Two year oral use of chlorhexidine in man. II. The effect on the salivary bacterial flora. *J Periodontal Res*. 1976;11:145–152.
14. Minah GE, DePaola LG, Overholser CD, et al. Effects of 6 months use of an antiseptic mouthrinse on supragingival dental plaque microflora. *J Clin Periodontol*. 1989;16:347–352.
15. Jones RD, Jampani HB, Newman JL, Lee AS. Triclosan: A review of effectiveness and safety in health care settings. *Am J Infect Control*. 2000;28:184–196.
16. Zambon JJ, Reynolds HS, Dunford RG, Bonta CY. Effect of a triclosan/copolymer/fluoride dentifrice on the oral microflora. *Am J Dent*. 1990;(3 spec no.):S27–34.
17. Walker C, Borden LC, Zambon JJ, Bonta CY, De-

Vizio W, Volpe AR. The effects of a 0.3% triclosan-containing dentifrice on the microbial composition of supragingival plaque. *J Clin Periodontol.* 1994;21:334–341.
18. Zambon JJ, Reynolds HS, Dunford RG, et al. Microbial alterations in supragingival dental plaque in response to a triclosan-containing dentifrice. *Oral Microbiol Immunol.* 1995;10:247–255.
19. Haraszthy VI, Sreenivasan PK, Zambon JJ. Community-level assessment of dental plaque bacteria susceptibility to triclosan over 19 years. *BMC Oral Health.* 2014;14:61.
20. Cullinan MP, Bird PS, Heng NC, West MJ, Seymour GJ. No evidence of triclosan-resistant bacteria following long-term use of triclosan-containing toothpaste. *J Periodontal Res.* 2014;49:220–225.
21. Rodricks JV, Swenberg JA, Borzelleca JF, Maronpot RR, Shipp AM. Triclosan: a critical review of the experimental data and development of margins of safety for consumer products. *Crit Rev Toxicol.* 2010;40:422–484.
22. Barkvoll P, Rolla G. Triclosan protects the skin against dermatitis caused by sodium lauryl sulphate exposure. *J Clin Periodontol.* 1994;21:717–719.
23. Langeveld WT, Veldhuizen EJ, Burt SA. Synergy between essential oil components and antibiotics: a review. *Crit Rev Microbiol.* 2014;40:76–94.
24. Fine DH, Furgang D, Barnett ML, et al. Effect of an essential oil-containing antiseptic mouthrinse on plaque and salivary *Streptococcus mutans* levels. *J Clin Periodontol.* 2000;27:157–161.
25. Meiller TF, Kelley JI, Jabra-Rizk MA, Depaola LG, Baqui AA, Falkler WA, Jr. In vitro studies of the efficacy of antimicrobials against fungi. *Oral Surg Oral Med Oral Pathol Oral Radiol Endod.* 2001;91:663–670.
26. DePaola LG, Minah GE, Leupold RJ, Faraone KL, Elias SA. The effect of antiseptic mouthrinses on oral microbial flora and denture stomatitis. *Clin Prev Dent.* 1986;8:3–8.
27. DePaola LG, Minah GE, Elias SA, Eastwood GW, Walters RA. Clinical and microbial evaluation of treatment regimens to reduce denture stomatitis. *Int J Prosthodont.* 1990;3:369–374.
28. White DJ. An alcohol-free therapeutic mouthrinse with cetylpyridinium chloride (CPC)—the latest advance in preventive care: Crest pro-health rinse. *Am J Dent.* 2005;18(spec no.):3A–8A.
29. Johnson N. Tobacco use and oral cancer: a global perspective. *J Dent Educ.* 2001;65:328–339.
30. Sturgis EM, Cinciripini PM. Trends in head and neck cancer incidence in relation to smoking prevalence: an emerging epidemic of human papillomavirus-associated cancers? *Cancer.* 2007;110:1429–1435.
31. Lopes CF, de Angelis BB, Prudente HM, de Souza BV, Cardoso SV, de Azambuja Ribeiro RI. Concomitant consumption of marijuana, alcohol and tobacco in oral squamous cell carcinoma development and progression: recent advances and challenges. *Arch Oral Biol.* 2012;57:1026–1033.
32. Currie S, Farrah C. Alcohol-containing mouthwash and oral cancer risk: a review of current evidence. *OA Alcohol.* 2014;10:1–4.
33. Ciancio S. Alcohol in mouthrinse: lack of association with cancer. *Biol Ther Dent.* 1993;9:1–2.
34. Silverman S Jr, Wilder R. Antimicrobial mouthrinse as part of a comprehensive oral care regimen. Safety and compliance factors. *J Am Dent Assoc.* 2006;137(suppl):22S–26S.
35. Van Leeuwen MP, Slot DE, Van der Weijden GA. The effect of an essential-oils mouthrinse as compared to a vehicle solution on plaque and gingival inflammation: a systematic review and meta-analysis. *Int J Dent Hyg.* 2014;12:160–167.
36. Haffajee AD, Yaskell T, Socransky SS. Antimicrobial effectiveness of an herbal mouthrinse compared with an essential oil and a chlorhexidine mouthrinse. *J Am Dent Assoc.* 2008;139:606–611.
37. Bernstein D, Schiff G, Echler G, Prince A, Feller M, Briner W. In vitro virucidal effectiveness of a 0.12%-chlorhexidine gluconate mouthrinse. *J Dent Res.* 1990;69:874–876.
38. Baqui AA, Kelley JI, Jabra-Rizk MA, Depaola LG, Falkler WA, Meiller TF. In vitro effect of oral antiseptics on human immunodeficiency virus-1 and herpes simplex virus type 1. *J Clin Periodontol.* 2001;28:610–616.
39. Giuliana G, Pizzo G, Milici ME, Musotto GC, Giangreco R. In vitro antifungal properties of mouthrinses containing antimicrobial agents. *J Periodontol.* 1997;68:729–733.
40. Giuliana G, Pizzo G, Milici ME, Giangreco R. In vitro activities of antimicrobial agents against candida species. *Oral Surg Oral Med Oral Pathol Oral Radiol Endod.* 1999;87:44–49.
41. Ellepola AN, Samaranayake LP. Oral candidal infections and antimycotics. *Crit Rev Oral Biol Med.* 2000;11:172–198.
42. Ciancio SG. Nonsurgical chemical periodontal therapy. *Periodontol 2000.* 1995;9:27–37.
43. Auschill TM, Hein N, Hellwig E, Follo M, Sculean A, Arweiler NB. Effect of two antimicrobial agents on early in situ biofilm formation. *J Clin Periodontol.* 2005;32:147–152.
44. Quintas V, Prada-Lopez I, Donos N, Suarez-Quintanilla D, Tomas I. In situ neutralisation of the antibacterial effect of 0.2% chlorhexidine on salivary microbiota: quantification of substantivity. *Arch Oral Biol.* 2015;60:1109–1116.
45. Gunsolley JC. A meta-analysis of six-month studies of antiplaque and antigingivitis agents. *J Am Dent*

Assoc. 2006;137:1649–1657.
46. Stoeken JE, Paraskevas S, van der Weijden GA. The long-term effect of a mouthrinse containing essential oils on dental plaque and gingivitis: a systematic review. *J Periodontol.* 2007;78:1218–1228.
47. Serrano J, Escribano M, Roldan S, Martin C, Herrera D. Efficacy of adjunctive anti-plaque chemical agents in managing gingivitis: a systematic review and meta-analysis. *J Clin Periodontol.* 2015;42(suppl 16):S106–S138.
48. Van Strydonck DA, Slot DE, Van der Velden U, Van der Weijden F. Effect of a chlorhexidine mouthrinse on plaque, gingival inflammation and staining in gingivitis patients: a systematic review. *J Clin Periodontol.* 2012;39:1042–1055.
49. Haps S, Slot DE, Berchier CE, Van der Weijden GA. The effect of cetylpyridinium chloride-containing mouth rinses as adjuncts to toothbrushing on plaque and parameters of gingival inflammation: a systematic review. *Int J Dent Hyg.* 2008;6:290–303.
50. Gunsolley JC. Clinical efficacy of antimicrobial mouthrinses. *J Dent.* 2010;38(suppl 1):S6–10.
51. Ouhayoun JP. Penetrating the plaque biofilm: impact of essential oil mouthwash. *J Clin Periodontol.* 2003;30(suppl 5):10–12.
52. Araujo MW, Charles CA, Weinstein RB, et al. Meta-analysis of the effect of an essential oil-containing mouthrinse on gingivitis and plaque. *J Am Dent Assoc.* 2015;146:610–622.
53. Kuehl FA, Jr, Humes JL, Egan RW, Ham EA, Beveridge GC, Van Arman CG. Role of prostaglandin endoperoxide PGG2 in inflammatory processes. *Nature.* 1977;265(5590):170–173.
54. Pan P, Barnett ML, Coelho J, Brogdon C, Finnegan MB. Determination of the in situ bactericidal activity of an essential oil mouthrinse using a vital stain method. *J Clin Periodontol.* 2000;27:256–261.
55. Fine DH, Furgang D, Barnett ML. Comparative antimicrobial activities of antiseptic mouthrinses against isogenic planktonic and biofilm forms of *Actinobacillus actinomycetemcomitans. J Clin Periodontol.* 2001;28:697–700.
56. Ross NM, Charles CH, Dills SS. Long-term effects of Listerine antiseptic on dental plaque and gingivitis. *J Clin Dent.* 1989;1(4):92–95.
57. Whitaker EJ, Pham K, Feik D, Rams TE, Barnett ML, Pan P. Effect of an essential oil-containing antiseptic mouthrinse on induction of platelet aggregation by oral bacteria in vitro. *J Clin Periodontol.* 2000;27:370–373.
58. Charles CH, Pan PC, Sturdivant L, Vincent JW. In vivo antimicrobial activity of an essential oil-containing mouthrinse on interproximal plaque bacteria. *J Clin Dent.* 2000;11:94–97.

59. Tinanoff N. Progress regarding the use of stannous fluoride in clinical dentistry. *J Clin Dent.* 1995;6(spec no.):37–40.
60. Walters PA, Biesbrock AR, Bartizek RD. Benefits of sodium hexametaphosphate-containing chewing gum for extrinsic stain inhibition. *J Dent Hyg.* 2004;78:8.
61. Mankodi S, Bartizek RD, Winston JL, Biesbrock AR, McClanahan SF, He T. Anti-gingivitis efficacy of a stabilized 0.454% stannous fluoride/sodium hexametaphosphate dentifrice. *J Clin Periodontol.* 2005;32:75–80.
62. Mallat M, Mankodi S, Bauroth K, Bsoul SA, Bartizek RD, He T. A controlled 6-month clinical trial to study the effects of a stannous fluoride dentifrice on gingivitis. *J Clin Periodontol.* 2007;34:762–767.
63. Paraskevas S, van der Weijden GA. A review of the effects of stannous fluoride on gingivitis. *J Clin Periodontol.* 2006;33:1–13.
64. Nabi N, Mukerjee C, Schmid R, Gaffar A. In vitro and in vivo studies on triclosan/PVM/MA copolymer/NaF combination as an anti-plaque agent. *Am J Dent.* 1989;(2 spec no.):197–206.
65. Modeer T, Bengtsson A, Rolla G. Triclosan reduces prostaglandin biosynthesis in human gingival fibroblasts challenged with interleukin-1 in vitro. *J Clin Periodontol.* 1996;23:927–933.
66. Mustafa M, Bakhiet M, Wondimu B, Modeer T. Effect of triclosan on interferon-gamma production and major histocompatibility complex class II expression in human gingival fibroblasts. *J Clin Periodontol.* 2000;27:733–737.
67. Mustafa M, Wondimu B, Yucel-Lindberg T, Kats-Hallstrom AT, Jonsson AS, Modeer T. Triclosan reduces microsomal prostaglandin E synthase-1 expression in human gingival fibroblasts. *J Clin Periodontol.* 2005;32:6–11.
68. Wallet MA, Calderon N, Alonso TR, et al. Triclosan alters antimicrobial and inflammatory responses of epithelial cells. *Oral Dis.* 2013;19:296–302.
69. Davies RM, Ellwood RP, Davies GM. The effectiveness of a toothpaste containing triclosan and polyvinyl-methyl ether maleic acid copolymer in improving plaque control and gingival health: a systematic review. *J Clin Periodontol.* 2004;31:1029–1033.
70. Rosling B, Dahlen G, Volpe A, Furuichi Y, Ramberg P, Lindhe J. Effect of triclosan on the subgingival microbiota of periodontitis-susceptible subjects. *J Clin Periodontol.* 1997;24:881–887.
71. Lanzos I, Herrera D, Santos S, et al. Mucositis in irradiated cancer patients: effects of an antiseptic mouthrinse. *Med Oral Patol Oral Cir Bucal.* 2010;15:e732–738.
72. Worthington HV, Clarkson JE, Bryan G, et al. Interventions for preventing oral mucositis for pa-

tients with cancer receiving treatment. *Cochrane Database Syst Rev.* 2011;(4):CD000978.

73. Salim N, Silikas N, Satterthwaite JD, Moore C, Ramage G, Rautemaa R. Chlorhexidine-impregnated PEM/THFM polymer exhibits superior activity to fluconazole-impregnated polymer against *Candida albicans* biofilm formation. *Int J Antimicrob Agents.* 2013;41:193–196.

74. Daly B, Sharif MO, Newton T, Jones K, Worthington HV. Local interventions for the management of alveolar osteitis (dry socket). *Cochrane Database Syst Rev.* 2012;(12):CD006968.

75. Wilson W, Taubert KA, Gewitz M, et al. Prevention of infective endocarditis: guidelines from the American Heart Association: a guideline from the American Heart Association Rheumatic Fever, Endocarditis, and Kawasaki Disease Committee, Council on Cardiovascular Disease in the Young, and the Council on Clinical Cardiology, Council on Cardiovascular Surgery and Anesthesia, and the Quality of Care and Outcomes Research Interdisciplinary Working Group. *Circulation.* 2007;116:1736–1754.

76. Fedorowicz Z, Aljufairi H, Nasser M, Outhouse TL, Pedrazzi V. Mouthrinses for the treatment of halitosis. *Cochrane Database Syst Rev.* 2008;(4):CD006701.

77. Loesche WJ, Kazor C. Microbiology and treatment of halitosis. *Periodontol 2000.* 2002;28:256–279.

78. Shi Z, Xie H, Wang P, et al. Oral hygiene care for critically ill patients to prevent ventilator-associated pneumonia. *Cochrane Database Syst Rev.* 2013;(8):CD008367.

INDEX

Please note: tables, figures, and boxes are indicated by an italicized "*t*", "*f*", or "*b*", respectively.

A

A1C test/levels, 44*t*, 45–47, 209–211, 211*t*, 216
AAP Task Force Report, 71–72, 74
abfraction, 114, 114*f*, 116, 161
abrasion
    defined, 108
    etiology, 108–110
    examples, 109*f*, 110*f*
    prevention, 110–111
    role in dentin hypersensitivity, 161, 161*t*
abuse, recognizing and reporting, 202
ACP (amorphous calcium phosphate), 168, 251
acquired immunodeficiency syndrome (AIDS), 124
Actinobacillus actinomycetemcomitans, 264
Actinomyces viscosus, 264
ADA Seal of Acceptance criteria, 258*f*
adverse pregnancy outcomes, evidence supporting oral-systemic link, 213–214
Agency for Healthcare Research and Quality (AHRQ), 17–18
    grades of recommendation, 18*t*
    levels of scientific evidence, 18*t*
Aggregatibacter actinomycetemcomitans, 71, 212
AGREE (Appraisal of Guidelines Research and Evaluation), 12*t*
AHA/ASA My Life Check–Life's Simple 7, 41
AHA Committee on Rheumatic Fever, Endocarditis, and Kawasaki Disease, 41
AHRQ (Agency for Healthcare Research and Quality). *See* Agency for Healthcare Research and Quality
AIDS (acquired immunodeficiency syndrome), 124
American Academy of Pediatric Dentistry's Clinical Practice Guidelines, 50–51
American Academy of Periodontology Workshop on Periodontal Regeneration and Tissue Engineering, 106
amorphous calcium phosphate (ACP), 168, 251
amoxicillin (AMX), 80
anticholinergic drugs, 177
antimicrobials/antibiotics
    antimicrobial dentifrice, 89
    antimicrobial mouthrinses, 89–90
    locally delivered, 79–80
    systemic, 80
antioxidants, 90
Appraisal of Guidelines Research and Evaluation (AGREE), 12*t*
arginine, 65
arginine-based desensitizing prophylaxis paste, 169
ASD (autism spectrum disorders), 229–230
attrition
    defined, 107
    etiology, 107–108
    examples, 107*f*
    prevention, 108
    role in dentin hypersensitivity, 161, 161*t*
autism spectrum disorders (ASD), 229–230
autoimmune diseases, 177, 183, 184–187

B

bacterial fluorescence, 60–61, 60*b*
Bacteroides forsythus, 147
Bacteroides species, 264
bad breath, 146
behavior and psychological interventions. *See* biopsychosocial patient care; special care dentistry
biofilms
    ecological plaque hypothesis, 62
    inflammatory response to, 208–210. *See also* oral-systemic health
    interdental biofilm removal, 87–89, 87*f*
    modifying composition of, 64, 65*b*
    non-fluoride management strategies, 249–252
    powered interdental cleaning devices, 87–89, 88*f*
    prebiotics and, 65
    probiotics and, 64–65
    quantifying, 60–61
    role of nature vs. nurture in, 65*b*
    selective targeted antimicrobial peptides, 66
    smart signaling systems in, 64
biomedical model of disease, 23
biopsychosocial patient care, 23–35
    application to clinical practice
        common psychological conditions, 31–32
        common risk factors and links to systemic health, 29
        disease prevention across the lifespan, 28
        health literacy in the context of dental appointments, 31
        integrating desired behavior into patient lifestyles, 30
        interpersonal communication, 30–31
        process of disease prevention, 28
        respectful patient communication, 31
        simplified communication, 31
        trying new behaviors vs. establishing healthy habits, 29–30
        using teach-back method, 31
    benefits of, 32–33
    Chairside Checklist, 32, 33–35
    defined, 23
    goal of, 23
    key considerations
        common risk factor approach, 24–25
        health literacy, 24
        motivational interviewing, 28
        quality of life, 24
        social cognitive theory, 25–26, 25*f*
        social determinants of health, 23–24
        socioeconomic gradient and poverty, 24
        stress and coping, 26–27

transtheoretical model, 27–28
understanding and influencing health behavior, 25
See also special care dentistry
Bradshaw, D. I., 62
bulimia nervosa, 111–113, 112*f*

C

calcium glycerophosphate, 63
calcium sodium phosphosilicate, 169
CAMBRA (Caries Management by Risk Assessment), 51, 63
Campbell Collaboration, 12
Candid. albicans, 262
Candida species, 260–262, 263
cardiovascular disease and stroke
    age-standardized prevalence estimates for ideal cardiovascular health, 40*f*
    AHA definition of cardiovascular health, 39*t*
    AHA prevalence of health metrics, 40*f*
    deaths in U.S., 38*f*
    evidence supporting oral-systemic link, 212–213
    incidence, symptoms and risk factors, 37–41
    risk assessment, 41
CARE (Customizable Assessment and Risk Evaluator) Tools, 50
care-resistant behavior (CRB), 223
caries
    case studies in
        adolescent patients, 66–67
        deterioration of dentition in adolescent patients, 67–68*f*
        diabetes mellitus complications, 69*f*
        elderly patients, 67–68, 69*f*
        oral-systemic health, 68–70, 69*f*
    demineralization and remineralization process, 236, 236*f*
    diagnosis and detection, 238
    fluoride therapies, 62–63, 238
    incidence and symptoms of, 50
    lifestyles promoting, 64
    non-fluoride interventions, 63–64
    paradigm shifts in etiology, 61–62
    risk assessment, 50–51, 63–64
        for birth to 5 years of age, 51*t*
        Caries Management by Risk Assessment (CAMBRA), 51, 63
        for children 6 and older, 52*t*
    risk factors for, 50, 57, 57*b*, 58–59, 58*b*
    role of biofilms, 64–66
        nature vs. nurture, 65*b*
    role of prevention, 57–58, 66
    trends and challenges in prevention
        Dunedin, New Zealand study, 58–59, 63
        early detection of caries, 59–60, 60*f*
        nonoperative caries treatment programs, 59
        pathogenesis of caries, 59
        quantification of dental plaque, 60–61
        WHO database conclusions, 61

Caries Management by Risk Assessment (CAMBRA), 51, 63
case-control study design, 5–6, 6*f*
casein phosphopeptide (CPP), 168
casein phosphopeptide–amorphous calcium phosphate (CPP-ACP), 63–64
case report/case series studies, 4, 4*f*
CASP (Critical Appraisal Skills Programme), 12*t*
Cavistat toothpaste, 252
CBCT (cone-beam computed tomography), 73–74
CDA Foundation, 51
Centre for Evidence-Based Medicine, 12*t*, 16–17
    CEBM table for diagnosis, 16*t*
    CEBM table for prognosis, 17*t*
    CEBM table for therapy, prevention, etiology, harm, 16*t*
CEOM (combination essential oil mouthrinse)
    application to clinical practice, 264–265
    composition of preventive chemotherapeutic mouthrinses, 262*t*
    efficacy of, 89, 260–262
cetylpyridinium chloride (CPC), 89, 264
cevimeline, 180
Chairside Checklist (for biopsychosocial patient care), 32, 33–35
chemotherapeutic agents, 257–268
    application to clinical practice
        cetylpyridinium chloride (CPC), 264
        chlorhexidine (CHX), 263–264
        combination essential oil, 264–265
        stannous fluoride with sodium hexametaphosphate, 265
        triclosan and PVM/MA, 266
    benefits of, 266–268
        strength of supporting evidence, 267*t*
    clinical evaluation of, 257–259, 258*f*
    defined, 257
    effect on microbial diversity, 260–262
    effect on oral mucosal tissues, 262–263
        composition of preventive chemotherapeutic mouthrinses, 262*t*
    overview of active agents, 259
        major strategies for effective chemotherapeutic agents, 259*t*
    safety of active agents, 259–260, 260*f*
chewing tobacco, 104–105
children and adolescents
    caries risk assessment, for children 6 and older, 52*t*
    fluoride use in
        benefits of professional interventions, 240–241
        caries experience in children who brush once or less vs. twice or more, 239*f*
        dietary supplements, 240
        fluoride varnish, 241, 241*f*
        gels and foams, 240
        mouthrinses, 240
        products available, 238, 239*f*
        toothpaste prescriptions, 242

INDEX

toothpastes, 238–239
mouthrinses for, 239f, 240
toothbrushing in, 239
toothpastes for, 238–239, 239f
chlorhexidine gluconate (CHX)
   application to clinical practice, 263–264
   composition of preventive chemotherapeutic mouthrinses, 262t
   efficacy of, 79–80, 89–90, 260–262
   in root caries prevention, 250
CINAHL (Cumulative Index of Nursing and Allied Health Literature), 2t
clinical decision making, 14
   See also evidence-based practice
clinical practice guidelines (CPGs), 15, 15t
Cochrane Collaboration, 2t, 13, 18–19, 19t, 63
cohort studies, 6–7, 7f, 8f
Colgate Maximum Cavity Protection Plus Sugar Acid Neutralizer, 251–252
Colgate Pro-Relief, 170f
Colgate Sensitive Toothpaste, 170f
Colgate Total Rinse, 262t
combination essential oil mouthrinse (CEOM)
   application to clinical practice, 264–265
   composition of preventive chemotherapeutic mouthrinses, 262t
   efficacy of, 89, 260–262
common risk factor approach, 24–25
communication, role in patient care, 30–31
cone-beam computed tomography (CBCT), 73–74
consistency, 223–224
CONSORT, 12t, 13
contingent/noncontingent escape, 223
conventional staged debridement (CSD), 77
COREQ, 12t, 13
CPC (cetylpyridinium chloride), 89, 264
CPGs (clinical practice guidelines), 15, 15t
CPP (casein phosphopeptide), 168
CPP-ACP (casein phosphopeptide–amorphous calcium phosphate), 63–64, 168, 252
CRB (care-resistant behavior), 223
Crest Pro Health Multi-Protection, 262t
Critical Appraisal Skills Programme (CASP), 12t
cross-sectional study design, 4–5, 5f
CSD (conventional staged debridement), 77
Cumulative Index of Nursing and Allied Health Literature (CINAHL), 2t
Customizable Assessment and Risk Evaluator (CARE) Tools, 50

D

damage prevention. *See* oral tissue damage
DARE (Database of Abstracts of Reviews of Effects), 2t
Dean, H. Trendley, 235
Decayed, Missing, Filled Surfaces (DMFS) Index, 59
demineralization/remineralization process, 59, 236, 236f, 247–249
DenPlan Excel/PreVisor Patient Assessment (DEPPA), 52
dental caries. *See* caries
dental endoscopy, 77
dental floss, 87
dental fluorosis (enamel mottling), 235, 235f
Dental Traumatology (journal), 196
dentin hypersensitivity, 160–171
   diagnosis
      air blast stimuli response, 165f, 166f
      aspects and elements of, 163–164
      differential diagnosis, 165–166
      oral examination, 164
      patient history, 164
      stimuli response testing, 164–165
      Yeaple probe stimuli response, 165f
   epidemiology, 160
   etiology, 160–161
      Brännström's Theory, 160f
   overview of, 171
   pathogenesis, 162–163
      enamel loss, 162f
      odontoblast and dentinal tubules, 163f
      scanning electron micrograph images, 163f
   patient management and interventions
      arginine technology sealing of dentinal tubules, 169f
      considerations for, 169–171
      major products available for, 170t
      options for, 171t
      preventive strategies, 166–167
      therapeutic interventions, 167–169, 167f
   risk factors, 161–162
      frequently encountered conditions associated with tooth sensitivity, 161t
      questions for patients experiencing dentin hypersensitivity, 161t
Dentition Risk System (DRS), 52
DEPPA (DenPlan Excel/PreVisor Patient Assessment), 52
diabetes mellitus
   awareness, treatment and control in adults, 42f
   case studies in, 68–70, 69f
   evidence supporting oral-systemic link, 209–212, 211t
   guiding principles for care, 44t
   incidence, symptoms and risk factors, 41–43
   risk assessment, 43–47, 70
      ADA assessment tool, 45f
      Finnish Diabetes Risk Score, 46f
DMFS (Decayed, Missing, Filled Surfaces) Index, 59
double-blind study design, 9
doxycycline, 79–80
DRS (Dentition Risk System), 52
dry mouth (xerostomia)
   case studies in
      female with autoimmune diseases, 184–187, 184t, 185f, 185t, 186f, 187f
      male receiving radiation therapy, 187–189, 188f,

188*t*, 189*f*
diagnosis
flow rates of whole saliva, 177*t*
salivary gland hypofunction, 176
xerostomia, 176
epidemiology, 177
prevalence of xerostomia and salivary gland hypofunction, 177*t*
etiology
age, 177
common systemic disorders associated with dry mouth, 178*t*
medication, 177
radiation therapy, 178
systemic disorders, 177–178
incidence, symptoms and risk factors, 53
overview, 175
pathogenesis, 175
contributors to salivary secretion, 176*f*
control of salivary secretion, 175*f*
patient management considerations, 182–183
prevention, 179–180
saliva substitutes, 181–182, 182*t*
risk assessment, 53
hyposalivation with xerostomia screening tool, 54*f*
role in caries progression, 247–248
therapeutic interventions, saliva stimulants, 180–181
Dunedin, New Zealand prevention study, 58–59, 63
dyskeratosis congenita, 124

E

EBD (evidence-based dentistry), 1
See also evidence-based practice
EBDM (evidence-based decision-making), 1
See also evidence-based practice
ecological plaque hypothesis, 62
EDS (excessive daytime sleepiness), 47
See also sleep-related breathing disorders
Effectiveness and Efficiency: Random Reflections on Health Service (Cochrane), 18
electronic nicotine delivery systems (ENDS), 124
Ellis class I and II injuries, 193
Embase, 2*t*
enamel mottling (dental fluorosis), 235, 235*f*
endogenic erosion
due to bulimia, 112*f*
due to GERD, 112*f*
etiology, 111–112
prevention, 112–113
ENDS (electronic nicotine delivery systems), 124
Engel, G. L., 23
erbium–yttrium aluminium garnet (Er:YAG) laser, 76
erosion
defined, 111
endogenic, 111–113, 112*f*
exogenic, 113–114, 113*f*

role in dentin hypersensitivity, 161, 161*t*
Er:YAG (erbium–yttrium aluminium garnet) laser, 76
erythromycin, 80
escape extinction, 224
essential oil rinses. *See* combination essential oil mouthrinse
European Health Literacy Survey, 24
evidence-based decision-making (EBDM), 1
See also evidence-based practice
evidence-based dentistry (EBD), 1
See also evidence-based practice
Evidence-Based Dentistry for the Dental Hygienist (Frantsve-Hawley), 12*t*
Evidence-based Dentistry: Managing Information for Better Practice (Richards, et. al.), 12*t*
evidence-based practice, 1–20
applying evidence to practice, 19–20
challenges in adopting
accessing information, 2–3
keeping up with literature, 2
locating best evidence, 3
resources to assist with critical appraisal, 12*t*
understanding research methodology, 3
clinical practice guidelines, 15, 15*t*
defined, 1
grading scientific evidence
Agency for Healthcare Research and Quality, 17–18
AHRQ grades of recommendation, 18*t*
AHRQ levels of scientific evidence, 18*t*
CEBM table for therapy, prevention, etiology, harm, 16*t*
CEBM tables for diagnosis, 16*t*, 17*t*
Centre for Evidence-Based Medicine, 16–17
Cochrane Collaboration, 18–19
Cochrane collaboration key principles, 19*t*
GRADE system, 17, 17*t*
overview of, 15–16
levels of evidence, 13–14
hierarchy of preappraised evidence, 14*f*
resources supporting clinical decision making, 14*t*
locating best evidence, 2*t*
model, 1*f*
overview of, 20
steps of, 13, 13*f*
study designs
case-control, 5–6, 6*f*
case report/case series, 4, 4*f*
cohort studies, 6–7
cohort studies: prospective, 7*f*
cohort studies: retrospective chart review, 8*f*
cross-sectional, 4–5, 5*f*
experimental studies, 8–10
guidelines for reporting, 13
hierarchy of, 3*f*
meta-analyses, 11–12, 11*f*
nonexperimental intervention, 8, 8*f*

qualitative studies, 10
randomized controlled trial: active control, 10*f*
randomized controlled trial: placebo control, 9*f*
registering systematic reviews and meta-analyses, 12–13
surveys and interviews, 3–4
systematic reviews, 10–11
excessive daytime sleepiness (EDS), 47
See also sleep-related breathing disorders
exogenic erosion
etiology, 113
examples, 113*f*
prevention, 113–114
experimental studies, 8–10
extraoral halitosis, 147
case studies in, 155–157, 156*f*
classification, categories of oral malodor, 147*t*
pathogenesis, 148
See also oral malodor

F

Fanconi's anemia, 124
Finnish Diabetes Risk Score (FINDRISC), 43
fluorescence, 60–61, 60*b*
fluorides
in adults and older adults
evidence for use, 238*f*, 242–243
midlevel providers and, 243
population-based interventions, 243
benefits of, 235–236
in children and adolescents
benefits of professional interventions, 240–241
caries experience in children who brush once or less vs. twice or more, 239*f*
dietary supplements, 240
fluoride varnish, 241, 241*f*
gels and foams, 240
mouthrinses, 240
products available, 238, 239*f*
toothpaste prescriptions, 241–242
toothpastes, 238–239
delivery methods, 236–237
dietary intake of, 235
efficacy of, 59, 62–63
future directions and best practices, 243–244
history of, 235
enamel mottling (dental fluorosis), 235, 235*f*
life course approach to, 237–238, 238*f*
caries detection and diagnosis, 238
using fluorides to prevent and treat caries, 238
optimal delivery, 237
optimal level, 235
overview of, 244
risks of use, 237
topical effect of, 236
demineralization and remineralization, 236*f*
fluorosis, 239
FMD (full-mouth disinfection), 77

FMPA (Frankfort Mandibular-Plane Angle), 195
FMSRP (full-mouth scaling and root planing), 76–77
focal infections, 208
foreshadowing, 223
Frankfort Mandibular-Plane Angle (FMPA), 195
frenal pull, influence on gingival recession, 104
full-mouth disinfection (FMD), 77
full-mouth scaling and root planing (FMSRP), 76–77
Fusobacterium nucleatum, 147–148, 148*f*

G

gastroesophageal reflux disease (GERD), 111–112, 112*f*
GC America MI Paste, 170*f*
GERD (gastroesophageal reflux disease), 111–112, 112*f*
geriatric patients
aggressive prevention, 226
clinical prevention, 225
conservative prevention, 225
empirical prevention, 225
fluoride use in, 242–243
guidelines for preventive dentistry, 224
influence of medical condition, 224
oral physiology changes in, 57–58
predictive prevention, 225
preventive care considerations, 230–231
team approach to preventive care, 224–225
gingival recession
effects of oral piercings, 105
effects of tobacco use, 104–105
epidemiology, 97–99
etiology, 99–101
examples, 98*f*, 99*f*, 100*f*, 101*f*
pathogenesis, 105–106
prevention and therapy, 106
role in dentin hypersensitivity, 161, 161*t*
gingivitis
case studies in, 91, 91*f*
classification, 72*t*
defined, 71, 208
epidemiology, 72–74
etiology and pathogenesis, 73
See also periodontal diseases
gingivitis artefacta, 97
glycated hemoglobin. *See* A1C test/levels
glycine powder air polishing (GPAP), 77–78, 78*f*
Google Scholar, 2*t*
GRADE (Grading of Recommendations, Assessment, Development, and Evaluation) system, 17, 17*t*
graft-versus-host disease (GVHD), 124
Guidelines for the Management of Patients with Periodontal Diseases (AAP), 52

H

habits, establishing, 29–30
Halimeter, 150
halitophobia, 147, 147*t*

halitosis, 146
    See also oral malodor
hard tissue damage. See under oral tissue damage
HbA1c. See A1C test/levels
head and neck cancers (HNCs)
    case studies in
        adolescent male using tobacco, 138–140
        young female with low health literacy, 140–141
    diagnostic tests, 128–131
        images and CT scan of tongue cancer, 130f
        images and CT scan of tonsillar cancer, 129f
        selected methods for detection and diagnosis, 130t
    epidemiology, 121–122
        new cases, deaths, and 5-year relative survival, 122f
        number of new cases by race/ethnicity and sex, 123t
        percent of deaths by age group, 123f
        percent of new cases by age group, 122f
    etiology and risk factors, 122–124, 123t
        levels of evidence for increased risk, 124t
    future epidemiological trends, 136–137
    future research efforts, 137–138
    incidence of, 121
    MASCC/ISOO practice guidelines, 144–145
    pathogenesis, 124–126
        cancer in situ, 127f
        cervical metastasis of left tonsil and tongue base, 126f
        common locations of head/neck cancers, 125t
        erythroplakia and mixed lesions, 127f
        HPV oncoproteins E6 and E7, 126f
        leukoplakia of tongue, 127f
        molecular biological and histopathologic comparisons, 125t
        SCC of posterior oropharyngeal wall, 126f
        SCC of upper lip, 127f
        tonsillar cancer, 125f, 126f
    patient management and interventions
        behavioral change stages in tobacco cessation, 133f
        considerations for, 135–136
        interventions prior to treatment, 132–134
        levels of evidence for interventions to reduce risk, 131t
        preventive strategies, 131–132
        special considerations, 136
        therapeutic interventions, 134–135
    role in dry mouth, 179
    role of oral health professionals, 121, 138
    signs and symptoms, 126–128
        comparison of HNCs by etiology, 128t
        symptoms of OPCs, 128t
    See also oral and pharyngeal cancer
Health Improvement in Dental Practice (HIDEP), 52
health literacy
    defined, 24
    role in interpersonal communication, 31
    role in patient care, 24, 31
Health Technology Assessment Database, 2t
HeartScore electronic risk assessment system, 41
herbal patches, 90
heterogeneous studies, 12
HIDEP (Health Improvement in Dental Practice), 52
HNCs (head and neck cancers). See head and neck cancers
homogeneous studies, 12
HPV-associated cancer
    diagnosis, 129–131
    etiology and risk factors, 123–124
        comparison of HNCs by etiology, 128t
        molecular biological and histopathologic comparisons, 125t
    future directions and best practices, 136–137
    future research efforts, 137–138
    HPV susceptibility testing, 50
    pathogenesis, 125
        HPV oncoproteins E6 and E7, 126f
    risk reduction, 141t
    survival rates, 121
    therapeutic interventions, 134–135
    vaccination against, 131–132, 136–137
    viruses included, 49
    See also head and neck cancers; oral and pharyngeal cancer
Human Microbiome Project, 62
hydrodynamic theory (of dentin hypersensitivity), 160
hydroxyapatite, 60
hypersensitivity. See dentin hypersensitivity

I

IADT (International Association of Dental Traumatology), 196–197
ICMJE (International Committee of Medical Journal Editors), 13
implants. See peri-implant diseases
IMRT (intensity modulated radiation therapy), 179
INSPIRE, 12t, 13
intentional abuse, recognition and reporting, 202
International Association of Dental Traumatology (IADT), 196–197
International Committee of Medical Journal Editors (ICMJE), 13
interpersonal communication, role in patient care, 30–31
intraoral chemotherapeutics, 259
    See also chemotherapeutic agents
intraoral halitosis
    case studies in, 154–155, 155f
    classification, categories of oral malodor, 147t
    defined, 147
    pathogenesis, 147–148
        detection of volatile sulphur compounds from P. gingivalis and F. nucleatum, 148f
        volatile malodorous contributors to, 148t

See also oral malodor
intrinsic fluorescence, 60, 60*b*
irrigation, supra- and subgingival, 78–79, 88*f*

L

Lactobacillus species, 250
laser technology, 76
LILACS (Literature from Latin America and the Caribbean), 2*t*
Listerine, 262*t*
local and systemic therapies, 79
longitudinal study design, 7

M

maintenance and recall, 80–81
    for implant-borne restorations, 84–86*t*
    for tooth-borne restorations, 82–83*t*
malodor. *See* oral malodor
Marsh, P. D., 62
MASCC/ISOO practice guidelines for oral mucositis, 144–145
McKay, Frederick, 62
mechanical therapy, 75–76
meta-analyses, 11–13, 11*f*
metronidazole (MET), 80
MFP (sodium monofluorophosphate), 169
MI (motivational interviewing), 28, 133
MIC (minimal inhibitory concentration) level, 79, 260
minimally invasive dentistry, 59
minocycline, 79–80
MOOSE, 12*t*, 13
motivational interviewing (MI), 28, 133
mouth protectors, 199–201, 200*f*, 201*f*
mouthrinses
    antimicrobial, 89–90
    arginine-based desensitizing prophylaxis, 169*f*
    for children and adolescents, 239*f*, 240
    oral malodor and, 153
My Life Check–Life's Simple 7, 41

N

nanoparticulate hydroxyapatite, 63
nanotechnology/nanoparticulate materials, 66
National Diabetes Education Program (NDEP), 43, 44*t*
National Information Center on Health Services Research and Health Care Technology (NICHSR), 2*t*
National Institutes of Health, accessing information through, 2–3
NCCL (noncarious cervical lesions), 114
Nd:YAG (neodymium–yttrium aluminium garnet) laser, 76
neurodegenerative diseases, 228
Nexo approach, 59
NICHSR (National Information Center on Health Services Research and Health Care Technology), 2*t*
NOCTP (nonoperative caries treatment program), 59
noncarious cervical lesions (NCCL), 114
nonexperimental intervention study design, 8, 8*f*

non-fluoride remineralization
    benefits of, 246
    calcium-based remineralization, 251–252, 251*f*
    casein phosphopeptide–amorphous calcium phosphate, 63–64
    demineralization/remineralization process, 59, 248–249, 248*f*
    overview of, 252–253
    patient assessment, 246
    progression of caries formation, 246–247, 247*f*
    role of dental plaque in caries, 246–247
    stimulating salivary flow, 251
    targeted antimicrobial therapies, 249–251
    traditional approaches, 249
nonoperative caries treatment program (NOCTP), 59
NovaMin toothpaste, 169, 170*f*
nutrition, 91

O

obesity, 91
obstructive sleep apnea (OSA), 47, 107–108, 111
    See also sleep-related breathing disorders
odds ratio (OR), 6
OHRQOL (oral health-related quality of life), 24
OPC (oral and pharyngeal cancer). *See* oral and pharyngeal cancer
oral and pharyngeal cancer (OPC)
    diagnosis, 129–131
    epidemiology, 121
    incidence, symptoms and risk factors, 48–49, 128, 128*t*
    mouthrinses and, 263
    risk assessment, 49–50
        CARE (Customizable Assessment and Risk Evaluator) Tools, 50
        Health Canada self-assessment quiz, 49*t*
        PreViser Oral Cancer Risk Assessment, 49
    See also head and neck cancers
OralChroma portable gas chromatograph, 150*f*, 151*f*, 155*f*, 156*f*
Oral Health Information Suite, 53
oral health-related quality of life (OHRQOL), 24
oral malodor, 146–157
    assessment
        Halimeter, 150
        history and evaluation, 149
        instrumental assessment, 150–151
        OralChroma portable gas chromatograph, 150*f*, 151*f*, 155*f*, 156*f*
        organoleptic measurement, 149–150, 150*t*
        saliva quantity and quality, 149
        Winkel Tongue Coating Index, 149, 149*f*, 150*f*
    case studies in
        female with extraoral halitosis, 155–157, 156*f*
        male with intraoral halitosis, 154–155, 155*f*
    classification, 147
        categories of oral malodor, 147*t*
    defined, 146

epidemiology, 146–147
   age distribution of patients attending private halitosis assessment clinic, 146*f*
management and treatment
   masking odor, 153
   mouthrinses, 153
   multistep approach to, 152
   options for, 151, 151*t*
   prevention, 154
   probiotics, 153
   referral to specialists, 154
   tongue scraping, 152, 152*f*
   toothpaste additives, 152, 153*t*
   treatment matrix, 152*t*
pathogenesis of extraoral halitosis, 148
pathogenesis of intraoral halitosis, 147–148
   detection of volatile sulphur compounds from *P. gingivalis* and *F. nucleatum*, 148*f*
   volatile malodorous contributors to, 148*t*
oral mucositis, MASCC/ISOO practice guidelines, 144–145
Oral Pathology CARE Tool, 50
oral piercings, 97–98, 98*f*, 100–101, 105–106, 116, 195
oral-systemic health, 207–218
   adverse pregnancy outcomes, 213–214
   application to clinical practice, 215–217
   cardiovascular disease, 212–213
   diabetes, 209–212
      effect of periodontal treatment on glycemic control, 211, 211*t*
   evidence supporting oral-systemic links, 207–208, 207*t*
   key considerations, 208–209
   overview of, 217–218
oral tissue damage, 97–116
   hard tissues
      abfraction, 114, 114*f*
      abrasion, 108–111, 109*f*, 110*f*
      attrition, 107–108, 107*f*
      endogenic erosion, 111–113, 112*f*
      erosion, 111
      exogenic erosion, 101*f*, 113–114, 113*f*
      multifactorial etiology, 114–115, 115*f*
      oral piercings, 98*f*
      overview of, 106–107
   overview of, 115–116
   soft tissues
      appliance-related recession, 100*f*, 101*f*, 103*f*
      chemical irritation, 105*f*
      epidemiology, 97–99
      etiology, 99–105
      gingival recession, 98*f*, 99*f*, 101*f*
      iatrogenic damage, 106
      pathogenesis, 105
      prevention and therapy, 106
      toothbrush trauma, 98*f*, 100*f*, 102*f*
      traumatic lesions, 105*f*
orofacial injuries, 192–204

case studies in
   sports-related TDI, 203–204, 204*f*
   thumbsucking, 203, 203*f*
epidemiology, 192–193
   complicated fracture in 10-year-old girl, 192*f*
   complicated fracture of left maxillary incisor, 193*f*
   palatal displacement resulting in traumatic occlusion, 193*f*
intentional abuse, 202
management, 196–197
   BB gun pellet embedded in soft tissues, 198*f*
   enamel-dentin fracture with tooth fragment, 198*f*
   tooth fragment embedded in tongue, 198*f*
   trauma bin contents, 196*t*
   trauma bin example, 196*f*
   trauma record example, 199*t*
overview, 192
prevention
   interceptive orthodontics, 201–202
   mouth protectors, 199–201, 200*f*, 201*f*
   overview of, 197–199
risk factors, 194–196
   increased overjet and flared maxillary incisors, 195*f*
sequelae, 193–194
   inflammatory root resorption, 194*f*
   results of necrosis, 194*f*
orthodontic treatment, influence on gingival recession, 103–104
OSA (obstructive sleep apnea). *See* obstructive sleep apnea

P

p53 tumor suppressor, 125
Paroex, 262*t*
patient behavior. *See* biopsychosocial patient care; special care dentistry
patient lifestyle
   cariogenic lifestyles, 64
   integrating desired behavior into, 30
   periodontal diseases and
      nutrition and obesity, 91
      stress and psychological factors, 91
      tobacco use, 90–91
PDT (photodynamic therapy diode), 76
pediatric dentistry. *See* children and adolescents
peptide–cetylpyridinium chloride combinations, 250
Peridex, 262*t*
peri-implant diseases
   case studies in, 92, 92*f*
   classification, 74
   defined, 74
   diagnosis, 74
   epidemiology, 74–75
   pathogenesis, 75
   risk assessment, 75

INDEX

subgingival air polishing, 78
Periodontal Assessment Tool, 53
periodontal diseases
  case studies in
    gingivitis in adolescent female, 91, 91*f*
    peri-implantitis in geriatric male, 92, 92*f*
    periodontitis in adult male, 92, 92*f*
  defined, 208
  diagnostic testing of, 73–74
  etiology and pathogenesis, 73
  gingivitis
    case studies in, 91, 91*f*
    classification, 72*t*
    defined, 71, 208
    epidemiology, 72–74
    etiology and pathogenesis, 73
  incidence, symptoms and risk factors, 51–52
  patient lifestyle and
    nutrition and obesity, 91
    stress and psychological factors, 91
    tobacco use, 90–91
  peri-implant diseases
    case studies in, 92, 92*f*
    classification, 74
    defined, 74
    diagnosis, 74
    epidemiology, 74–75
    pathogenesis, 75
    risk assessment, 75
    subgingival air polishing, 78
  periodontitis
    case studies in, 92, 92*f*
    chronic vs. aggressive, 71–72
    Classification System for Periodontal Diseases and Conditions (AAP), 71, 72*t*
    defined, 71, 208
    diagnosis, 71
    epidemiology of chronic, 73
    etiology and pathogenesis, 73
    guidelines for determining severity, 72*t*
    International Workshop for a Classification of Periodontal Diseases and Conditions, 71
    Task Force Report (AAP), 71–72
  prognosis and risk assessment, 74
  risk assessment, 52–53
    DenPlan Excel/PreVisor Patient Assessment (DEPPA), 52
    Dentition Risk System (DRS), 52
    Health Improvement in Dental Practice (HIDEP), 52
    Periodontal Risk Assessment (PRA), 52
    Periodontal Risk Calculator (PRC), 53
    Risk Assessment-Based Individualized Treatment (RABIT), 52
  treatments and strategies, at-home
    antimicrobial dentifrice, 89
    antimicrobial mouthrinses, 89–90
    antioxidants, 90
    herbal patches, 90
    interdental biofilm removal, 87, 87*f*
    powered interdental cleaning devices, 87–89, 88*f*
    probiotics, 90
    recommendations for, 81–83
    toothbrushes, 83–87, 86*f*
  treatments and strategies, in-office
    dental endoscopy, 77
    full-mouth disinfection, 76–77
    laser technology, 76
    local and systemic therapies, 79
    locally delivered antimicrobials/antibiotics, 79–80
    maintenance and recall, 80–81
    maintenance and recall for implant-borne restorations, 84–86*t*
    maintenance and recall for tooth-borne restorations, 82–83*t*
    mechanical therapy, 75–76
    subgingival air polishing, 77–78, 78*f*
    supra- and subgingival irrigation, 78–79, 88*f*
    systemic antibiotics, 80
Periodontal Risk Assessment (PRA), 52
Periodontal Risk Calculator (PRC), 53
periodontitis. *See under* periodontal diseases
photodynamic therapy diode (PDT), 76
PICO format, 13
piercings. *See* oral piercings
pilocarpine, 180
polyvinylmethyl ether/maleic acid copolymer (PVM/MA), 266
Porphyromonas gingivalis, 71, 147–148, 148*f*, 212
poverty, as determinant of health, 24
  See also biopsychosocial patient care
PRA (Periodontal Risk Assessment), 52
PRC (Periodontal Risk Calculator), 53
preappraised research, 14, 14*f*
prebiotics, 65
predator bacteria, 65
pregnancy outcomes, evidence supporting oral-systemic link, 213–214
prevalence studies, 4
Prevent Diabetes STAT toolkit, 43
prevention across the lifespan
  biopsychosocial patient care, 23–35
  caries, 57–70
  chemotherapeutic agents, 257–268
  dentin hypersensitivity, 160–171
  dry mouth (xerostomia), 175–189
  evidence-based practice, 1–20
  fluorides, 235–244
  head and neck cancers, 121–142
  MASCC/ISOO oral mucositis guidelines, 144–145
  non-fluoride remineralization, 246–253
  oral malodor, 146–157
  oral-systemic health, 207–218
  oral tissue damage, 91–116
  orofacial injuries, 192–204

periodontal diseases, 71–92
risk assessment, 37–54
special care dentistry, 221–231
PreViser Oral Cancer Risk Assessment, 49
Prevotella intermedia, 147
primary research, 14
PRISMA, 12t, 13
probiotics, 64–65, 90, 153
prospective study design, 6–7
PROSPERO, 13
PscyINFO, 2t
pseudohalitosis, 147, 147t
psychological conditions, effect on patient care, 31–32
publication bias, 11
PubMed, 2t
PVM/MA (polyvinylmethyl ether/maleic acid copolymer), 266

Q

QLF (quantitative light fluorescence), 60–61
QOL (quality of life), 24
quadrant scaling and root planing (Q-SRP), 77
qualitative studies, 10
quality of life (QOL), 24
quantitative light fluorescence (QLF), 60–61

R

RABIT (Risk Assessment-Based Individualized Treatment), 52
radiation therapy
　role in dry mouth, 178, 179
　therapeutic interventions, 183
RAGE (receptor for advanced glycation end products), 209–210
randomized controlled trials (RCTs), 9–10, 12, 13
　active control design, 10f
　placebo control design, 9f
rate ratio (RR), 6
recall. *See* maintenance and recall
recall bias, 6
receptor for advanced glycation end products (RAGE), 209–210
RECORD, 12t, 13
red disclosing tablets, 60
relative rate, 6
relative risk, 6
remineralization therapies. *See* fluorides; non-fluoride remineralization
Replacement Theory, 64
retrospective study design, 5, 7
risk assessment, 37–54
　defined, 37
　for oral health
　　caries, 50–51, 51t, 52t, 63–64
　　oral cancer, 48–50, 49t
　　peri-implant diseases, 75
　　periodontal disease, 51–53, 74

xerostomia, 53, 54f
overview of, 53–54
for systemic health
　cardiovascular disease and stroke, 37–41, 38f, 39t, 40f
　diabetes mellitus, 41–47, 42f, 44t, 45f, 46f, 70
　goals of, 37
　sleep-related breathing disorders, 47–48, 47f, 48t
Risk Assessment-Based Individualized Treatment (RABIT), 52
risk ratio, 6
role modeling, 223–224
RR (rate ratio), 6

S

salivary gland hypofunction (SGH)
　case studies in, 184–187
　defined, 175
　diagnosis, 176
　epidemiology, 177, 177t
　etiology, 177–178
salivary gland transfer (SGT), 179
salivary precipitin, 247
scaling and root planing (SRP)
　adjunct therapies, 76
　efficacy of, 75–76
　FMSRP (full-mouth scaling and root planing), 76–77
SciELO (Scientific Electronic Library Online, in Spanish), 2t
scientific evidence
　applying to practice, 19–20
　grading
　　Agency for Healthcare Research and Quality, 17–18
　　AHRQ grades of recommendation, 18t
　　AHRQ levels of scientific evidence, 18t
　　CEBM table for therapy, prevention, etiology, harm, 16t
　　CEBM tables for diagnosis, 16t, 17t
　　Centre for Evidence-Based Medicine, 16–17
　　Cochrane Collaboration, 18–19
　　Cochrane collaboration key principles, 19t
　　GRADE system, 17, 17t
　　overview of, 15–16
　levels of, 13–14
　　hierarchy of preappraised evidence, 14f
　　resources supporting clinical decision making, 14t
Scope, 262t
SCORE (Systemic Coronary Risk Evaluation), 41
Screening Tool for Hyposalivation with Xerostomia, 53–54, 54f
SCT (social cognitive theory), 25–26, 25f
SDD (subantimicrobial dose doxycycline), 80
secondary research, 14
Seikaly Jha procedure (SJP), 179
selective targeted antimicrobial peptides (STAMPs),

66, 250
self-efficacy, 25
Sensodyne Toothpaste, 170f
sensory disorders, 228–229
SGH (salivary gland hypofunction). *See* salivary gland hypofunction
SGT (salivary gland transfer), 179
shaping, 223
single-blind study design, 9
6S Hierarchy of Preappraised Evidence, 14, 14f
Sjögren's syndrome, 177, 183, 184–187
SJP (Seikaly Jha procedure), 179
sleep-related breathing disorders
    incidence, symptoms and risk factors, 47–48
    Mallampati Classification, 47f
    risk assessment, 48
        STOP-Bang questionnaire, 48, 48t
        STOP questionnaire, 48, 48t
smokeless tobacco, 104–105
SnF2 (stannous fluoride with sodium hexametaphosphate), 265
snuff, 104–105
social cognitive theory (SCT), 25–26, 25f
social determinants of health, 23–24
    See also biopsychosocial patient care
soda beverages, 113–114
sodium monofluorophosphate (MFP), 169
soft tissue damage. *See under* oral tissue damage
special care dentistry, 221–231
    application to clinical practice, 231
    barriers to care in special needs patients, 221
    behavior and psychological interventions
        approaches to, 222
        benefits of, 222
        consistency and role modeling, 223–224
        contingent and noncontingent escape, 223
        escape extinction, 224
        shaping through successive approximation, 223
        systematic desensitization, 222–223
    care delivery problems
        patients with autism spectrum disorders, 229–230
        patients with neurodegenerative diseases, 228
        patients with sensory disorders, 228–229
        patients with speech and language impairments, 229
    geriatric patients
        aggressive prevention, 226
        clinical prevention, 225
        conservative prevention, 225
        empirical prevention, 225
        guidelines for preventive dentistry, 224
        influence of medical condition, 224
        predictive prevention, 225
        preventive care considerations, 230–231
        team approach to preventive care, 224–225
    importance of preventive care, 221–222
    populations included, 221

preventive care considerations
    adjuvant interventions, 226–227
    dietary considerations, 227–228
    first and annual visits, 226
    home care and family involvement, 228
    impact of systemic or psychological declines, 227
    periodic preventive maintenance, 226
speech and language impairments, 229
SRP (scaling and root planing). *See* scaling and root planing
STAMPs (selective targeted antimicrobial peptides), 66, 250
stannous fluoride with sodium hexametaphosphate (SnF2), 265
STARD, 12t, 13
Stichting Center for Evidence-Based Management (CEBMa), 12t
STOP-Bang questionnaire, 48, 48t
STOP questionnaire, 48, 48t
Streptococcus gordonii, 65
Streptococcus mutans, 62, 64, 250, 261, 264–265
Streptococcus salivarius K12, 153
Streptococcus sanguinis, 65, 250–251, 264
stress and coping, effect on health, 26–27, 91
STROBE, 12t, 13
study designs
    case-control, 5–6, 6f
    case report/case series, 4, 4f
    cohort, 6–7
        prospective, 7f
        retrospective, 8f
    cross-sectional, 4–5, 5f
    experimental, 8–10
    hierarchy of, 3f
    meta-analyses, 11–12, 11f
    nonexperimental intervention, 8, 8f
    qualitative, 10
    randomized controlled trials (RCTs)
        active control, 10f
        placebo control, 9f
    registering systematic reviews and meta-analyses, 12–13
    surveys and interviews, 3–4
    systematic reviews, 10–11
subantimicrobial dose doxycycline (SDD), 80
subgingival air polishing, 77–78, 78f
successive approximation, 223
supra- and subgingival irrigation, 78–79, 88f
surveys and interviews, 3–4
systematic desensitization, 222–223
systematic reviews, 10–11, 12–13
Systemic Coronary Risk Evaluation (SCORE), 41

T

Take Action to Prevent Diabetes: A Toolkit for the Prevention of Type 2 Diabetes in Europe, 43
TDIs (traumatic dental injuries). *See* traumatic dental

injuries
teach-back method, 31
tell-show-do method, 223
temporary halitosis, 147, 147*t*
tetracycline, 80
3D conformal radiation therapy, 179
Tiel-Culemborg study, 59
tissue damage. *See* oral tissue damage
tobacco use, 90–91, 104–105, 132–133, 133*f*
tongue scraping, oral malodor and, 152, 152*f*
toothbrushes, 83–87, 86*f*
toothbrushing
 in children and adolescents, 239
 effects of improper technique, 102
 gingival injury due to, 101–102
 influence on gingival recession, 102–103
 recommendations for, 106
toothpastes
 acid-neutralizing, 251
 arginine-based desensitizing prophylaxis paste, 169, 170*f*
 arginine bicarbonate/calcium carbonate, 252
 for children and adolescents, 238–239, 239*f*
 oral malodor and, 152, 153*t*
 prescription fluoride, 242
transtheoretical model (TTM), 27–28
traumatic dental injuries (TDIs)
 case studies in, 203–204, 204*f*
 epidemiology, 192–193
 management, 196–197
  BB gun pellet embedded in soft tissues, 198*f*
  enamel-dentin fracture with tooth fragment, 198*f*
  tooth fragment embedded in tongue, 198*f*
  trauma bin contents, 196*t*
  trauma bin example, 196*f*
  trauma record example, 199*t*
 overview of, 192
 prevention, 197–202
  interceptive orthodontics, 201–202
  mouth protectors, 199–201, 200*f*, 201*f*
 risk factors, 194–196
 sequelae, 193–194
traumatic lesions, 104–105
TREND, 12*t*, 13
Treponema denticola, 147
tricalcium phosphate, 63
triclosan/copolymer, 250, 261, 266
TRIP (Turning Research Into Practice), 2*t*
Tristan da Cunha (British colony), 58*b*
TTM (transtheoretical model), 27–28
21 Cities study, 235

U

University of Oxford Critical Appraisal Tools, 12*t*
University of South Australia Critical Appraisal Tools, 12*t*

V

visualization, 223

W

Winkel Tongue Coating Index, 149, 149*f*, 150*f*

X

xerostomia. *See* dry mouth